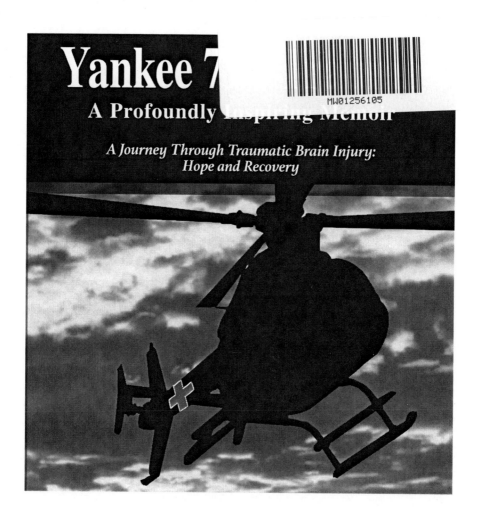

Yankee 7

A Profoundly Inspiring Memoir

A Journey Through Traumatic Brain Injury:
Hope and Recovery

Elizabeth A. Scott

Yankee 794 Trauma
A Profoundly Inspiring Memoir
A Journey Through Traumatic Brain Injury: Hope and Recovery

Cover design by Joshua A. Suggs
Wedding photos by Joni Dusek, Sarasota. Used with permission.

For information regarding permissions, call 941.922.2662
or contact us at our website:

www.peppertreepublishing.com or write to:

The Peppertree Press, LLC
Attention: Publisher
1269 First Street, Suite 7
Sarasota, Florida 34236

ISBN: 9781614934394

Library of Congress Control Number: 2016936153

Printed March 2016

Contributors

Barbara S. Scott

Cover Design by Joshua A. Suggs

Editing:
Barbara Flewelling
Joseph Anthony Schroeder

"FAITH is a place of mystery, where we find the courage to believe in what we cannot see and the strength to let go of our fear and uncertainty."

Brene Brown

Hello Elizabeth and Barb. What a journey the two of you have traveled. My daughter is now 19 yrs old and is 13 months post TBI... she is my beautiful miracle.

Congratulations to you both on the publication of your story... you were spot on when you wrote that people may find it difficult to put their stories down on paper so to speak. I love to write myself but my emotions make it impossible when it comes to what we are going through. So thank you for being brave enough to tackle this I am sure there were many times when it was not easy and you have my absolute admiration! I intend to share your book with other family members who don't "get it" in the hope they will be more understanding. Education is key! Love and prayers to you both.

–Railli Porter

Elizabeth I have cried with every page. Your knowledge as a nurse makes this an invaluable book for medical professionals as well as survivors and their families. Your love shines through every written word and your faith in God is like a neon light guiding us all through the journey. This is a masterpiece my friend a masterpiece of blood, sweat, tears and triumph! I feel so blessed to read and get a glimpse of Barb's journey through you. Amazing job and countless others will benefit from both your love and your knowledge.

Warmest,

–Debbie Wilson

This book is so honest to the core. It's a mother's fight to save her daughter after she suffered a Traumatic Brain Injury. The mother also had to fight to save her own life. Not once, but twice! What a Fierce Momma Bear! As a Traumatic Brain Injury Survivor myself, what her daughter was fighting to survive and needed her mother in order to Thrive was beyond horrific. Thank God her mother had the strength to fight through it all for her daughter.

This is the True Story of Both Their Fights!
–Jennifer Stokley (TBI Survivor/Thriver)

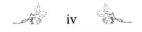

Dedication

This book is dedicated to:
God's Team of Medical Angels
The men and women who save lives every day.
They are our police, firefighters, and medical personnel.
Putting yourselves in harm's way.

To each of you who were "on scene."
at *the* pivotal moment.
God appeared and said,
"It's your time to act."

Each of you
showed up, showed courage,
made the right judgment calls.

Each of you
was **"in the right place at the right time."**

Each of you
did what you do so selflessly every day.
If not for you, the outcome
would have been very different.

Miracles happen to all of us.
You only have to reach out your hand and heart.
Have faith and ask God.

When you are a believer,
and are unable to ask,
God shows up anyway.

I look back and marvel at how events unfolded
that clearly might have resulted
in my daughter's untimely death.

It was not to be,
because God was there.
He was working through each of you,
and God declared,
"Not now my Child.
Your work on Earth is not finished."

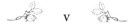

Yankee 794 Trauma

_ℒ_

This book is dedicated to each 9-1-1 responder.
The people who answered the call.

Each of you
know in your heart,
you choose your field as
you're inspired path in Life.

Each of you
knew that you had a gift
you wanted and needed to share with the world.

Each of you
made a significant contribution to doing
your part in saving my daughter's life.

How many others are there that you that saved?
How many never got the chance to come back and say

"Thank You!"

Firefighters and 9-1-1 responders
The Unsung Heroes
Each of you is on God's team.

Every day you impact so many lives,
in ways you may not realize — and can't imagine.
Too often people, for many reasons,
can't come back to say

"Thank You!"

Each of you,
in your way,
possesses a gift from God.

The dedication, talents, tenacity, perseverance, compassion, hope, optimism,
and skill you possess, ***changes lives.***

_ℒ_

YOU MAKE A DIFFERENCE!

Dedication

Cedar Hammock Fire Department

**5200 – 26th Street West
Bradenton, Florida 34207**

Division Chief Administrator Alexander Lobeto
(Supervisor on scene at Barb's 9-1-1 call 12/29/10)
**Lt. Vincent "Mike" Soper
FF-1 Ryan French
FF-4 James Taylor
FF-1 Justin L. Jackson
FF-1 Jason S. Moore**

The two men who were in the ambulance
that took Barb from impact scene
delivering her to Bayflite alive.
**Kenneth Bland – Paramedic
Bryan Boley – EMT**

**YOU HAVE OUR UNDYING GRATITUDE.
WE THANK YOU.**

Bayflite Staff

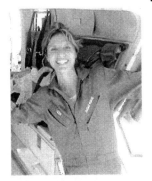

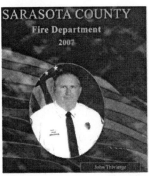

Patricia "Patty" Klein R.N.
Flight Nurse

John Thivierge, **Paramedic**
Battalion Chief (Retired)
Sarasota (Fl.) Fire Department

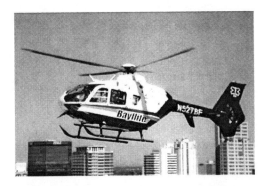

**To the helicopter pilot whose skill enabled everyone
to arrive on the scene and then safely to Bayfront
Medical Center, St. Petersburg, Florida**

༈

To those on duty at the pre-dawn hours of 12/29/10:

Bayfront Emergency Department, St. Petersburg, Florida

The Bay Area Surgical Associates, St. Petersburg, Florida

Dr. Nicholas Price M.D. Trauma and Acute Care — SURGEON

Dr. Brian S. Hedrick D.O. EMERGENCY MEDICINE

Dr. Thomas J. Stengel M.D. NEUROSURGEON

Dedication

Dr. Steven G. Epstein MD Trauma and Acute Care
Dr. Amy J. Koler MD Trauma and Acute Care
Dr. Robert G. Hamilton MD Orthopedic

**To the dedicated Nursing Staff, Technicians, and
Social Workers in Neuro-ICU Bayfront Medical Center.**

♃

HealthSouth RidgeLake Hospital
HealthSouth Rehabilitation Hospital
Heartland Rehabilitation
Sarasota, Florida

After Barb Returned Home

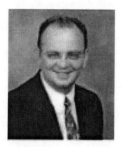

Dr. Craig Trigueiro M.D. — "Dr. T."
Family Practice — Bradenton, Florida

Dr. Trigueiro, semi-retired at time of publication, specialized in providing ongoing comprehensive medical care for patients of all ages, in some cases providing lifelong care. In the provision of general medical care, Dr. Trigueiro treated patients for a wide range of ailments and conditions, usually acting as the point of the first contact and referred patients to a specialist if necessary – AKA: *a primary care provider.*

"Dr. T" has been Barb's caring friend for many years, and we credit him with guiding her through every step of her long-term recovery.

Yankee 794 Trauma

> IMPOSSIBLE IS JUST A BIG WORD THROWN AROUND BY SMALL MEN WHO FIND IT EASIER TO LIVE IN THE WORLD THEY'VE BEEN GIVEN, THAN TO EXPLORE THE POWER THEY HAVE TO CHANGE IT. IMPOSSIBLE IS NOT A FACT. IT'S AN OPINION. IMPOSSIBLE IS NOT A DECLARATION. IT'S A DARE. IMPOSSIBLE IS POTENTIAL. IMPOSSIBLE IS TEMPORARY.
>
> IMPOSSIBLE IS NOTHING.

Dr. Frank Loh MD Neurologist & Electrodiagnostic Medicine

Dr. David S. Tsai MD Physical Medicine & Rehabilitation

Dr. James M. McGovern, Psy. D.
Licensed Clinical Neuropsychology, ABPP-CN

Dr. Eric L. Berman MD Neuro-Ophthalmologist & Oculoplastic Surgery

Dr. John Shelton MD Ear, Nose and Throat and Head,
Neck, and Sinus Surgery

Dr. Ivan E. Rascon-Aguilar, M.D. Gastroenterology

Dr. James L. Slocum, M.D. Geriatric Psychiatry – Sarasota, Florida

Dr. James W. Raniolo D.O. Emergency Medicine

❧

Neil W. Scott, ESQ.
Attorney-At-Law, Sarasota, Florida, *a credit to his profession, and leader in our community. Whose compassion, gentle nudging, and expertise, kept me moving forward when I thought I was too overwhelmed. If not for your willing and expert advice, and guidance, through the legal process — our ship would have sunk.*

David Cornish, ESQ.
(Barbara's Attorney) Attorney-At-Law, Venice, Florida

❧

M.D. Stevens

THE MIKEY CENTER for Hyperbaric Therapy Sarasota, Florida

You have become a trusted and valued friend and mentor, who loved us through this. You were the inspiration for so many, and for the prequel to this book **The Search for Judith Ann** *(2016)*

X

Dedication

𝓛

Valerie Shaw
Patient Access Services Coordinator Bayfront
Medical Center, St. Petersburg, Florida

𝓛

INTERMEDIA PRODUCTIONS

James L. Flynn – Executive Producer
1234 – 2nd Street – Sarasota, Florida 34236
www.intermediaproductions

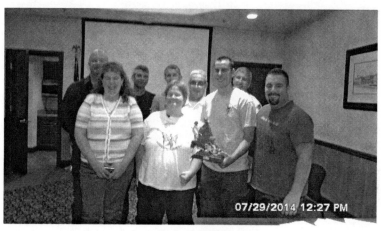

August 2014

**Barb (middle front) with sister Andrea (left) and her 9-1-1 First Responder
Team from Cedar Hammock Fire Station, Bradenton, Florida**

"To love someone fiercely,
To believe in something with your whole heart
To celebrate a fleeting moment in time
To fully engage in a life
that doesn't come with garentees –
These are risks that involve Vulnerability
and often Pain …
I'm learning that recognizing and leaning into
the discomfort of Vulnerability
Teaches us how to live with Joy, Gratitude and Grace."

Brene Brown

Foreword

When you are a child, the world is a surprising place all the time. It is not possible to see how your actions, and those of others, result in outcomes that will have predictable consequences, and what result you may find.

As a child, that wide-eyed innocence allowed you to believe *"all things are possible"* even when the adults surrounding you can see that your predicted outcome, is not likely to be the result. No matter how much you, the child, might *"wish on a star"* to make it so, others who have already traveled that same path can predict it is not to be.

A child's mind has no knowledge of things to come, or the ability to predict the outcome of a journey of a 10,000 days, that begins with one step. It is that wide-eyed enthusiasm that *"all things are possible"* that has made Walt Disney's empire so appealing to so many, for so long. It is why fantasy and sci-fi, and other popular entertainment thrive.

I believe, perhaps it is the nature of human intelligence that allows that *"all things are possible"* and to move on that premise. It is at the core of how the U.S. made it in 1969 when everyone tuned in to see three American astronauts land on the Moon. We saw Neil Armstrong step out of the space capsule and declare,

"That's one small step for Man, one giant leap for Mankind."

Indeed! That event, celebrated around the world, made everyone proud to be an American, and revert to our childhoods and declare,

"If a man can get to the moon, anything is possible!"

Neil Armstrong is unequivocally an American hero. His bravery and skill earned him the honor of the first human to ever set foot on the Moon. As a result, Neil Armstrong has been looked to for insight into the human condition, as well as commentary on the state of technology and space exploration.

Did you know that Neil Armstrong also is quoted as saying,

"I think we're going to the Moon because it's in the nature of the human being to face challenges. We're required to do these things just as salmon swim upstream."

"Mystery creates wonder and wonder is the basis of man's desire to understand."

"Man was given an inquisitive nature, and that manifests itself in our desire to take that next step, to seek out the next great

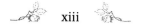

adventure. Going to the Moon wasn't really a question; it was the next step in the evolution of our knowledge, of our understanding. It was necessary to explore the limits of our technology and set the stage for what mankind could achieve in the future."

Neil Armstrong
(1920 – 2012)

A child's mind is to be envied for not understanding what may and may not be possible. It is wonderful to view the world through *"anything is possible"* and *"nothing is impossible"* eyes. Not having the foresight to see down the road and predict the result of actions people can expect when they make a choice, good or bad.

However, as children grow into adulthood, that *should* change. You *should* know that certain decisions and actions, predict specific results in many cases though some results will surprise you even late in life.

I came to understand that moment in time, which shifted The Universe as I knew it. That moment impacted my life with such alarming trepidation, and perilous force, that nothing would ever be as it was.

The molecules in my life had shifted, in one brief moment, which changes not only me, but the world around me – forever.

The same was true with Neil Armstrong's walk on the moon. America turned on their TV to watch history in the making and even though we were not there, *we knew*. It effected each as a witness. There was that palpable moment July 20, 1969 *"before"* he stepped out of Apollo 11, and that moment *"after"* he stepped out. It changed the world, as we thought we saw it.

There are few moments in our personal lifetime that can claim such an impact. The collision this event created sent shockwaves reverberating like shouting into The Grand Canyon, and listening to see how long it would be before my silent screams could be heard no more.

A person knows, instinctively,
when such a catastrophic event occurs.
In one lifetime, it only happens a handful of times.

You can run, but you cannot hide. You know the exact time these two worlds collided, even if you were not standing there, a witness to the moment of impact. This calamity was the catalyst that catapulted me into a time-warp where for a period, life seemed to be playing out in slow motion.

An event so unexpected and so impactful that we look back and realize that nothing anyone would have said or done could have prepared me.

There is *that journey that must be traveled alone.* Your reactions, feelings, and responses, will be unlike anyone around you. Your emotional fingerprint and the resolve to persevere may be so significant, that it taps into the core of who you are — the person that you have prepared to become your entire life.

All your senses are heightened, and you know with absolute certainty and resolve, that this will be unlike any challenge you have faced in your lifetime or are likely ever to face again. This sensation can be described in the same way as Neil Armstrong described standing on the Moon when he was quoted as saying, **"I put up my thumb and it blotted out the planet Earth."**

That moment created is like a tsunami, coming out of nowhere, with no real time to prepare.

I found myself swept along, attempting retreat, seeking a place to hide, knowing that this event screams *"be afraid, be very afraid."*

I found myself lost to the clamor of meaningless activity and noise around me. As sweeping, swirling unseen tides carried me along, I seemed to be caught in a whirlpool of emotions.

I found myself surveying the unparalleled damage I could only begin to envision, radiating in every direction. I wonder if Life as I knew it could ever be the same. Deep in my soul, I knew it would not.

Then I reminded myself that sometimes **you have to step up and step out.** For the inspired thinker, who believes that God Almighty understands that **thinking "inside the box" means confinement** in the world where one is supposed to be "confined to the norm."

Rule breakers do not confine themselves to reason or fitting a mold. God Almighty is "a Rule Breaker". He cannot be confined to the boxes many Christians choose to confine Him.

Those "boxes of limitations" are man's perception. We simply must remember that <u>God</u> is in <u>charge</u>.

We must surrender to His will
and allow God to do what He is designed to do.

🙐

**"And Jesus said unto them,
Because of your unbelief:
for verily I say unto you
if you have faith as a grain of mustard seed,
ye shall say unto the mountain
remove hence to yonder place, and it shall remove;
and nothing shall be impossible unto you."
Matthew 17:20 (KJV)**

🙐

Innocent child-like faith will bring
you to a place where God can
have his way in your life.
A spark can set a forest on fire.
It is about perception and stepping out
into the truth that only
God can provide.

As I begin to walk thru the tragedy unfolding in our lives, and encounter the destruction that was left behind, I found new and formally unseen devastation around my family. It seemed to me that there were unseen dangers lurking at every turn in the road. Every fiber of my being told me that every thought, every feeling, and every belief system that made me who I was, would be tested, in a way I had never been tested before.

🙐

**The only certainty left for me
was to reach into was faith in my Creator.**

🙐

"You may encounter many defeats,
but you must not be defeated.
In fact, it may be necessary to encounter the defeats, so you
can know who you are, what
you can rise from, how you
can still come out of it."

Maya Angelou

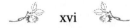 xvi

Table of Contents

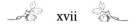

Table of Contents

God has a reason for allowing
things to happen. We may never
understand His wisdom, but we
simply have to trust His will.

Psalms 37:5 (NLT)

Gratitude unlocks the fullness of life.
It turns what we have into enough,
and more. It turns denial into
acceptance, chaos to order, confusion
to clarity. It can turn a meal into a
feast, a house into a home, a stranger
into a friend. Gratitude makes sense
of our past, brings peace for today,
and creates a vision for tomorrow.

Melody Beattie

Create An Attitude of Gratitude.

When your life is in motion you will
come up against obstacles. Sometimes
they will knock you down. Get up
with determination. When you get
bold God shows up and does miracles.
Believe in God for the supernatural
and it will manifest.

CHAPTER 1

Where Is Barb?

I am a very deliberate and articulate thinker and learned early in my nursing career to pace myself, be deliberate, assess the situation, and do not hurry.

There was no way I could have been prepared for what we were about to face. There was no indication that this day would bring uninvited news; that would devastate and challenge my life, and that of both my daughter and her siblings. That day everything in my existence would take an unexpected detour, effectively rerouting our lives forever.

It is impossible to find the words to describe this type of life-altering experience when it happens. I suspect that is why more people do not try to write down their journey when their lives are turned up side down. It is my hope I can do it justice, as I write this memoir to inspire as well as inform and educate.

I was employed on Siesta Key in Sarasota, Florida, and was expected at work at 2 PM. It was beautiful sunny Florida weather, listening to the radio, confident that my life was finally on track. I had been at work for approximately 10 minutes when my phone rang. It was Andrea, my oldest daughter.

"Mom? Have you heard from Barb?"

"No, why? " I quizzed.

It seemed to be an odd question.

We did not talk every day. Barb, my middle child, was the most independent person I knew. I raised her that way! I had thought nothing about not hearing from her since Christmas Day when we all had dinner together.

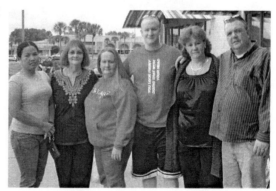

Christmas Day 2009 – Chona (Mark's wife), me, Barb, Mark, Andrea (my eldest daughter), and her husband Alan Shields

Andrea continued, *"I tried to call, and she is not answering. Some of her friends have also called her phone. She isn't answering her phone. That's weird! It goes to voicemail. I can't understand why she isn't answering."*

As our conversation unfolded, she continued, *"I heard there was a bad wreck out on 53rd Avenue last night, and the person was flown to Bayfront..."*

Bayfront Medical Center, was the only **Level One Trauma Center** in our area at the time and is located in the larger metropolitan area of St. Petersburg, Florida, north of the small town of Bradenton, Florida, where we lived.

I could not comprehend how the two statements were connected. It was obvious that Andrea had not connected the two events either, and yet, *why did she say that to me?* The fact was that 53rd Ave, was in the middle of town, six blocks from where Barb lived. She drove by there all the time.

My daughter, Barb, worked 60 hours a week. She had a full-time job at Pinnacle Medical Center in urgent care (a state-of-the-art sub-acute walk-in medical facility), *plus* she worked at two home health agencies part-time. Her occupation was, in effect, her life. Most people saw her as a confident, well-put-together, sweet and giving spirit.

If anyone has asked me to describe her, I would have had to say *she was a Gift from God*, one of the most amazing creature ever put on this Earth. Then again, I am her mother!

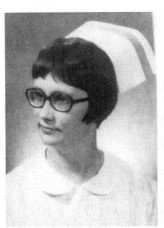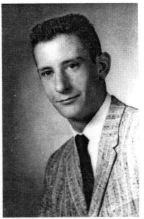

Barb's parents. Betty in 1971 and David's HS grad. 1965.

Barb had always been my little red-headed "spitfire" and a tomboy to boot! When she was 2-3, we affectionately referred to her as "Pig Pen" after the Charlie Brown cartoon. I could get her clean and dressed to go out to play. Five minutes later she would look like a dirt cloud had attacked her!

Among her accomplishments had been competitive gymnastics for several years around ages 8-13. We previously lived in Springfield, Missouri., and her

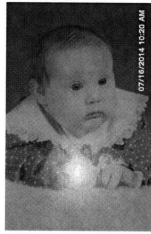
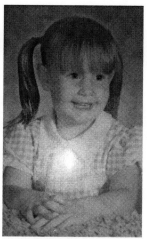

Barb in 1972 at 3 mo. Old

Barb in 1976 – age 4

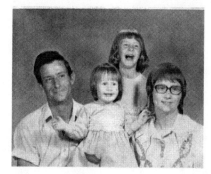

Taken in 1974. Barb was 2 and Andrea was 6.

team took Missouri State Championship when she was 12. She was quite an athlete!

She had later been a high school cheerleader. When the football or basketball team scored,

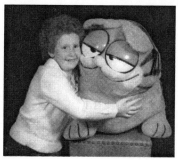

Barb was able to do five back hand springs and cartwheels to celebrate. The crowd would go crazy.

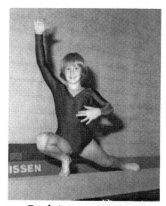

Barb in gymnastics – age 12.

Barb age 12 with her Garfield.

 3

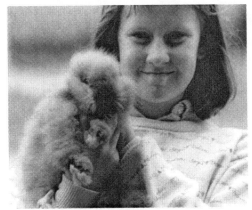
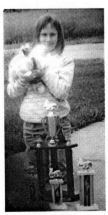

As members of the ARBA (American Rabbit Breeder's Association), Barb shows her rabbits at youth shows. Her favorites were the Netherland Dwarfs, Holland Lops, and English Angoras. Barb age 14 in 1986, when one of her English Angora won lots of awards and ribbons. The awards included the honor of winning Best-In-Show with this baby at an ARBA show!

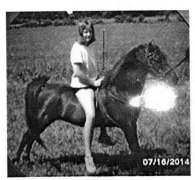
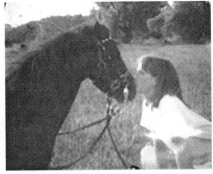

Barb with her Walking Pony Stallion, Lucky. His sire was a National Grand Champion. He was her 14th birthday present.

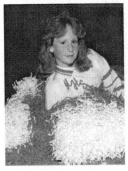

The summer we moved to Florida was 1988, and she turned 16. She felt like a fish-out-of-water. Her old high school, in Everton, Mo. was small. There were 53 in her class. When she transferred to Manatee High School, Bradenton, FL, there were 530 students in her graduating class.

Bradenton, Florida is latitude 27.46 N and longitude 83.58 W. It is a sleepy blue-collar town of 54,000 nestled

Barb as a cheerleader
– age 14.

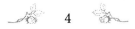

a few miles south of Tampa, and just north of Sarasota, on the west coast of Florida in Manatee County on the Tamiami Trail. I-75 skirts west of the town.

Annual high temperature: 82.3°F
Annual low temperature: 64.4°F
Average temperature: 73.35°F
Average annual precipitation - rainfall: 56.21 inch
Downside: Hurricanes

It benefits include:
(1) world-class beaches for a great vacation in winter
(2) two-hour drive to Orlando and all the attractions there
(3) the world headquarters to Tropicana
(4) spring training home of the Pittsburg Pirates
(5) Red Barn Flea Market – 1000 vendors
(6) semi-tropical climate
(7) one state university
(8) one vocational institute
(9) zero murders in the town in 2010

As long as I have made it my home the residents have been friendly, easy-going and down-to-earth, giving people.

That being said, it had culture shock for Barb when we first relocated. In time, her resilient spirit adjusted, and in addition to her school work, she decided to go to work at Publix, a large grocery store chain in the south, as a cashier part-time.

When she contracted Mononucleosis (sometimes called "Kissing Disease") which comes from having a compromised immune system, her white blood count went through the roof. She was in bed for a month, mostly sleeping. Somehow she still managed to keep her grades up.

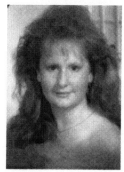
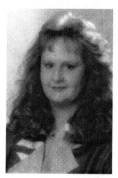

Barbara Suzanne Scott – Class of 1990   *Barb in 1994*

"Tenacious" is one word that comes to mind when people asked me about my daughter, Barb.

"Okay, Andrea, let me see if I can find out anything, I will call you. If you find out anything, you call me." I told her.

I had just hung up the phone when it rang again.

Mrs. Scott?" came the voice.

"Yes?"

"This is Shelley at Pinnacle Medical Center. I am Barb's supervisor at work. Barb was due at work at 2:00, and it is now 2:20. She hasn't shown up for her shift. She is never late for work."

Barb had worked at Pinnacle Medical Center as charge nurse for the past few years. She was very accomplished at her job and loved the challenge. Her co-workers were more like an extended family, and her job was a lot of fun, too! Nursing was her life. Barb always said that was what she loved about her job. You never knew what was coming in the door next. All their physicians were Emergency and Trauma trained and certified.

I think Shelley said some other things, but by this time, the churning in my stomach told me it was time for *red flags*. My body was shaking, my heart began pounding, and mind was racing.

SOMETHING WAS WRONG!

I was completely unsuccessful in locating a phone book, so my next thought was to call a good friend. He might be able to help find some information. I hit the speed dial button and to my relief, he answered.

"Andrea called me. Barb isn't answering her phone. Her friends have called, and it keeps going to voicemail. Then Shelley called me from work, and Barb didn't show up for her shift. You know that's not like her! Andrea said something (to me) about a bad wreck out on 53rd early this morning, and they took the driver to Bayfront. I don't know if one has anything to do with the other. Something isn't right. I can't find a phone book here at work. Can you call and see what you can find out?"

My daughter was not one to disappear. She has lots of friends and family she talked to all the time. *Was this all a big misunderstanding, I thought.*

My nursing training had conditioned me that you stay calm in a crisis, and I tried to practice that. However, when it's your kid, it's hard to practice what you preach, because you are emotionally involved.

Chapter 1

Andrea commented that her last text from Barb was at 2:30 AM, after she left her night shift, and she was on her way to Ryan's to watch a movie.

Ten agonizing minutes later my friend called me back.

"They have Barb at Bayfront in ER. She was in an accident last night and has been admitted as "a Jane Doe" early this morning... and from what I was able to find out, her condition is Critical. It does not look good."

His voice cracked.

My stomach dropped.

My mind was spinning.

"I will meet you in Bradenton at Alan and Andrea's as soon as I can get permission to leave," I told him.

I hung up the phone and called my employer, the son of the lady I was staying with. He assured me it was fine for me to leave — not to worry. He was on his way over to his mom's, who had early-stage Alzheimer's. She was not at risk to wander off... yet.

Pulling out of the driveway and heading north from Siesta Key, I was in Andrea's driveway in Bradenton by 3:15 PM. All four of us piled into their car and headed north to Bayfront Medical Center in St. Petersburg, Florida, 45 minutes away. I was thankful not to be driving.

Bayfront was the closest **Level 1 Trauma Center** in our area, at that time. I saw it as "good and bad news." There are three superb hospitals in the immediate vicinity that she could have been transported to, but none were classified as *Level 1 Trauma Centers.*

The fact that the 9-1-1 first responders assessed her condition onsite and called Bayflite, meant *there were life-threatening injuries.* Bayfront was 15-20 minutes *by helicopter.* That in itself was terrifying, especially in the face of having no additional information on her condition.

What would we find when we arrived?

Andrea mentioned as we drove across the Sunshine Skyway Bridge (a landmark that connects North Tampa Bay to South Tampa Bay, the shortest route to St. Petersburg, Fl.), that "someone" had said Ryan might have seen her last night.

I called Ryan from the peak of the Sunshine Skyway Bridge.He explained that she was on her way over to his place to watch a movie, *but never got there.* I explained what was happening.

His immediate reaction was remorseful and emotional.

"When she didn't show up, I should have gone looking for her. If I had gone to look for her, maybe she would be okay now!"

I told him that we would keep him informed when we knew more after reaching Bayfront.

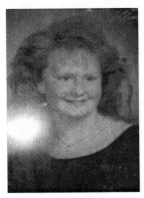

HS Graduation 1990

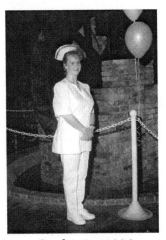

Graduation 1996

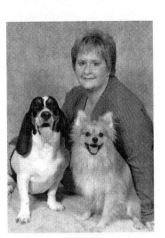

2004 – Daisy & Bodie with Barb

 8

CHAPTER 2

Patience Is the Ability to Tolerate Delay

Minutes later the four of us drove into the parking garage and walked across the street to Bayfront Medical Center, in St. Petersburg, Florida. My adrenalin was in overdrive. My inner voice kept reminding my brain to stay calm. However, I questioned how much that helped. It was as though my mind and my body were working independently of one another.

Someone asked for directions to the emergency room, and we ended up on an elevator. It was as though I was in an altered state of consciousness, aware of my surroundings but feeling numb. I heard sounds, however, I was not comprehending the meaning of them.

As the elevator door opened, we were facing a never-ending hallway, which was filled with echoing, noise, and chatter. It would lead to the E.R. Inside; my head was screaming,

"I can't imagine how being in a Level One Trauma ER can be good! "

I remember my legs carried me down that hall, and every step I took, brought me closer to *a sense of dread*, spiraling down into the depths of my soul.

Many of us know that God can do anything. There are those who do not understand that God is willing. I happen to be one of those who know

God is willing when you ask Him.

As we approached ER, I saw a patient on a gurney in the hallway. I could not help but notice the one lone person from a distance. It was obvious that they had been grievously injured. I glimpsed and briefly assessed them, as my long-time nursing background kicked in. Whatever they had experienced, the injuries were extensive and severe, *maybe near-fatal.* There were hospital personnel working there around **the Life Support Unit**, which was keeping the person alive — at least *for the moment.* There did not seem to be any family present. I was comforted by the fact that the person was not alone.

My mind flashed back to the day I faced a sinister scenario with my

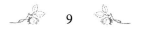

husband David in 1978. David was only 30 and healthy, but he had developed a brain aneurysm, that blew out.

A brain aneurysm is not even on the short list of suspects in an otherwise healthy 30-year-old man. After 45 minutes in ER, a spinal tap revealed gross amounts of bright red blood.

I had been eight months pregnant with our son Mark, our third child, when his family discovered him unconscious, and he was taken to an ER. It happened on a Sunday morning while he and the girls were visiting his parent's farm near Boonville, Missouri. He had complained of a headache and gone outside to get some air. It was Barb, age 5, who found her dad and could not wake him up. Alarmed, his family immediately took him to the nearest hospital.

When a diagnosis was *finally* determined later that morning, and his heart arrested at 5:00 PM, he was placed on life support. *Only then* was a brain scan done, revealing he was "brain dead." It was April 9, 1978 and our family was catapulted into "legal limbo."

The following three days were etched into my memory, as we agonized over choices that needed to be made. That traumatic event ended with his death.

Again I turned my attention to finding out what was happening with my daughter I had yet to find. I figured she was still back in one of the ER bays or had already been moved upstairs.

Either way I needed answers.

As I turned, we were approached by a nurse. I asked about my daughter by name. The nurse looked at me and then looked over at the patient on the gurney in the hall.

"She is waiting for a room in Neuro-ICU on the 5th floor."

The nurse then looked toward the person on the gurney, *again*, indicating that the person in the hallway was Barb. It took a minute to "grasp" that she was referring to Barb — my Barb, my daughter. Everything was moving in slow motion, as I pivoted to look squarely at the patient I had previously noticed — *and dismissed.*

From the depth of my soul I wanted to cry out, *"No! You have made a mistake. THIS can't be MY daughter!"*

I was speechless. Obviously I had misunderstood her!

I focused my attention on the person on the gurney *in disbelief.* I turned again to look at the nurse. I wondered if she had *understood* whom I had inquired about. Again, she motioned me to the only person in the hall. I paused, took a deep breath, and felt like I was going to freeze in my tracks.

With slow and deliberate steps, I walked closer to the gurney and looked into the face. Her eyes were closed. *I felt like I was under water and couldn't breathe* – yet I was eerily calm. I knew that falling apart was not an option, at least not for me, and (above all) **not now.**

She was on Life Support!

NO GOD – PLEASE — NO!!!

Moving closer my eyes examined her face, and I focused, looking more deliberately at her. I looked at her face *again*, and my mind wanted to resist believing. Her eyes were turning black and blue. *My knees wanted to buckle.*

Four days ago she was bright bouncy, bubbly young lady. We had opened Christmas gifts and were laughing with her sister and her brother (who had Skyped in from Iraq). She had years of a promising life ahead of her.

Suddenly, her entire life was in jeopardy.

I looked at her hands, and I knew those hands. I spotted an ID bracelet that clearly identified her. I understood "the bigger picture" of what it meant. *Fear on steroids gripped me.* It took every ounce of energy I had to keep going.

All I could think of was to turn this over to God. He will direct our path.

I glanced up at a clock on the wall. The time was 4:30 PM, and I learned the accident had occurred at 2:41 AM. I realized that she had been in ER for *more than 12 hours.*

Who is so critically injured that they spend 12 hours in ER without dying or going to surgery?

Barb was hurt last night, and I was at home sleeping when *this* happened. **The Mom knows.** She has a dream or is startled awake. Isn't that how it is supposed to work?

I stayed asleep all night and woke up feeling no sense of impending doom. What was my problem?

I felt to the core of my soul I should have known "when it happened" or that *something* had happened.

The truth is that in real life, it does not happen that way, at least it didn't for me. There were many times later, that I went over and over that night, but nothing alerted me. Eventually, I would realize I was beating myself up over something I could do nothing about.

The four of us stood in the hall next to Barb *speechless*, for what seemed like an eternity. It was as though we were standing over her, *trying to guard her against any more harm*. The obvious was exactly that. There was nothing to be said until we knew more. We waited in a vacuum for information. My mind would have raced… but to where?

"Stand firm," I told myself, *"and don't let go…"*

I look back now and realize it was probably no more than 10 minutes waiting for them to transport her to fifth-floor NEURO-ICU. I tried to talk to her, but, of course, it was all quite futile.

She was completely unresponsive.

There is no appropriate way to respond when you are staring into the face of *one of the most incredible human beings you have ever known*, and communicating is impossible. There is no way to let her know that we were there. Quite the opposite, she is lying helpless on a gurney in a hospital corridor on life support, dangling between life and death – and *her future is completely uncertain*.

Knowing if she had a future was all in God's hands.

I knew that certain circumstances might make living worse than dying. *Did Barb go without oxygen to her brain, and if so, how long? If she had been deprived of oxygen to her brain for too long, the prognosis was bleak at best, even if she survived.*

I reflected on David, her dad, being on life support, and how that had ended with his death 33 years earlier — after three days. *Was I going to be faced with that choice again?* I refused to allow my mind to go there. I kept telling that to myself over and over,

There was no need to seek out The Chapel in the hospital. All I needed to do was to call on my God, where I stood. He was already with me, waiting for my request:

Prayer is a surrender to Hope.

𝒜

"Please God,
I humbly come to you now,
to ask you to watch over my daughter
and bring her back to us.

I am powerless over this.

You know her, and the lives she has touched.

You can heal her.
Patience is the ability to tolerate delay.
God, please help me with this!

I am her mother,
and I now surrender her into your loving arms.
Do with her what you will."

Amen.

𝒜

CHAPTER 3

Without You, My Daughter Will Die!

The transport people arrived and announced they were taking Barb upstairs to Neuro-ICU on the 5th floor. My eyes glued themselves to her Ambu bag, as they disconnected her from *Life Support*. Right at that moment, *it was the only thing keeping her alive.*

I watched the guy take my daughter's Ambu bag *and her life* in his hands. He was assisting her breathing and began systematic compressions (deflate and inflate) it. Every 4-5 pumps, *he would miss a beat!* When I would see him miss a beat, all I wanted to do was scream. *"Let me have the bag! At least I can count… and I have rhythm!* **Don't you understand without you doing what you are doing, my daughter will die!"**

I was trying to keep my composure, so I remained silent and stoic, following him every pump down the hall. I caught myself biting my lip to keep quiet.

We finally stepped into the elevator, and up to the 5th floor we ascended. I watched the guy compressing and *missing every 4th - 5th beat. By now, I am trying not to come unglued from the floor. Every muscle, nerve, and fiber of my being was tensing and protesting.*

I was willing my daughter to live!

When the elevator opened, we marched down another seemingly never-ending hallway and turned a corner. Big double doors led into Neuro-ICU. Her cubicle was 519.

As we entered ICU, her cubicle was momentarily quiet. Then suddenly a flood of professionals began turning on multiple machines and hooking up a line of life to Barb's body, getting her settled into what could be the last room she would ever enter.

I wanted this to all be a horrible nightmare!
Of course, that never happened.

Later, I read the report from Bayflite. Each patient is given an ID or alias before they can be identified when Bayflite is called. That stays with them regardless of when their name is attached to their chart.

Barb's assigned alias was "TRAUMA, YANKEE 794."

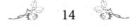

Chapter 3

A portion of her report read as follows: *"This patient arrived at a remote LZ (landing zone) via MCEMS (Manatee County EMS) Ambulance. MCEMS stated that the patient was a driver of a vehicle that struck a tree at a high rate of speed. It was undetermined if the patient was restrained prior to the collision. This patient was unresponsive. Limited information was available…"*

Later, we went to the scene of the accident with the investigator. He had 25 years of experience and went over all the details. After examining her car, he concluded that Barb did, indeed, have her seatbelt fastened.

He told me, *"You see that?"*

He pointed at her seatbelt, now lying on the ground as it hung out of her car. *"That is how I know she had her seat belt on. If not, it would have been snugged up against the inside of her car wall of her T-bar. **That is all that was between her and death.** I am always amazed at how people can find the only tree within 500 yards, and manage to hit that tree. If your daughter had not been wearing her seatbelt, she would have been **dead on impact."***

His words sent chills up and down my spine *"…**dead on impact.**"*

Barb was alone in the car. I thanked God for that. No one else was involved or injured. It was 2:41 AM and the road was deserted. She had sent her last text to her sister, Andrea at 2:30 AM. She was on her way over to her friend Ryan's. She did not have to be at work until 2:00 PM, twelve hours later. She needed some down time, and they had agreed they would relax and watch a movie.

Barb was employed full time by Pinnacle Medical Center in urgent care, a state-of-the-art, doctor-owned, walk-in clinic on 75th Street in Bradenton (FL). She had worked there for more than six years and the last four she had been Charge Nurse. That is quite unusual when you consider that she was an LPN. She had been working 60 hours a week forever, between her official position, and the two part-time home health care jobs she held. Her occupation had become her life.

We later heard that two guys pulled up just after she was propelled into a 50 MPH impact with a tree and called 9-1-1. If not for that, she might have remained unnoticed for an hour or more, and "The Golden Hour" would have passed.

Golden Hour Principle (Wikipedia)

In emergency medicine, the golden hour (also known as golden time) refers to a period lasting for one hour, or less, following traumatic injury being sustained by a casualty or medical emergency, during which there is the highest likelihood that prompt medical treatment will prevent death.

It is well established that the patient's chances of survival are greatest if they receive care within a short period after a severe injury; however, there is no evidence to suggest that survival rates drop off after 60 minutes. Some have come to use the term to refer to the core principle of rapid intervention in trauma cases, rather than the narrow meaning of a critical one-hour period.

Barb was exhausted and simply fell asleep at the wheel.

"There is no other direction for me to go in other than *within* at this point."

Alania Marissette

"Love recognizes no barriers.
It jumps hurtles, leaps fences,
penetrates walls
To arrive at its destination
full of hope."

Maya Angelou

CHAPTER 4

Trauma Alert

The Cedar Hammock Fire/Rescue is one block down the street and around the corner, so when they were called, they responded within seconds of dispatch calling.

2:41 EST DP - Dispatch:
Kenneth Bland (Paramedic) and Bryan Boley (EMT)
2:44 EST – En Route
2:46 EST — AR – Arrived

2:47 EST — WP — Patient Contact / ALS
Assessment Preformed YES
2:48 EST — Assess Lung Sounds:
Left Lung Sounds: Clear Right Lung Sounds:
Clear SKIN Color: Normal / Pink Moisture: Normal/Dry
Temp: Normal, Cap Refill: 2 Seconds
Pupils: L: Mid-Position R: Mid-Position

GCS: (*) 3 – **No Response** – 1 – Motor: **No Response**
1 – Verbal: any Response
Vital Signs: SBP / Radial
Pulse 110 Regular
R-Rate: 25 Regular Respiratory Efforts: Normal
2:52 EST — DEVICE: NonRetreater Mask LPM: 15
2:53 EST — Assess Lung Sounds Left Lung Sounds: Clear
Right Lung Sounds: Clear
SKIN Color: Normal/Pink – Moisture: Normal/Dry
Temp: Normal Cap Refill <2 Seconds
Pupils L Left: Mid-position
Right: Mid Position PERL: Not Assessed

GCS: 3 (NOTE: GCS = <u>Glasgow Coma Scale</u>: first documented)
To be explained
Eye: No Responses - 1
Motor: No Response – 1
Verbal: No Response – 1 SBP/DBP: / Radial Pulse 115 Regular
R-Rate: 25 Assisted Respiratory Effect: Normal

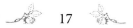

2:57 EST - SPLINT
PULSE PRIOR: Present
SENSATION PRIOR: Present
MOTOR PRIOR: Present
PULSE AFTER: Present
SENSATION AFTER: Present
MOTOR AFTER: Present
Type: LSB/CC/CID/Straps

3:00 EST — Assess Lung Sounds:
Left Lung Clear
Right Lung Sounds:
Clear ASSESSMENT:
SKIN Color: Normal / Pink- Moisture: Normal/Dry –
Temp: Normal Cap Refill <2 seconds
Pupils: L: Mid-Position
R: Mid-Position
PERL: Not Assessed

GCS: 3 (Glasgow Coma Scale)
Eye: No Response – 1
Motor: a Response – 1
Verbal: No Response
OXYGEN: DEVICE Bag Valve Mask LPM: 15
Notes: ASSISTED VENTILATION
VITAL SIGNS: SBP / DBP: Radial Pulse: 108 regular – Resp. R. 19
Assisted: ECG Rhythm: ST – *Sinus Tachycardia* (rapid heart rate)
Respiratory Effort: Normal Entropy: Not Observed

3:01 EST — IV PERIPHERAL
IV SITE: LA – Left Anticubital
IV SOLUTION: NS DROPS/MIN DROPS/CC GUAGE: 14 TOTAL CC's:
SCCESS Y/N No
ATTEMPTS: 3 Notes: 18G x 2
3:05 EST — MediVac Arrived
3:05 EST — BG-BLOOD GLUCOSE
SITE: I.V. MG/DL: 162
3:15 EST — Left Lung Sounds: Clear
Right Lung Sounds: Clear
SKIN Color: Normal / Pink – Moisture: Normal/Dry
Temp: Normal Cap Refill: <2 Seconds Pupils:

L: Mid-Position – R: Mid-Position
PERL: Not Assess

GCS: 3 (Glasgow Coma Scale)
Eye: No response
1 Motor: No response
1 Verbal: No Response

Note: VENTILATED BY BAYFLITE STAFF
3:15 EST — VITAL SIGNS SBP/DBP. 110/86
Method: Automatic Cuff ECG Monitor
Pulse: 105 Regular – R-Rate: 15
Assisted ECG Rhythm: ST – *Sinus Tachycardia*
3:20 EST — MediVac Departed

TRANSPORT INFORMATION

Dispatch Times	Date	Clinical Times
Time of Call	12/29/10	02:49 ARE
Incident	12/29/10	02:49 EST
Time of Dispatch	12/29/10	02:50 ARE
Rendezvous	12/29/10	03:17 EST
Time Enrooted	12/29/10	02:56 AM
Depart with Patient	12/29/10	03:25 EST
Arrival on Scene	12/29/10	03:06 ARE
Accepting Unit	12/29/10	03:43 EST
Depart Scene	12/29/10	03:29 ARE
Sign over	12/29/10	03:44 EST
Arrive Facility	12/19/10	03:40 AM

Regulatory: **First responder was Manatee County EMS,**
Bradenton, Florida
The second responder was:
BAYFLITE 2 (out of Sarasota, Florida)
Other Service Agencies: Fire Dept., Law Enforcement
Intent of Injuries: Unintentional
Mechanism of Injury: Blunt
Injury was caused by: Motor Vehicle traffic

TRAUMA ALERT ACTIVATED: GCS < 12
Valuables: Clothing and valuables left with Trauma room staff.
Fluids: Enrooted 250.0 cc
Prior to Arrival / Crew Assessment/Intervention / Physical Exam

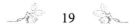

Reason for Transport:
The level of care required is not available at patient's location.
Receiving Level of Care: Level 2
Transport: County/Regional or State protocols
recommend air transport.

Patient Consent: IMPLIED: Patient unconscious or incapable
Incident: **There was a significant intrusion.**
Loss of Consciousness. Extrication required.

> "Some of our greatest obstacles can be
> our best teachers."
>
> Jonas Elrod

> "You may not control all the
> events that happen to you,
> But you can decide not to be
> reduced by them."
>
> Maya Angelou

> "I can be changed by what happens to
> me, but I refuse to be reduced by it."
>
> Maya Angelou

John Thivierge's Report

Trauma, Yankee 794

December 29, 2010

Flight Number: 5-10-62752
My name is John Thivierge.

On December 28, 2010, I was a flight paramedic on **Bayflite 2**, based in Sarasota, FL at Dove Field off of Fruitville Rd.

My shift started at 6:00 pm and was to end on the 29th at 6:00 pm. This particular shift was an interesting and challenging shift because it was my first shift back at Bayflite 2 after surgery approximately 2 months prior. Having been away from the base for 2 months I was eager to get back to work and work with one of the three flight nurses, I was usually scheduled with.

The first half of my shift, until the end of her shift at 7:00 am, I spent working with *Patricia (Patti) Klein, RN*. When I arrived at **Bayflite 2** (about 5:30 pm) we were immediately toned out for first of four flights that evening until the end of my partners shift at 7:00 am.

This particular flight (Trauma, Yankee 794) was our third flight since I came into work. The first two flights were into Sarasota and Manatee County (Florida) to assist their EMS agencies.

At 02:56 am **Bayflite 2** received a call from our Dispatch Center, to respond to Manatee County. Since Patti and I were already awake, and completing documentation from our two previous flights, we immediately prepared for the flight by gathering of flight helmets, PFD's (personal flotation devices), blood, and medications.

Our pilot that evening had already performed his preflight weather check, safety check and was rapidly starting the helicopter for the flight.

Patti and I then proceeded to the aircraft, and conducted our walk around, as part of our preflight check. Following our preflight checks, we secured ourselves into our seats and belted in (The configuration for the flight that evening was the pilot in the right front seat, Thivierge in the left front seat and Klein in the right aft position, behind the pilot.)

At 02:56 am the pilot safely lifted the helicopter off the ground, and we

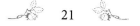

quickly transitioned to forward flight. I immediately called our Dispatch Center, and gave the information of *"Lifted with 3 souls and 120 minutes of fuel."*

The Dispatch Center responded back **"Bayflite 2**, heading 321 degrees for 18 nautical miles. Respond to Manatee County for an MVC positive Trauma Alert, patient back to Bayfront". The information was then verbally repeated back to the Dispatch Center.

During the flight, the landing zone (LZ) crew provided information on the LZ, and *they reported that the patient would be delayed to the LZ due to extensive extrication to remove the patient from the vehicle.*

This particular flight had the LZ set up in Bradenton, FL. This is a common LZ for responses into that area of Manatee County. The patient report was obtained from the Manatee County EMS unit treating the patient (***Barbara - referred to as the patient***, because we did not have information on her name until a later time).

During the flight to the LZ, there was no other information, and we proceeded to go on final approach and landed safely at 03:06 am.

Patti and I were cleared by the pilot to exit the aircraft, and we removed the stretcher, medication bag, and airway bag, and proceeded to wait on the scene until the ambulance arrived from a remote location.

On arrival of the ambulance, Patti quickly entered and received a short report from the EMS crew. *EMS reported a motor vehicle collision with a tree head-on.*

The patient was noted to be unresponsive, did not have a patent intravenous site, and that *she was unable to protect her airway*, even while she was breathing on her own, and *would require intubation for failure to oxygenate properly* on an oxygen mask, and to protect her airway.

The patient was bound on a long spine board with her head secured by head-blocks, and she was strapped to the board for spinal motion restriction. A quick head-to-toe assessment was performed by Patti while I was setting up for intubation.

The assessment revealed that the patient was unresponsive, pupils were dilated equally, there was bleeding from the nose, her trachea was midline, the chest symmetry was normal, lung sounds were clear, and breathing was labored and rapid. The abdomen, pelvis, and upper and lower extremities revealed no significant life-threatening trauma. The heart rhythm was sinus tachycardia and oxygen saturation 90% on high flow oxygen.

Chapter 5

An IV site was unable to be found immediately, and *a decision was made to use an intraosseous (1)* (I/O) needle, and give medications directly to the veins via the bone.*

The patient then had an *I/O inserted into the left humeral head*, and secured by Patti. We were now able to give the patient IV fluids, a sedative (Etomidate) and a paralytic (Succinylcholine) was given by Patti to facilitate intubation.

The patient was then intubated by me, John Thivierge, and the tube was secured. The patient's oxygen saturation then improved to 95%, and she could be ventilated more efficiently.

Patti then gave a longer acting paralytic (Zemuron) to prevent the patient from breathing on her own and start moving during flight. Patti also administered medication for pain (Fentanyl).

We then moved the patient to the aircraft and *loaded for a flight to Bayfront Medical Center in St. Petersburg, Florida, the closest Level I Trauma Center.*

After we had lifted the LZ, we made sure that the patient had warm blankets applied, ear plugs placed, and that she was maintaining her vital signs and airway status.

During the flight to Bayfront, *I placed an orogastric* (O/G) tube into the patient's stomach to prevent secretions, and emesis (blood and stomach contents) from coming out of the stomach, and interfering with the airway, or compromising any other treatment.*

While the O/G tube was inserted, Patti advised the Trauma Room that we were transporting a positive trauma alert and advised them of our findings, treatment and ETA (estimated time of arrival).

We landed on the roof of Bayfront Medical Center at 03:40 am, and *quickly removed the patient from the helicopter*, and took the elevator from the roof (7 floors above the Trauma Room) *to the waiting trauma team* in the trauma room.

At 03:44 am the patient was transferred to the trauma room staff and Drs. Brian S. Hedrick, Emergency Medicine, and Nicholas W. Price, Trauma and Critical Care, with a report of assessment, treatments and condition update.

We then secured supplies, medications and prepared the helicopter for the next flight that would be coming in, before our shift ended. Following this flight, we received one more flight before the end of Patti's shift at 07:00 am.

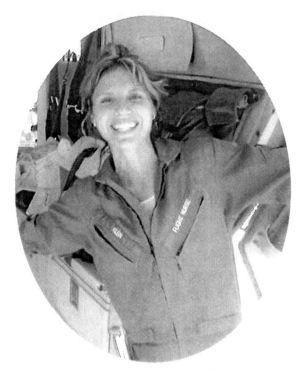

PATRICIA "Patti" KLEIN
May 9, 1971 – Dec. 30, 2010

Please note that on the morning of December 30, 2010, at 9:00 am Patti Klein was killed in a single-vehicle auto crash at the northbound off ramp from I-75 at Bee Ridge Rd in Sarasota. She was killed instantly in the crash.

I was at the scene, and it was a devastating crash.

Patti was truly a professional. I enjoyed working with and miss to this day.

The care that she gave Barbara, and every patient she encountered, was some of the best care I have ever seen given.

Credentials of John Thivierge as of December 29, 2010:
Battalion Chief/ Paramedic for Sarasota County Fire Department (Full-time)
24 years' experience Flight Paramedic-
Bayflite 2/ Bayfront Medical Center (Part-time)
7 years' experience
State of Florida Certified Paramedic JA9616

Chapter 5

Intraosseous infusion: From Wikipedia, the free encyclopedia)

Intraosseous infusion (IO) is the process of injecting directly into the marrow of a bone to provide a non-collapsible entry point into the systemic venous system.[1] This technique is used in emergency situations to provide fluids and medication when intravenous access is not available or not feasible. A comparison of intravenous (IV), intramuscular (IM), and intraosseous (IO) routes of administration concluded that the intraosseous route is demonstrably superior to intramuscular and comparable to intravenous administration (in delivering pediatric anesthetic drugs.)

Procedure

The needle is injected through the bone's hard cortex and into the soft marrow interior which allows immediate access to the vascular system. An IO infusion can be used on an adult or pediatric patients when traditional methods of vascular access are difficult or impossible. Often the anteromedial aspect of the upper tibia is used as it lies under the skin and can easily be palpated and located. The anterior aspect of the femur, the superior iliac crest and the head of the humorous are other sites that can be used.

Tracheal intubation, usually simply referred to as intubation, is the placement of a flexible plastic tube into the trachea (windpipe) to maintain an open airway or to serve as a conduit through which to administer certain drugs. It is frequently performed in critically injured, ill or anesthetized patients to facilitate ventilation of the lungs, including mechanical ventilation, and to prevent the possibility of asphyxiation or airway obstruction.

Major Trauma includes the following categories:

Physiologic Status
(1) Patients with multi-system blunt or penetrating trauma and unstable vital signs.

Anatomical Injuries
(2) Patients with known or suspected anatomical injuries and stable or normal vital signs.

Mechanism of Injury
(3) Patients who are involved in "high energy" event with a risk for severe injury despite stable or healthy vital signs. Once these patients

are identified, an appropriate systems response should be activated. Triage occurs at both the pre-hospital and hospital level.

DISCLAIMER:

Note To Readers

Chapter 6 *is quoted from medical records. It is an accurate timeline and account of what occurred when Barb was delivered to Bayfront Medical Center.*

If you have a background in understanding medical terminology, you will find this interesting and informative.

My goal:

To report minute-by-minute, how my daughter was accessed and diagnosed with life-threatening injuries for those who will find this interesting. The majority of the time when a person is critically injured and taken to a Level One Trauma Center, the family and friends arrive and are completely unaware of what that person has been through.

Chapter 6 is copied directly from Barb's medical records for accuracy. For some of my readers, this may be a very enlightening and informative chapter. However, to do footnotes on each and every procedure and machine would take up entirely too much space here.

If you are a person with no knowledge of medical terminology, and no interest in the events that unfolded in Bayfront Medical Center ER, prior to Barb being diagnosed and admitted, *you may wish to skip this chapter.*

I give a very down-to-earth lay person's account of what all these medical terms boil down to in Chapter 9.

Elizabeth A. Scott

> "PEACE does not mean to be in a
> place where there is no noise, trouble,
> or hard work. It means to be in the
> midst of those things and still
> be calm in your heart."
>
> (Unknown)

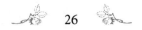

CHAPTER 6

Completely Unresponsive

The report by Bayflite revealed the following:
Non-verbal, unconscious, unresponsive,
Loss of consciousness.
Both right and left pupils dilated.
Breathing: Labored
Sinus Tachycardia (meaning rapid heartbeat).
3:19 AM — Airway Management: 12/29/10
3:42 AM — Received in Bayfront ER

Diagnostic orders by Dr. Price included:
(1) Trauma Pack

Dec. 29, 2010
3:45 AM – The patient is a 38-year old white female, who was a driver in a motor vehicle accident, unsure if she was restrained. She was intubated at the scene due to decreasing level of consciousness and transported as a trauma alert *. They were unable to get venous access. They did interosseous (3) access.

On arrival, the patient was completely unresponsive

CT of the brain shows:
(1) *subarachnoid hemorrhage* throughout the right temporal lobe.
(2) *basilar skull fractures.*

CT of the check was:
(1) negative for aortic (6) injury
(2) bilateral upper rib fractures
(3) bilateral lung contusions* (bruising)

CT of the upper abdomen was negative, but there is fluid or blood in the pelvis. Solid organs appear negative

CT of the C-spine shows: **hemorrhage around the spinal cord,** but no evidence of any acute spinal fractures

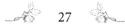

PLAN: Continue with resuscitation with fluids.

<u>Neurosurgery consult</u>

Low volume ventilation with ileal CD (Continuous Delivery) and Nexium IV, SCD' (Sequential Compression Device) to the legs. I also have to insert a high right central venous line in the right femoral vein for access... Nicholas W. Price MD

3:58 AM — A central line was installed in her R-groin by Dr. Price
4:10 AM — A Urinary Foley Catheter was placed.
5:05 AM — Neuro-Surgeon (Dr. Stengel) is called due to:
(1) Abnormal CT scan
(2) Abnormal Radiology Findings
(3) Multiple ICH (Inter-Cranial hemorrhage)
(4) Fractured Skull
(5) C-Spine hemorrhage
(6) Blood in abdomen

5:15 AM — Bp 94/palp Respirations up to 50.

6:20 AM — Order by Dr. Price to: **<u>ADMIT to hospital</u>**

<u>ADMISSION DIAGNOSIS:</u>
MBI (Multiple Body Injury)
CHI (Closed Head Injury),
ICH (Intercranial Hemorrhage)
Assessment reveals: FAILURE TO OXYGENATE, Failure to Protect Airway, Failure to Ventilate

Patient prepared for Oral intubation.

Oral-gastric Tube placed.
15G x 3 in EZ-10 placed in Left Humorous (arm).

Between 3:17 and 3:40 her GCS scored dropped from 8 to 4... not good.

Her **Glasgow Coma Scores** between 3:17 and 3:40 **remained at 3**.
At 3:21 she was given a medication that sedated and paralyzed her. And then there was her ***Glasgow Coma Score.***

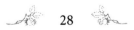

Chapter 6

The Glasgow Coma Scale:

Measures level of consciousness, especially after head injury. It is a quick, practical standardized (universal) system for assessing the degree of consciousness, predicting the duration and ultimate outcome of coma, primarily in patients involving eye opening, verbal responses, and motor responses, all of which are evaluated to a rank order that indicates the level of consciousness, and degree of consciousness, is assessed numerically by the best response.

The results may provide a visual representation of the improvement, stability or deterioration of consciousness, which is critical to predicting the eventual outcome of coma... each parameter can also be used as an overall objective measurement with impairment, 3 compatible with brain death, and 7 usually accepted as an indicator for certain diagnostic tests and treatments...

The scale has consistency even when used with varied experience. A scoring system for evaluating the severity of traumatic brain injury, which measures 3 parameters —- motor responses, verbal responses and 0 (brain death) to a maximum score of 15 for a normal cerebral function.

Glasgow Coma Scale

The eye-opening part of the **Glasgow Coma Scale** has four scores:

Elements of the scale

Eye

Does not open eyes. Opens eyes in response to painful stimuli. Opens eyes in response to voice, Opens eyes spontaneously

Verbal

Makes no sounds Incomprehensible sounds. Utters inappropriate words Confused, disoriented. Oriented, converses normally

Motor

Makes no movements. Extension to painful stimuli (decerebrate response) Abnormal flexion to painful stimuli (decorticate response). Flexion / Withdrawal to painful stimuli. Localizes painful stimuli. Obeys commands

Note that a motor response in any limb is acceptable.

[2] The scale is composed of three tests: eye, verbal and motor responses. The three values separately as well as their sum are considered. The lowest possible GCS (the sum) is 3 (deep coma or death), while the highest is 15 (fully awake person).

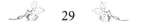

Yankee 794 Trauma

Eye response

There are four grades starting with the most severe:

1. No eye opening

2. Eye opening in response to pain stimulus.
(a peripheral pain stimulus, such as squeezing the
lunula area of the patient's fingernail is more effective
than a central stimulus such as a trapezius
squeeze, due to a grimacing effect).[3]

3. Eye opening to speech. (Not to be confused with the awakening
of a sleeping person; such patients receive a score of 4, not 3.)

4. Eyes opening spontaneously

Verbal response (V)[edit]

There are five grades starting with the most severe:

1. No verbal response

2. Incomprehensible sounds. (Moaning but no words.)

3. Inappropriate words. (Random or exclamatory articulated speech,
but no conversational exchange. Speaks words but no sentences.)

4. Confused. (The patient responds to questions coherently
but there is some disorientation and confusion.)

5. Oriented. Patient responds coherently and appropriately to
questions such as the patient's name and age,
where they are and why, the year, month, etc.)

Motor response (M)

There are six grades:

1. No motor response

2. Decerebrate posturing accentuated by pain
(extensor response: adduction of arm, internal rotation
of shoulder, pronation of forearm and extension
at elbow, flexion of wrist and fingers,
leg extension, plantarflexion of foot)

3. Decorticate posturing accentuated by pain (flexor response:
internal rotation of shoulder, flexion of forearm and wrist
with clenched fist, leg extension, plantarflexion of foot)

4. Withdrawal from pain (Absence of abnormal posturing;
unable to lift hand past chin with supra-orbital pain
but does pull away when nailbed is pinched)

5. Localizes to pain (Purposeful movements towards painful
stimuli; e.g., brings hand up beyond chin
when supra-orbital pressure applied.)

6. Obeys commands (The patient does simple things as asked.)

The best verbal response part of the test has five scores:
- 5 is given if the patient is oriented and can speak coherently.
- 4 indicates that the patient is disoriented but can speak coherently.
- 3 means the patient uses inappropriate words or incoherent language.
- 2 is given if the patient makes incomprehensible sounds.
- 1 indicates that the patient gives no verbal response at all.

The best motor response test has six scores:
- 6 means the patient can move his arms and legs in response to verbal commands.
- A score between 5 and 2 is given if the patient shows movement in response to a variety of stimuli, including pain.
- 1 indicates that the patient shows no movement in response to stimuli.

Barb's Glasgow Scale was a consistent 3… which in truth is as low as you can score without being dead. There is "medical humor" around ER's that goes like this "A tree has a Glasgow Coma Score of 3."

3:42 Barb arrived at Bayfront Medical Center and **admitted into the care of Dr. Nicholas Price M.D., Trauma Surgeon, and Dr. Brian Hedrick D.O. The Emergency Room attending.**

She was unresponsive with hypoxia (inadequate oxygen).
It was noted that a small laceration to the left frontal/temporal had been treated and bleeding controlled. Her oxygen SAT (Saturation Rates) were way down (never good.)

The initial Trauma Surgeon's report read in part

Chief Complaint: MVC trauma* (*Motor Vehicle Trauma)

First seen 3:42 AM
HISTORY OF PRESENT ILLNESS:
This patient is a 38-year-old white female, who was the driver in a motor accident, unsure if she was restrained. She was intubated at the scene due to decreasing level of consciousness and transported as a trauma alert.

On arrival, *the patient was completely unresponsive…* I have no other history.

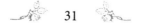

Yankee 794 Trauma

3:42 Small laceration on left front/temporal scalp/bleeding controlled

3:54 CT Abdomen and Pelvis with Contrast
Initial finding: …extensive bilateral pulmonary consolidation consistent with Pulmonary contusion (bruising)
Multiple acute rib fractures.

3:56 Right groin CVL* placed by Dr. Price
3:58 Labs sent – Pt. SAT rate down
3:58 Chest 1V
4:10 Foley catheter placed
4:15 Backboard D/C
4:18 C-Collar D/C
4:19 ET Tube* in place.
NG Tube* in place.

There are rib fractures the right
There is a fracture of the right clavicle…
Pulmonary contusions bilaterally (lung bruising both sides)

4:20 Prep for CT scan…
(1) right clavicle comminuted (shattered) fracture…
(2) bilateral first rib fractures…
(3) multiple left posterior rib fractures…
(4) rib fractures at the 4th and 5th level.

4:44 CT Brain w/o Contract
(1) Posttraumatic subarachnoid hemorrhage in the right temporal lobe…
(2) Hemorrhage adjacent to the right temporal bone…
(3) Subarachnoid hemorrhage…
(4) Linear horizontal fracture through the greater wing of the sphenoid is bilaterally that includes the right sphenoid sinus.

4:44 CT Brain with Contrast
(1) There may be acute hyper dense hemorrhage within the cervical spinal
(2) Canal and basal cistern…
(3) Fractures of ribs, right clavicle, skull base
(4) Right mastoid and left pterygoid;
(5) Probable cervical spinal fluid acute hemorrhage.

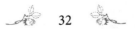

Chapter 6

4:44 CT of The Head Without Contrast
IMPRESSIONS:
Posttraumatic subarachnoid hemorrhage in the right temporal lobe… linear horizontal fracture through the greater wing of the sphenoid bilaterally that includes the right sphenoid sinus.

4:48 CT of Cervical Spine w/o Contrast
IMPRESSIONS: No obvious acute cervical spine fracture; Acute fractures of both 1st ribs, right clavicle, skull base, and right mastoid and pterygoids; possible cervical spinal fluid acute hemorrhage.
4:54 CT Cervical Spine with Contrast reported (in part): …acute mid right clavicular fracture… endotracheal tube and enteric catheter which appears to be in good position…

4:57 CT Abdominal and Pelvis with Contrast
IMPRESSIONS:
Probable cervical spinal fluid acute hemorrhage.

There are acute fractures minimally displaced of the medial and lateral pterygoid on the left. There may be dislocation at the left temporomandibular joint incompletely imaged.

Acute nondisplaced fracture also suspected at the anterior right middle cranial fossa skull base with associated intracranial emphysema.

There are right tympanic cavity and mastoid air cell effusion with a probable acute right temporal bone fracture.

There is an acute fracture of the proximal first left rib…
There may be an acute hyper dense hemorrhage within the cervical spinal and basal cisterns; acute fractures of both first ribs, right clavicle, skull base, right mastoid and left pterygoids; probable cervical spinal fluid acute hemorrhage."

CT scan stated:
There are noted to be small pleural effusions (bilaterally).
There appear to be pulmonary contusions bilaterally. This is most pronounced on the right.

CT Cervical Spine w/o Contrast
…acute mid right clavicular fracture.

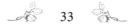

33

An endotracheal tube and enteric catheter which appears to be in good position.
There may be dislocation at the left temporomandibular joint incompletely imaged...
Acute nondisplaced fracture also suspected at the anterior right middle cranial fossa skull base with associated intracranial emphysema.

There is a right temporal bone fracture.
There is an acute fracture of the proximal first left rib.
NO acute cervical spine fracture or facet malalignment.
There may be hyperdense hemorrhage within the cervical spinal canal and basal cisterns.

IMPRESSIONS:
(1) No obvious acute spine fracture;
(2) acute fractures of both first ribs,
(3) right clavicle, skull base,
(4) right mastoid and left pterygoids;
(5) probable cervical spinal fluid acute hemorrhage.

4:54 Procedure: CT Abdomen and Pelvis with contrast or
(1) Injury in upper right quadrant about the inferior vena cava
(2) 4 cm hyper dense or enhancing round hepatic mass
(3) Vascular abnormality verses atypical acute injury.

IMPRESSIONS:
Hemoperitoneum and retroperitoneal soft tissue stranding

5:02 Angio Thorax –
CTA of Patchy consolidation with and w/o Contrast
IMPRESSIONS:
(1) Multiple bilateral rib fractures
(2) Increased attenuation in the anterior mediastinum may represent venous hemorrhage
(3) Negative for evident of aortic dissection or pseudo-aneurysm
(4) Patchy consolidation in both lungs most consistent with bilateral pulmonary contusions.
(5) Negative for pneumothorax or plural effusion.
(6) Comminuted (shattered) right clavicle fracture.

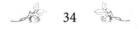

5:02 PROCEDURE — CTA of the chest with and w/o Contrast

IMPRESSIONS:
(1) Multiple bilateral rib fractures.
(2) Increased attention in the anterior mediastinum may represent venous hemorrhage.
(3) Negative for evidence of aortic dissection or pseudo-aneurysm.
(4) Patchy consolidation in both lungs most consistent with pulmonary contusions.
(5) Negative for pneumothorax or plural effusion.

Procedure: CTA of the chest with and w/o Contrast
IMPRESSIONS:
(1) Multiple bilateral rib fractures
(2) Patchy consolidation in both lungs most consistent with bilateral pulmonary contusions.
(3) Comminuted right clavicle fracture.

Procedure: CTA of the chest with and w/o Contrast
IMPRESSIONS:
(1) Multiple bilateral rib fractures
(2) Patchy consolidation in both lungs most consistent with bilateral pulmonary contusions.
(3) Comminuted right clavicle fracture.

5:05 Dr. Brian Hedrick D.O., the ER doctor, and Dr. Nicholas Price M.D., the Trauma Surgeon, were made aware of initial CT findings as per CT tech — **"diffuse" blood in the head.**
Called Dr. Thomas Stengel **(Neuro-Surgeon) for consultation.**

5:06 — CT of the Brain reported
"…There is **posttraumatic subarachnoid hemorrhage in the right temporal lobe…**

Procedure: CTA of the chest with and w/o Contrast
IMPRESSIONS:
(1) Multiple bilateral rib fractures
(2) Patchy consolidation in both lungs most consistent with bilateral pulmonary contusions.
(3) Comminuted right clavicle fracture.

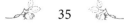

(4) Axial hemorrhage adjacent to the right temporal bone...

There is a horizontal linear fracture through the greater wing of the left sphenoid that appears to cross the midline and involves the sphenoid sinus and the right greater wing of sphenoid.

There is a left lateral pterygoid plate fracture.
There is a small nondisplaced fracture right parietal bone with adjacent pneumocephalus.

Question nondisplaced fracture through the right mastoid air cells.
There is a small amount of pneumocephalus in the right middle cranial fossa inferiorly.

No other skull fractures were found.

5:20 Dr. Price was informed that patient's respiration fracture right parietal bone with adjacent pneumocephalus are up to 50 per minute and BP is 94/palp (meaning lower number was questionable).

5:35 Radiology called with a report of abnormal CT abdominal/pelvis results. Dr. Price asked for a repeat abdominal scan to double check.

6:20 Dr. Price writes ADMIT orders.
By now she had been given 2100 cc of IV fluids and her urinary/gastric output was 1375 cc.

14:50 PM H and P

FINAL REPORT
(1) Subarachnoid hemorrhage throughout the right temporal lobe
(2) Basilar skull fracture
(3) Bilateral upper rib fractures
(4) Bilateral lung contusions
(5) Fluid or blood in pelvis
(6) C-spine shows hemorrhage around spinal cord, but no evidence of any acute spinal fractures.

Initial blood gases from her upper extremity shows pH 7.18,
Base deficit -11.6, p02 49, hemoglobin 13.

Plan: Continue with resuscitation with fluids.
Neurosurgery consult
Low volume ventilation with ileac CD and Nexium IV
SCD's to the legs.

I also had to insert a high right central venous line* in the right femoral vein
for access.
Dr. Nicholas W. Price MD

11:34 AM — CT Brain w/o Contrast
IMPRESSIONS:
(1) Interval evolutionary changes identified within hemorrhagic
(2) Contusions to the right temporal lobe with acute subarachnoid blood,
(3) Small right subdural and intraventricular hemorrhage noted.
(4) Ventricular size is stable.
(5) Tiny hemorrhage focuses also identified within the subcortical white
matter of the high life parietal lobe.
(6) Multiple skull base fracture extending to the right petrous temporal bone
sphenoid bone are again noted.

13:30 I was asked by staff to try to locate NOK* (*next-of-kin) for this patient,
who arrived earlier, in search (brother)- no phone listed, (mother) - no
phone listed, (sister) — phone number incorrect, (mother) — phone number
incorrect
I used whitepages.com – no phone numbers listed for above. I called FHP/
Manatee County and was told an officer has already gone by patient's address
and left card have not heard back. They will keep us updated if they receive a
call.
Chaplain Chanchal
(Note: Family all had cell phones.)

13:37 CT Angio Head
(1) Fracture through the right temporal bone and bilateral greater wing of the
sphenoid bone with fracture line extending into the sphenoid sinus.
(2) Fracture through the body of the pterygoid bone,
(3) Fracture of both left medial and lateral pterygoid plates.
(4) Fracture of the bony nasal septum

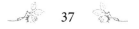

13:37 CT Angio Neck

(1) **Numerous skull base fractures** involving the greater wing of the sphenoid bone bilaterally, both pterygoid plates and left parietal bone with extension into the sphenoid sinus…
(2) Soft tissue density alone the superior aspect of the left orbit with a small focus on the air. This may represent edema or sub periosteal hematoma with a minimal inferior displacement of the superior rectus muscle.

NOTE: By the time Barb was admitted to Neuro-ICU, and we were with her it was 5:00 PM (17:00 EST), the diagnoses were piling up beyond comprehension, although, *at the time, I had no idea what they were.* I had not seen any of the reports, so the extent of her injuries was still a mystery to me.

Later, I was able to obtain the full picture, and that information would take me to another whole level of fear, I had yet to experience.

"Even in darkness it is
possible to create light."

Elie Wiesel

"Having courage does not mean
that we are unafraid. Having courage
and showing courage means
we face our fears."

Maya Angelou

ALIVE
"We are wired to be brave; that's why
we never feel more alive than when
we're being courageous."

Brene Brown

CHAPTER 7

Things to Remember: What Happens Immediately After the Injury?

November 3, 2015

What happens to the brain at the point of injury?

Traumatic brain injury (TBI) refers to damage or destruction of brain tissue due to a blow to the head, resulting from an assault, a car crash, a gunshot wound, a fall, or the like.

In closed head injury, damage occurs because the person receives a blow to the head that whips the head forward and back or from side to side (as in a car crash), causing the brain to collide at high velocity with the bony skull in which it is housed. This jarring bruises brain tissue and tears blood vessels, particularly where the inside surface of the skull is rough and uneven; damage occurs at (and sometimes opposite) the point of impact. Thus, specific areas of the brain – most often the frontal and temporal lobes – are damaged. This focal damage often can be detected through MRI and CAT scans.

http://media.songkhoe24.vn/archive/images/

2015/04/23/105746_stv2.jpg

In closed head injury, the rapid movement of the brain can also stretch and injure neuronal axons – the long threadlike arms of nerve cells in the brain that link cells to one another, that link various parts of the brain to each other and that link the brain to the rest of the body.

This widespread axonal injury interrupts functional communication within and between various brain regions and sometimes between the brain and other body parts. However, this type of diffuse damage typically cannot be detected by currently available imaging technology (but with new developments, this may change).

Its existence is very clear, however, in the widespread effects it has on the individual's functioning.

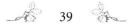

In sum, after a closed head injury, damage can occur both in specific brain areas (due to bruising and bleeding) and also be found throughout the brain (due to stretched or destroyed axons).

The results of a closed head injury tend to affect broad areas of the individual's functioning, primarily due to the diffuse axonal injury.

The extent of damage is correlated with the force of the blow to the head; for example, a head forced into a car windshield at high speed will tend to sustain more tissue damage than when the car is traveling at a slower speed.

Open head injury, the second type of TBI, occurs when the skull is penetrated, for example by a bullet. Damage following open head injuries tends to be focal, not diffuse, and the implications for subsequent impairment tend, also, to be focal and limited. However, such injuries can be as severe as closed head injuries, depending on the destructive path of the bullet or another invasive object within the brain.

What happens immediately after TBI?

Immediately following TBI, two types of effects are seen. First, brain tissue reacts to trauma and to tissue damage with a series of biochemical and other physiological responses. Substances that once were safely housed within the cells now flood the brain. These processes further damage and destroy brain cells, in what is called secondary cell death.

The second type of effect is seen in the individual's functioning. For those with more severe injuries, loss of consciousness (LOC) occurs at the time of trauma, lasting from a few minutes or hours to several weeks or even months. Lengthy LOC is referred to as coma. In such severe injuries, the first few days after trauma may also produce adverse changes in respiration (breathing) and motor functions.

As an individual regains consciousness (those with the severest injuries may never do so), a variety of neurologically based symptoms may occur: irritability, aggression, and other problems. Post-traumatic amnesia (PTA) is also typically experienced when an injured person regains consciousness. PTA refers to the period when the individual feels a sense of confusion and disorientation – Where am I? What happened? – and an inability to remember recent events.

As time passes, these responses typically subside, and the brain and other body systems again approach physiological stability. But, unlike tissues such as bone or muscle, the neurons in the brain do not mend themselves. New nerves do not grow in ways that lead to full recovery. Certain areas of the brain remain damaged, and the functions that were controlled by those areas may emerge as challenges in the individual's life.

Before discussing in greater detail what happens to the person after injury, which depends to great extent on the severity of the injury, "severity" needs to be defined (in the next question).

What is meant by "severity of injury"?

Typically, "severity of injury" refers to the degree of brain tissue damage. Although the degree of such damage cannot be directly measured, it is estimated typically by measuring the duration of loss of consciousness (LOC) and the depth of coma (and sometimes by the length of PTA).

The scale most commonly used to measure the depth of coma is the **Glasgow Coma Scale (GCS).** The GCS is used to rate three aspects of functioning: eye opening, motor response, and verbal response. Individuals in deep coma score very low on all these aspects of functioning, while those less severely injured or recovering from coma score higher.

A Glasgow Coma Scale (GCS) score of 3 indicates the deepest level of coma, describing a person who is totally unresponsive. A score of 9 or more indicates that the individual is no longer in a coma, but is not fully alert. The highest score (15) refers to a person who is fully conscious.

The severity of the injury is typically categorized into three levels: mild (or minor), moderate and severe. A commonly used rule of thumb is that mild injury refers to LOC of less than 20 minutes and an initial GCS of 13-15. Typically, an initial GCS of 9-12 defines a moderate injury and 3-8 a severe injury.

Although initial "severity" measures may generally predict long-term impairment, initial severity scores do not correlate well with negative consequences in a person's life. The effects of TBI on individuals and the meaning of those results depend upon a wide variety of factors, only one of which is initial "severity of the injury."

How long does recovery take?

Recovery after injury is usually quite different for those with moderate-to-severe injuries versus those with mild injuries. And, as must be constantly kept in mind, recovery varies greatly from person to person. Thus, *recovery will not be the same for any two people with TBI.*

In mild TBI, one person may recover quickly and completely while another may experience significant challenges even several years after injury. (Recovery after mild TBI is discussed more fully in a later question, What Problems Emerge after a Mild TBI?)

In more severe injuries, recovery is a multistage process, which typically continues in a variety of ways for months and years. However, the length of this recovery process is not uniform, and the stages of recovery that are typical when considering the population as a whole may be very different for any specific individual. Stages may not proceed step-wise but may overlap, one stage with the next, or one or more stages may be skipped altogether. The early recovery process is discussed more fully in the next question.

How is recovery measured right after injury?

The progress seen during the immediate recovery period in individuals with severe to moderate TBI is often tracked using the Rancho Los Amigos Scale, which specifies eight levels – from the depths of coma to return to awareness and purposeful activity. These levels of recovery of functioning reflect processes within the brain, as it heals, stabilizes, and reorganizes itself to some extent.

Although the Rancho scale assumes that recovery will pass through eight stages, a small percentage of people with severe injuries remain stuck at Levels I to III for months or years. They remain in a coma or in a relatively unresponsive state and fail to return to purposeful, appropriate functioning.

Rancho Los Amigos Scale

- Level I (No Response): The individual is in a deep coma and does not respond to any stimuli.

- Level II (Generalized Response): The person sleeps most of the time, with periods of brief wakefulness. Responses and movements are largely reflexed not purposeful.

- Level III (Localized Response): The person is alert for lengthier periods. He/she reacts inconsistently to commands, but his/her responses are related to the type of stimulus presented. For example, noises will produce a listening response.

- Level IV (Confused and Agitated): As awareness increases, the individual's behavior reflects his/her sense of confusion and disorganization. Aggressive and/or silly behavior may be seen, with verbal abuse, agitated actions, and incoherent speech. The person's attention span is too short to allow full cooperation in treatment programs; and the person is unable to do basic tasks, such as eating, independently.

Chapter 7

- Level V (Confused, Inappropriate, Not Agitated): Simple commands are now followed consistently; the person's long-term memory is returning, and she/he can now carry out over-learned skills such as eating. The difficulty is evident in following complex commands, short-term memory, learning new skills, and concentrating for more than a few minutes.

- Level VI (Confused, Appropriate): The individual begins to show goal-directed behavior, but usually still needs direction. The person is more aware of his/her deficits, family members, and so forth. He/she can carry out more tasks independently and retains relearned skills from one occasion to the next.

- Level VII (Automatic, Appropriate): The individual performs daily routines automatically and is better able to learn new skills, although slower than before the injury. The person still has poor short-term memory; judgment and problem solving are still impaired.

- Level VIII (Purposeful, Appropriate): The person is able to function once more in the community. Impairments in cognitive, social, and emotional functioning, to a greater or lesser extent, may continue.

> "Power is the Alignment of your personality and your soul."
>
> Gary Zukav

> "Intuition is not a single way of knowing – it's our ability to hold space for uncertainty and our willingness to truth the many ways we've developed knowledge and insight, including instinct, experience, faith and reason."
>
> Dr. Brene Brown Ph.D.

CHAPTER 8

The Anatomy of the Brain

Elementary Guide: How The Brain Works

The human body is made up of a number of different types of organs, which help us grow and stay healthy. While all of these organs are important, the nervous system—which features the brain—is one of the most important. Without our brain, our ability to walk, talk, and the dress would be very difficult, if not impossible. People who are interested in learning more about the brain are should first understand its parts and the way those parts work. Knowing the responsibilities of the nervous system is also important for those who hope to learn more about this important part of the body. Brain Model.

Parts of the Brain

Currently, there are four individually-recognized parts of the brain. These include the cerebellum, cerebrum, brain stem, and limbic system. The biggest part of the brain is the cerebrum and is divided into the frontal, parietal, temporal, and occipital lobes. While these different parts of the brain do have their own functions, they must also work together to ensure optimal results in human health.

The Brain's Function

Unsurprisingly, the different parts of the brain have different jobs. For example, the cerebrum is responsible for thoughts, such as reasoning, planning, emotions, problem-solving, and perceptions. The cerebellum works to maintain balance, muscle tone, and gait. The brain stem is especially important since it is important for blood pressure, respiration, and heart rate. Finally, the limbic system controls hunger, thirst, memory, fear, and emotion. These different processes must often work together.

Functions of the Nervous System

The nervous system is the series of nerve cells that send messages back and forth between different parts of the body. As with the brain, there are a number of functions of the nervous system. Specifically, the nervous system provides a lot of information about the environment, such as temperature, smell, sound, and taste. Without the assistance of the nervous system, the brain would not be able to function properly.

http://nursingschool.org/kids-guide-to-how-the-brain-works/

Chapter 8

Right Temporal Lobe Functions
by Rudolph Hatfield,
Demand Media Google

The right temporal lobe is primarily involved in processing nonverbal information.

The two temporal lobes of the brain are divisions of the cerebral cortex located on the lower side of each cerebral hemisphere. The right temporal lobe has many different functions that complement left temporal lobe functions, and new information is being discovered all the time.

The primary functions of the right temporal lobe area nonverbal memory, nonverbal aspects of communication, aspects of pitch and sound location and certain aspects of personality.

Memory

The temporal lobes contain structures necessary for memory. The right temporal lobe is specialized to process nonverbal memories such as memory for pictures, visual scenes, familiar faces, routes or directions and music, but may also contribute to verbal memory, which is a primary left temporal lobe function. The temporal lobes do not store all of these memories but instead encode new information and relay it to other systems of the brain to be stored. Thus, if the right temporal lobe is severely damaged, the person may remember many previously learned scenes, pictures and music, but she will not be able to form new memories of these.

Nonverbal Communication

The right temporal lobe is important in prosody or the rhythm of one's speech. People with damage to the right temporal lobe often produce meaningful sentences, but they are choppy and uneven. The right temporal lobe is also important in decoding speech intonations, the changes in the tone of speech that give it different meanings in different contexts; decoding others' facial expressions, and interpreting sequences of visual and verbal information. Thus, people with right temporal lobe damage often have difficulty picking up social cues, understanding facial expressions, following tunes and melodies, inhibiting comments that might be offensive to others and understanding aspects of nonverbal communication — such as humor, expressed anger or sadness — in others.

Pitch

The auditory cortex, the portion of the brain that processes the sounds picked up by your ears, is located in the temporal lobes. The right auditory cortex processes most of the information from the left ear and vice versa; however, damage to the right auditory cortex does not result in a person being unable to process sounds from the left ear because each ear sends information to both hemispheres. The right auditory cortex does process information about the direction from which sounds come based on their differences in pitch; it also processes how high or low the pitch of these sounds is. People with right temporal lobe damage often have difficulty locating the source of sounds or determining changes in pitch.

Personality

The right temporal lobe is also involved in aspects of personality. Research on individuals with severe right temporal lobe damage indicates these people are often egocentric or unable to consider the perspectives of other people. They can be long-winded and emphatic when speaking, have trouble moving from one topic to another and can stick to one topic to the point of being inappropriate. They may display aggression and paranoia and are often obsessed with strict religious or moral concerns.

ᕫ

Lasting Love

Love is much more than a tender caress
And more than bright hours of happiness.
For a lasting love is made up of sharing
Both hours that are joyous and also despairing.

It's made up of patience
and deep understanding
And never of stubborn or selfish demanding.

It's made up of climbing the steep hills together
And facing with courage,
life's stormiest weather,
And nothing on earth or in heaven
can part a love
That has grown to be part of the heart.

And just like the sun and the stars and the sea
This love will go on through eternity.
For true love lives on when earth things die,
For it's part of the spirit that soars to the sky.

Author: Unknown

ᕫ

CHAPTER 9

Could My Daughter Be Dying?

꙳

11 Now faith is the substance of things hoped for,
the evidence of things not seen.
Hebrews 11:1 (KJV)

꙳

What I hadn't yet processed was that *my daughter might be dying.* The multiple fractures encompassing her skull were significant – life-altering. **Any one of the six (6) traumatic brain injuries (TBI's) *could have killed her.***

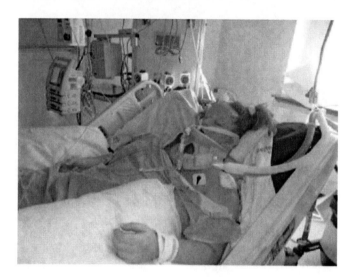

The capacious scanning ordered within hours after she was delivered in the arms of the incredible trauma team of Dr. Hedrick and Dr. Price told an unsettling story that unfolded as follows:

The entire upper front and sides of her face & chest had taken the brunt of the impact when her car slammed into the tree at nearly 50 MPH, attempting to propel her through the windshield. She should have been thrown from the car, and been DOA (dead on arrival) when the first responder team arrived.

(1) Her right Clavicle was not only fractured – it was shattered.

(2) Nearly all of the bones in her face were significantly fractured (from a broken nose to both eye sockets, and extending all the way to behind her right and left ear).

(3) Her 1st, 2nd, 3rd, 4th, and 5th ribs both right and left side were fractured.

(4) Both hips were fractured.

(5) Her left lung had collapsed for a time.

(6) She had gone into Stage 3 Hemorrhagic Shock.

We later determined that she *was* wearing her seatbelt, and *her seatbelt was all that separated her from life and certain and immediate death.*

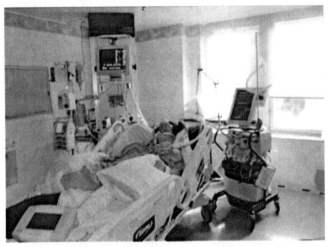

Dec. 30, 2010 Barb in ICU (on life support).

Dr. Stengel, her Neurosurgeon, introduced himself to me. He offered to answer any questions I might have, however, he did not volunteer any information.

Mostly I was speechless, which anyone who knows me will tell you *is extremely rare.* What question was I going to ask him? How could he help me to understand what had happened to Barb?

He was very calm and deliberate in the way he moved around my daughter's bed. It seemed reassuring. The only way I could possibly describe what I was feeling was **fear on steroids.**

At a loss for what I needed to ask, and to grasp for information, I tossed out *the one question* that seems to make sense, in all the chaos, *"How long do you think it will be before she begins to regain consciousness?"*

He looked up over his glasses from reading the monitor, and his eyes met mine. In a very compassionate, confident, and reassuring tone, *his answer gave me hope,*

"In about fifteen days, she should start to come out of this coma."

"Does she need surgery?" was my next question.

"There is no surgical intervention needed for her at this time." was his answer.

Frankly, that sounded to me like a politician's non-committal answer (when I look back now that I know the whole picture we were facing). Of course, I took that to mean that Barb had not suffered any broken bones. In the ensuing days, I would come to realize **I had asked the wrong question!**

What I wanted to know was, *did she have any broken bones*? Had I asked *that*, he would have given me a very different response. She has lots of broken bones. However, they could not be fixed by surgery. **Time and God were to be the healer here.**

The smell of fear and uncertainty was palatable, permeated the air like some sort of unpleasant sewer stench.

Not long after that he again addressed us. *"You folks need to go to the waiting room now, for a few minutes. I need to install an ICP* (Intracranial Pressure Probe) into your daughter's head. We have to measure the pressure in her brain, and see what the reading tells us for the next few days."*

"What are you looking for?" I inquired.

*"Once the ICP (*covered end of this chapter) is in, there will be a **purple line** you can follow on the monitor. If it shows a reading of more than 20, that is not good, especially for an extended period of time. If it stayed below 20, **that** is a good sign."*

As all four of us retreated down the long hallway to the ICU waiting room. I knew he was going to drill a hole in my daughter's already over-traumatized head.

I glanced around the waiting room. My eyes are stopping to analyze faces, one-by-one, and wondering why each was in this place at this time. What had their loved one experienced that brought them to ICU?

The smell of fear and uncertainty was palatable, permeated the air like some sort of unpleasant sewer stench.

I think, more than anything, I was trying to distract myself, as my anxiety level went through the roof!

For what seemed like an eternity we all sat waiting. When I could stand it no longer, after 45 minutes, I headed back to Barb's room with Andrea in hot pursuit.

As we entered Room 519, there was a probe sticking approximately 2 inches out of the upper left side of Barb's skull. One-quarter of her hair had been shaved. A good deal of her long gorgeous auburn hair was gone!

"Oh my gosh, Mom!" Andrea declared. "They shaved her head! Barb's going to be so upset, when she wakes up, and sees what they did!"

(This was a reference to the fact that Barb would let her hair grow for 4 years, and then, she would have it cut, and donate it to Locks of Love. Her hair was due to be cut again shortly.)

From the day the ICP was placed, I would watch that purple line, one of seven lines on the monitor. It would fluctuate between readings of 4 and 14. It never did hit 20 or above, and for that, I was very relieved and grateful. **It was an early sign that gave me Hope.**

What is Intracranial Pressure (ICP)?

Intracranial Pressure (ICP) is a vital way of monitoring the health and outcome of the brain after injury. The brain is encased in a non-flexible cover – the skull. Therefore, if there are changes which result in increased pressure, the fluid that surrounds the brain has nowhere to go.

The doctors in the emergency room and in acute care facilities in hospitals are continuously interested in whether or not this pressure has been raised.

In a healthy adult, the ICP is usually in the range of 0 to 10 mmHg, and any pressure greater than 20mmHg is abnormal. When ICP is greater than 40mmHg, there is almost always some neurological dysfunction (impairment of consciousness, problems breathing, pupil dilation, compression of the brain found on MRI) as well as impairment of the brain's electrical activity (an abnormal EEG). A pressure above 60mmHg is fatal while pressures between 20 and 40mmHg indicate a much poorer outcome for patients suffering from such pressure.

CHAPTER 10

Could Facebook be Therapeutic?

Isn't it odd how the human brain rationalize information? As we hung around the ICU waiting room, we began to hear whispers about a man down at the other end of the hall. He had taken a nose dive off the top of a 4-story ladder and landed *face first* on the concrete sidewalk below. The thought made my skin crawl. In truth, the trauma that Barb's head had suffered was probably nearly as severe. ***I was amazed her neck was not broken, resulting in a lifetime of paralysis.*** Thank God for small favors, I remember thinking.

> Any one of six (6) traumatic brain injuries could have killed her. I was amazed her neck was not broken, resulting in a lifetime of paralysis.

All of us had been entertaining ourselves with Facebook (FB) for some time. Each of us, including Barb, had a page. Never did I think it would become an integral part of my life until that day.

In coming days and weeks, my updates on FB kept everyone in the loop without me having to answer my phone when I needed to be dealing with medical issues at the hospital.

I began journaling on Barb's FB page immediately when I returned home from our first hospital visit!

The first post came from her friend, Ryan, even before I got home from the hospital. She had been on her way over to his house that night to watch a movie when the accident occurred. (From this point on some messages will be posted, but they won't necessarily include names. There were *so many* messages that I can't begin to reproduce all of them — so we are doing a few very significant ones.)

(Start of Facebook posts)

December 29, 2010 — Day 1 — 5:24 PM

Ryan: *To all friends of Barb. She was in a bad car accident last night. She has been Bayflited... I'm in contact with her mom... I will post more info as it becomes available... As of now, she is in I.C.U at Bayfront, St. Pete.*

6:28 PM Shelley: Barb you are a fighter. I'm thinking of you. I need you to come back to help with the City of Bradenton. U and I are the team for that! I enjoyed working with you. I 'm praying for u. Love you girl.

9:18 PM Christina: Barb, sending healing angels to watch over you. Praying for your speedy recovery. My thoughts and prayers are with you.

9:42 PM: **I am Barb's Mom, Elizabeth Scott.**

We have just come from, Bayfront Medical Center in St. Pete. Barb's was Bayflited and is in **critical condition with Traumatic Brain Injury (TBI), abdominal and chest injuries, and bleeding on the brain.** She is completely unresponsive right now. Please pray that she is okay. The Neurosurgeon says she is "stable" and only time will tell the outcome. She is in Neuro-ICU Room 519. Please send prayers and I will post any updates on her FB page.

Edward (her uncle): Your Grandma Betty, is praying for you and loves you very much!!!

Lisa: Praying for you. May God heal you and make you completely whole.

Stacy: My sister by another mister. My heart and prayers are with you!

Cassandra: Barb U are a fighter. I'm thinking of you. I need U to come back to help with the City of Bradenton. U and I are a team for that. I enjoy working with you. I am praying…

Carol: Barb, we are keeping you in our prayers. Hang in there… ((Hugs))

10:25 OMG, Barb! I am thinking of you and your family and praying for you all!!!

10:44 Barb, work won't be the same without you! You have to get better so we can see your beautiful smile again.

11:56 Barbie, this is your Aunt Janet, please get well. I'm praying for you. **KISSES and HUGS.**

Angela: Put up a fight Barb. Lots of prayers being said for you tonight!!!

Shelley: Barb, you're in our prayers. I know you are a fighter. Be strong. You're an essential part of our team, and the thing will not be the same without you.

11:39 PM — **Angie:** Barbara, and to all her family… My prayers go out to all of you. I graduated from Manatee High with Barb, and she has always taken such good care of me at Pinnacle. My heart aches for you all and I pray she will be okay. Please, oh Lord, take care of Barb. I love you Barb and may the Lord heal you and restore you to health. God Bless you all. A Hug from me.

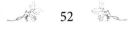

Chapter 10

11:45 PM – **Elizabeth Scott:** I had no idea what was going to be happening on a minute-by-minute or day-by-day basis. However, it was a good thing that Bayfront Medical Center exists for us in this emergency being the only Level One Trauma Center in our area (at the time). That night as we all tore ourselves away from the ICU, I was feeling completely overwhelmed.

We had no clue if Barb would live or die. All four of us came in one car, so other arrangements had to be made.

She had hundreds of people who were her FB "friends", and she brags that she knows all of them. I realized that they were waiting to hear something – any crumb of hope I could toss them as an update. It would be a far less hindrance if I could place the updates on her FB page than to have numerous phone calls creating interruptions to my time and day. I promise to keep the news coming by posting here as it is made available to me.

People had tried to call her and were alarmed that she was not answering her phone. As her mother, I felt it fell to me to post on her FB page and keep her family and friends informed of whatever news we had — *good or bad.*

Dec. 30, 2010 Kelli Stevens — Day 2 — 12:34 AM — I have spent 2 hours trying to figure out what everyone is talking about... should have thought to check here first. Barb... You are tough as nails... pull through this. We need you! We love you!

6:12 AM — Heavenly Father, please wrap your arms around Barbara... heal her and send her back to us... we all love and need her... we asked this in your son's precious name Jesus!!! Amen

7 AM **UPDATE** — Barb's purse and cell phone were left in her now-demolished vehicle when Bayflite airlifted her to Bayfront Medical Center. For 12 hours, none of us were notified she was in an accident. (The law was changed in 2010 in Florida to allow you to place next-of-kin in a database with FHP) The family only became alarmed after 2:10 PM when she could not be reached by her sister... and then by her supervisor at work (Pinnacle), Shelley, called me that Barb did not show up for work. She was never late for work, and by 2:20 PM this became a big red flag. Her only brother is currently in Iraq. He called me around 11 PM when he began seeing posts on her FB page. I updated him.

Dr. Stengel, her Neurosurgeon, says *it is too early to determine if Mark should come home from Iraq.* He promised to let me know if she takes a turn for the worse.

Nurses gave her a bath during the night, and she is showing *"localization"*—

meaning she is responding to stimulus, but NOT responding to verbal commands...

10:26 AM **UPDATE** — I spoke to the social worker, Mary Ann, at Bayfront Medical Center. Barb is responding to some physical stimulus and moving her lower extremities. She is not responding yet, in any other way including to voices.

Dr. Stengel is to call with the report on her M.R.I. No flowers or balloons allowed in Neuro-ICU., however, cards and letters are welcome and encouraged.

Bayfront Medical Center, 701 – 6th St. South, Room 219, St. Petersburg, Fl. 33701.

Let's fill her room so when she wakes, she knows how much she is loved. Elizabeth Scott (Barb's mom).

11:23 AM PRAYING THAT YOU GET BETTER FAST!! HANG IN THERE BARB. Our thoughts are with you!

Paul: You are an amazing woman Barb! Hang in there. We all know you can!

Lacey Dawn: Praying that you get better fast!! Hang in there Barb. Our thoughts are there with you. From the entire Scott family in Missouri.

11:24 AM Barb, you are in our prayers this morning as I reread the many posts on this page. Please know that you are loved by many, and you and your family are in our thought at this difficult time. See you soon!

3:19 PM **Paige:** Barbara, I pray that you heal and come back to us! We all love you so much! My son is looking at your photo, and he is talking about all the times you and I took him to the park for our walks! He is saying "I see Miss Barbara; there she is; can we go to the park now?" (He is 3.) I pray that we WILL go to the park again, soon!

4:03 PM: **Elizabeth Scott:** She is not (yet) responding to voices, but she is a fighter. I think by the weekend we might have more news on prognosis.

10:12 pm **UPDATE:** I have been waiting all day for the MRI results. Finally, I called the hospital tonight to get a report on Barb from Heather, her nurse. She opened her eyes once this evening... progress.

Also, the PA called from Dr. Stengel's office. She now reports that the MRI was done to confirm what Dr. Stengel thought was a bleed at her brain stem (which controls respiration) was not a bleed. The MRI was to double-check on what they thought they saw. It turns out **there is not a brain stem bleed,** which is surprising news, meaning her respiratory system is not compromised. Instead, what **they are now finding is that the left side of her head was impacted, which set her brain into a "slosh" causing a right temporal lobe bleed.** Time will heal this — her brain is bruised and is trying to fix itself.

Thank you, God! It will be a long recovery, but I think we may be heading in the right direction.

<u>Right Temporal Lobe Bleed</u>:

One of the primary functions of the temporal lobes is the recognition of speech, sound, and visual information. When your temporal lobe is not functioning properly, your ability to understand what people are saying or to understand visual information can be lost. The right and left lobes work together.

She is a fighter and Barb is trying to override the respirator. This is encouraging! It means her brain stem (though damaged) is functioning!!!

Her Neurological Assessments today are improved from yesterday. She is moving her arms and legs. Her vital signs are stable.

The probe in her brain measures 11 and down (20 and up is dangerous). She has a PICC Line (peripherally inserted central catheter (PICC), elongated catheter introduced through a vein in the arm, then through the subclavian vein into the superior vena cava or right atrium to administer parenteral fluids (as in hyperalimentation) or medications or to measure central venous pressure

Barb (in Mo.): Hey, Snicklefritz… hugs and prayers. Love you bunches. Get well soon.

Mitzie: Barb, my prayers are with you and your family! We miss you!

Shannon: OMG, Barb! I am thinking of you and your family. Praying for you all!!!

Jennifer: Barb we are all praying for a full recovery.

7:32 PM — **Andrea** (her sister): I want to thank everyone that is praying for my sister, and I'm also praying for her to get better very soon, although it will probably be a long recovery process. She is a fighter, and **I have all the faith in God right now, that she will pull through this. Only God can see the whole picture. I'm sure He has a plan.**

Jennifer: Barb, I'm praying for your full recovery.

Korey: Praying for you Barb! Get better soon, we all need and love you!

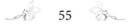

Barb's brother, Mark, is in the US Army in Iraq. We are asking the Red Cross for help in processing his request to come home. We have been working all day on this. He called, and I was at the hospital, and I was able to update him on her condition.

Dec. 31, 2010 — Day 3— 8:21 AM

UPDATE: Barb had an uneventful night. Her vitals are stable, her color is excellent, and she is warm to touch her hands and feet.

The Neurological assessment from Wednesday to Thursday is an 180-degree improvement!

I have been waiting all day for the MRI results. Finally, I called the hospital tonight on Barb and asked Heather, her nurse. Barb opened her eyes once this evening... progress. Shelley, Barb's supervisor (Pinnacle Medical Group) went to Bayfront to visit Barb, even though she is unresponsive, and on a lot of machines. After speaking with the medical staff at Bayfront, and "visiting" with Barb, she reported that they are very encouraged. **We feel confident in her sweet spirit, and steadfast determination will be restored.**

Shelley told me that *the staff has agreed to share Barb's hours to hold her job. It's called Spirit and Team Work.* This is a beautiful thing, and we all thank them for their confidence.

She is not yet responding to voices, but she is a fighter. I think by the weekend we might have more news on the prognosis.

Our family discovered today that she had AFLAC!!! That means that in addition to Blue Cross Blue Shield, all her hospitalization, her rehabs, and any disability are covered!!! *It means everything to me to know that she will get all the care she needs through her recovery.*

I spoke to a social worker, Mary Ann at Bayfront Medical Center. Barb responded to some physical stimulus and were moving her lower extremities.

Dr. Stengel is to call shortly with a report on her MRI. My concern now is that THIS is New Year's Eve day. If we do not get the paperwork signed this afternoon for my son to begin his journey home (from Iraq), it might take another couple of days for all the paperwork to be in place through the military. That would mean up to a week delay for him to arrive here.

The Red Cross paperwork is up in ICU for Dr. Price to sign and somehow it keeps missing him — getting delayed. *Until it is approved, no action can be taken* through The Red Cross and in turn, the US Army, *to allow my son's orders to be released, to come home.*

Chapter 10

UPDATE: I have been on the phone tirelessly, trying to alert the trauma doctors to the fact that *the paperwork that absolutely needs to be signed* is in Neuro-ICU, and an attending (doctor) has to authorize a release of the information, *to get my son home.* Finally, I was able to connect to "the trauma attending" who immediately passed the information on to Dr. Price. She called be back (almost immediately) to tell me that Dr. Price had just signed the paperwork, and it has now been faxed over to The Red Cross office locally for processing. I have been on FB-IM with my son throughout this ordeal and expected he will be in touch to give me his schedule for departure from Iraq through Kuwait to the US and home to us.

Edward (her uncle): We love you and are praying for you, that God will make you completely whole: Physically, mentally, and spiritually.

Tiffany: Barb, you are in my prayers this morning as I read the many posts on this page. Please know that you are loved by many, and you and your family are in our thoughts at this difficult time. See you soon.

12/31/2010 – Day 3 — 2:48 PM — We have not met Dr. Nicholas Price MD, her trauma doctor. Another CT scan was done today. Dr. Stengel, her neurosurgeon, reports her CT scan looks good. However, he cautions that the type of *Traumatic Brain Injury* (TBI) she sustained, involved a lot of damages that will not show up on any CT scan or MRI. He stated to me that in approximately 15 days or so if progress continues, he would anticipate they may replace the respirator with a trach, and then she will be weaned off of that… when she is ready. She had 2 units of blood today.

3:28 PM — Dr. Price inserted a right femoral triple lumen venous catheter.

WE NEED FRIENDS TO DONATE BLOOD.

Barb's blood type is "O" positive, but any kind of blood will be appreciated. Someone will benefit. It helps to hear that you all are out there loving Barb back to us. Dr. Stengel seems to be an excellent, compassionate doctor, with a terrific bedside manner.

8:26 PM New Year's Eve 2010 — My son has finally gotten information from the Red Cross we have been waiting for. With any luck, he is on his way home from Iraq to help his sister heal. Praise The Lord!

9:01 PM — Barbara, you are one very special woman to a lot of people. It is truly amazing to see such love and support one had in this world! You keep fighting this and get better; we have still got a lot of years to catch up on. I will keep you in my thoughts and prayers. Love and miss you so much!

Yankee 794 Trauma

10:39 PM Linda— Barbara and to all her family – My prayers go out to all of you —I graduated from Manatee HS with Barb, and she had always taken such good care of me at Pinnacle. My heart aches for you all, and I pray that she will be okay. Please oh Lord, take care of Barb. I Love You Barb, and may the Lord heal you and restore your health… God Bless You all. Give Barb a hug from me.

> "Every human being on the planet
> has their pain and their heartaches,
> and it is up to all of us to find our
> way back to the light."
>
> Diana Nyad

> "In the flush of love's light
> we dare be brave.
> And suddenly we see
> that love costs all we are
> And will ever be. Yet, it is only
> love which will set us free."

CHAPTER 11

New Year's Day 2011

January 1, 2011 – Day 4 —12 MN

HAPPY NEW YEAR to my precious daughter.

You won't remember ringing in the New Year, but we will be thinking of you. Sleep, knowing soon this will all be better, and 2011 will be a better year.

Your brother e-mailed that he will catch a plane home from Iraq to Kuwait in 5 hours, and certainly (with delays) he will be with you by Monday. **We love you!** Mom

By the time Barb has been at Bayfront for several days, there were get well cards arriving from many of her friends and family, and her window sill was filling up.

2:46 AM — Prayers will go up every day for Barb for a full recovery… we all need her back home with us. First and foremost with you, her family whom she loves, and her Pinnacle family who we all love and miss… and also those of you that are her dear friends!!! God is a merciful God, and He will see her through, and give each of you the strength you'll need to ensure the next precious months that lie ahead. **Hang in there Barb. You've got a loving family that will be there every step of your journey back home!!!!!!!!**

8:25 AM — Barb's brother, Mark, is finally on his way on emergency leave. We have not seen him since Christmas 2009. Her progress can be followed on this blog. Our family is holding vigil over her sweet spirit and praying she makes a full recovery. She has many injuries consistent with having her seat belt on. However, she is diagnosed with **Traumatic Brain Injury** (TBI), specifically a skull fracture on her left side, and **bleeding to her Right Temporal Lobe.** *Please pray for her recovery in 2011.*

8:55 AM **UPDATE:** Barb had an "uneventful" night. I am beginning to realize that "uneventful" could be one of the best words in the dictionary.

Dr. Price, her Trauma doctor (he was one of the first to see her when she was brought by Bayflite to Bayfront) is "old school" and still uses the term serious – however *Barb is still critical which means we are not backsliding. She is stable, and* **she is alive.**

The rest we will deal with when the time comes. With all her ribs broken and severely bruised lungs, she will be in a lot of physical pain for a long time when she is finally awake. *She has skull fractures and other injuries including two fractured hips.*

A special thanks to The Red Cross, as well as anyone else who helped to expedite my son getting Emergency Leave from Iraq to come home to his sister. He will be arriving from Iraq at 10:40 AM (1/3/11) at Tampa International Airport.

Our family will be overjoyed to see him, and take him immediately to Bayfront. No idea how long he will be here. *Thank you to everyone who are praying and keeping vigil. Please continue to send healing messages, thoughts, and prayers...*

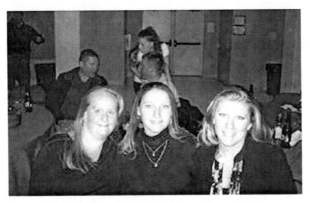

Taken: Pinnacle Christmas Party 2010
This photo was taken 5-6 days prior to the accident.
Barb Melanie Shelley

4:11 PM **UPDATE:** *Barb's condition had been upgraded from critical to serious today.* She is still medicated so her breathing can be assisted because her lungs are so bruised. *She is fighting the respirator* and is restless.

Mark has been on e-mail with me the past few days. It is an amazing thing... to be able to chat with him in a war zone and update my son in real time on Barb's condition. She is still hooked up to all types of equipment, but her vitals are stable. She is on a feeding tube.

Andrea (her sister) was there this AM. I had planned on going this afternoon but got tied up trying to get reports to bring my son home. It is now late afternoon on New Year's Eve; I am going up in the AM rather than be on the road tonight. Nothing can drag me out on the roads on New Year's Eve. It is too dangerous. Hundreds of people are reading our posts.

Chapter 11

Dr. Robert G. Hamilton M.D. Orthopedics wrote a consultation report which read: 9:32 AM "…The patient is unresponsive and is also intubated at this time. Trauma team accidentally found the right clavicle fracture on the chest x-ray…"

PHYSICAL EXAMINATION:

"The patient is intubated and not following commands. The skin is intact. There is no protrusion of the bone. Both of her bilateral lower extremities were intact. No ligamentous instability. "

PLAN:

We would like to repeat a dedicated right clavicle x-ray, AP, and oblique. Currently, the patient will be non-weight bearing with the right upper extremity. No surgical intervention needed at this time. We will further evaluate the patient's clavicle fracture in a week and repeat x-rays at that time."

13:25 PM — An RN inserted a PICC line in radiology with ultrasound guidance… Central access needed.

7:57 PM — *Little victories are now significant:* Today they removed her neck brace after concluding *there are no neck fractures.* Initially, they indicated they saw "something." How she had no neck injuries is a secret only God knows.

She had many broken ribs. Movement is sporadic and limited. So far no sign of pneumonia. There is always a possibility of pneumonia developing. *If pneumonia sets in because her immune system is comprised, this whole picture could still turn around. Her lungs are excessively bruised. If pneumonia were to become a problem and you can't breathe, your other injuries won't matter.* For now, it is good news.

January 2, 2011 – Day 5 — 3:56 PM UPDATE: I went to the hospital and stayed in Barb's room, talking to her. I am a nurse and know that families "hover" for their own needs when a patient is critical. It does not help the staff to do their work if you are in their way. I try to stay out of their way. I come, and I go.

She is unresponsive, but *I believe she hears.* Her nurse says, "no change in her condition" still critical – however, she also is not getting worse, and is holding her own.

Our family is very thankful for all the many notes here (on Facebook). Please remember to send cards and letters to her. They will mean so much when she wakes up. **It is comforting to know that my daughter has so many friends and family who love her.**

*PLEASE REMEMBER TO DONATE BLOOD IN
BARB'S NAME. SOMEONE WILL BENEFIT*

January 3, 2011 – Day 6 — 4:09 PM — **UPDATE:** TIA (Tampa International Airport) at 10:45 AM we picked up my son, Mark, who arrived on emergency leave from Iraq. It was so amazing to see my son walk off that plane all in one piece! He will be here for two weeks, extended if needed. The Army ordered him to return to Ft. Hood, Texas, and *not return to Iraq*, which may be the best news of all! We took him to Bayfront and Andrea (sister) met us there.

Barb spiked a temp of 104 during the night. Blood cultures have been sent to the lab. She is now on two state-of-the-art antibiotics. Dr. Stengel explained to me the ICP needs to be removed, because:

(1) her intracranial pressures are stable

(2) after 4 – 5 days the monitors start to show inaccurate or incorrect readings.

Shelley, Barb's supervisor at work, (as well as her friend) visited ICU again today and brought a number of get well cards. As she read the cards to Barb, she reported to me noticing tears coming from Barb's eyes. Shelley said she wiped the tears away and felt that Barb's reacted to her touching her face.

11:31 PM **UPDATE:** Last phone call to the unit. Barb's condition is unchanged. Temperature remains down. I call every night and every morning to see how she is.

This afternoon my daughter-in-law called. She is my son's bride since July 2010. They have not seen each other since he came home on leave in July, and he returned to Iraq mid-August. It was mid-afternoon. She stated, "I am at the airport (in Texas) and will be landing in Tampa at 10:24 PM tonight."

We were surprised and delighted! We will all drive to Tampa to welcome her. My son is exhausted. He has not slept since he left Iraq more than 72 hours ago. "Get some rest Mark! 'Sleeping Beauty' will need you when she wakes. Love, Mom"

Vancomycin 1.75 IV every 12 hours is the antibiotic she is receiving.

Dr. Stengel came into Barb's room. He explained that he was taking the ICP out. *"They are only accurate for about 5 days,"* he told me. *"Her readings never exceeded 14, and **that is a positive sign for her recovery!"***

At that time, I was grasping for any words of encouragement that would come my way. That gave me hope, even though I had no idea what the future held for my daughter.

Chapter 11

January 4, 2011 - Day 7 — 11:29 AM **UPDATE:** I finally was able to speak to Barb's nurse this morning after a 2nd call. Barb's condition is unchanged: Critical. Temp is normal.

There is no word as yet on what the blood cultures. They will reveal what state-of-the-art antibiotics will be effective until we have results… usually 72 hours.

As the medication wears off, she becomes increasingly agitated. This could be pain or brain injury ("neuro') —- most likely a combination. The nurse did tell me she feels confident that the numbers of broken ribs are significant —- five on each side, along with her shattered Clavicle and two fractured hips.

10:19 PM I spoke to Barb's nurse, Gloria, who reported that Barb opened her eyes once on the day shift. My son, Mark, his wife and my daughter, Andrea, were there this afternoon. There may have been others. I was unable to make it to the hospital, but will be there in the AM.

Temperature remains normal, and Barb remains stable. We are in a "holding pattern" right now while her brain "reboots" itself. It may be a few more days before we know more, or see any significant (outward) signs of progress.

In time, she will want to thank everyone for their concern and love. Temporary Power-of-Attorney and insurance issues are being considered, and we are seeking legal advice.

The Power of Prayer is pulling her back to us!

January 5, 2011 — Day 8 — 4:10 AM **FINDINGS:** The endotracheal tube, left-sided PICC Line, and gastric tube unchanged.

11:09 AM Nurses in Barb's unit report "no change" in her condition.

I have been contacted by Dan Newman, of the ***Florida Brain and Spinal Cord Injury Program*** in Sarasota/Manatee County (BSCIP). Margaret "Peggy" Giaranita, Lead Case Manager, for Barb through community-based programs through Florida Dept. of Health, and follow her case from now until Barb can return to work. Their website has much educational information on it. We will be working *intimately* with this organization to coordinate the care Barb needs, and targeting her needs individually.

Bayfront is a *Level I Trauma Center* and the best place for the care that she possibly be right now. The hospital's social worker, Mary Ann, and medical staff are required, by law, to work with these people to give her the absolute best care available.

My next step is to request the doctors to get Barb a "pressure relief mattress" so that she does not have skin breakdown.

UPDATE: 10:18 PM — Our family presented a united front keeping a meeting with Mary Ann, who has a Ph.D. and LCSW Critical Social Work. Some issues needed to be addressed. There were short-term and long-term possibilities to be discussed.

We all want Barb to come back however while we wait; many concerns need to be addressed and dealt with. Beyond that, all is conjecture and speculation.

Mary Ann made an observation that a crisis like this tears a family apart. They can't seem to get past the anger. Our family is drawn together, and this makes us united. We all looked at each other and knew which way we were heading… together.

> We will do what is required, one day at a time.
> Love had no boundaries.
> Love cannot be taken for granted.
> We must move heaven and earth to
> protect those we love.

10:26 PM - Today I walked into your room, and I took your hand in mine. I said to you, my daughter, *"You probably don't know this Barb, but a week ago you were in a terrible car accident. You have been sleeping since then. So many people are praying for you, and loving you back to us now. God is here with us. It's okay for you to come back to us. We will all be here when you are ready."*

God, grant me the serenity
To accept the things I cannot change,
The courage to change those things I can,
And the wisdom to know the difference. Amen
Reinhold Niebuhr (1882 – 1971)

January 6, 2011 - **Day 9 — 10:48 AM** - Ultrasound was done. Reason for Exam: Edema

Procedure: Venous Doppler, Right, and Left Lower Extremities Indications: Limb pain

Findings: There is normal compression, augmentation, and flow in the deep venous system…

Impressions: Exam negative for deep venous thrombosis (blood clots).

Mary Ann requested that I meet with her. I sat down in her office, directly outside of Neuro-ICU, and she began to explain to me that she was going to help me start the process of filling paperwork for Barb's Social Security Disability.

If it turned out that we didn't need it, that's okay. The process was a long one, and the hospital felt we should get going in case my daughter's recovery was a long one.

6:26 PM - Barb is the same. It seems redundant for me to keep saying *"critical but stable."* Keep checking. As soon as I have any news, I will post an update. If I am not posting, things remain the same.

January 7, 2011 – Day 10 — 6:28 EST - Radiology shows further improvement of aeration of both lungs.

8:29 EST - CT Brain w/o Contrast

Findings: There is expected evolution of blood products within the right temporal lobe. There is persistent hypodensity surrounding the right temporal lobe which may represent edema. There is a small amount of intraventricular blood product layering within occipital horn of the left lateral ventricle. There has been the resolution of blood products seen within the subarachnoid space. There may be a few blood products layering along the right tentorium. The ventricles are stable in size, shape, and position.

Impressions: *Evolution of blood product within the right temporal lobe with persistent hypodensity within the right temporal lobe probably representing contusions (bruising). A few subdural blood products are layering along with right tentorium.*

No significant interval change in small focus of intraventricular hemorrhage layering in the occipital horn of the left lateral ventricle.

Resolution of subarachnoid hemorrhage is seen in the suprasellar cistern.

No significant intervals change in skull fracture involving the mastoid portion of the right temporal bone...

10:38 AM There is no change in Barb's condition — critical/stable/no temp. Dr. Stengel, her neurosurgeon, told us Sunday to anticipate 10-14 days before she would begin to respond and so we are hopeful that "no news is good news."

Ryan and I will make the trip to Bayfront at noon. Barb was on her way to Ry's when the accident occurred. He has been asking to go see her. Until now we have been unable to coordinate our schedules. I fully anticipate after the weekend, we will begin to see more news and progress slow and steady.

All insurance paperwork had been approved, and we are moving forward one day at a time.

3:32 PM - Ryan and I returned from the hospital. I read Barb the get well cards that have arrived. Please keep them coming. They are lined up on her windowsill in her room. Each one is a treasured reminder of how much she is loved.

Ry talked to her, and she squeezed his hand. She is also much more animated than Wednesday. My son and his wife were there, and they also saw how much more active she is. We are all encouraged. Another CT scan was done this AM – microscopic change. She has no temperature today.

My daughter-in-law is flying back to Texas 11 AM Sat. so the whole family is having dinner together this evening. We will all miss Barb!

January 8, 2011 - Day 11 — 11 AM – I spoke to the nurse who turned Barb at 8 and 10. She reports that Barb opened her eyes both times!! They are trying to wean her off the ventilator. Her temperature is 100.4. We have requested an ophthalmologist to check her eyes. My son was at the hospital this morning.

10:30 PM — I spoke to the nurse assigned to Barb tonight. Her condition is primarily unchanged. I mentioned that the family has concerns about her right eye *again*. We are requesting an ophthalmologist exam her. Both her siblings and I have mentioned our concerns over the past few days to staff. I also asked to speak to Dr. Stengel around noon Sunday (1/9/11) regarding updates, while I am in the unit.

Thank you to everyone who had been concerned about and love Barb.

January 9, 2011 – Day 12 — **Barb's temperature is 103. MSSA Pneumonia.** She is reported as stable. The reports from the lab were coming back showing "many Staphylococcus aureus." I was very concerned that if she developed pneumonia (which would be common for this type of patient) her condition would significantly worsen, and she might be lost to us.

5:54 PM – My friend, Ray, drove up with me to Bayfront around 1 PM. Prior to us making this trip, we made our way over to the impound lot where Barb's 2006 Saturn Ion was taken. Ray has been a paint and body man for 40 years. He took one look at the way the roof was crumpled over the driver's head and remarked

"You see that roof? This car is totaled. It can't be fixed!"

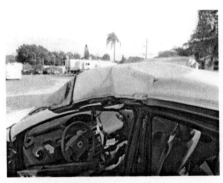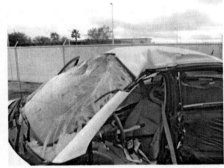

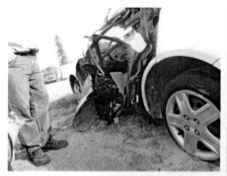
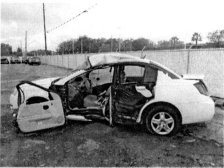
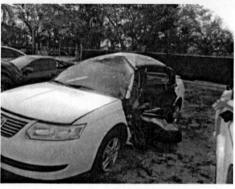

Then we walked around to see the driver's side, and his first remark was that the stabilizing post between the front and back door was "gone" (broken), where the impact actually occurred – *where my daughter's head was.*

One of the things that concerned us is that her air bags *never* deployed. We now have a much clearer picture what happened 12/29/10 at 2:41 AM when Barb was critically injured at 20th Street and 53rd Ave. (Bradenton, Fl.).

The accident happened in front of a church, and the tree she t-boned stands in testament to the impact on my daughter's now-demolished vehicle. Trying to understand exactly where her vehicle had impacted the tree, I eyed it. *Jaws of life were not used* to extract my daughter from her car. The damage you see in the photos was done due to the force with which her car impacted the tree she hit at nearly 50 MPH.

It is my understanding that she was unresponsive at the scene when Manatee EMS arrived, and *they called* Bayflite to send a medical helicopter to try to stabilize her and transport her to Bayfront Medical Center, so these excellent doctors could save her life. (Note: It is a strange thing, looking at her car, and where she was sitting in the driver's seat is demolished – T-bar detached. The front, back and passenger's side of the car are perfect… no damage.)

The nursing staff says although her condition is "unchanged", and she actually not responding, there are small, but encouraging signs. She is making progress toward the day she will start to regain consciousness. We all need to keep the visits and prayers coming her way.

January 10, 2011 – Day 13 — 1:36 PM Barb's temp 102.3. **Confirmed: MSSA** (Methicillin – Sensitive Staphylococcus Pneumonia). Barb remains stable today, although she did spike a temp of 103. They sent more cultures to the lab to see if they can isolate the culprit. They have placed her on a "cooling blanket". She has opened her eyes and responded to pain. Her condition remains essentially unchanged.

UPDATE: Lauren, Barb's nurse today, called. The trauma doctor has requested our family have a meeting with him at 9:30 AM, January 11th at Bayfront. We all plan to be there.

CHAPTER 12

Stable Isn't Good

January 11, 2011 — Day 14 — 7:58 PM - This is Barb's brother-in-law, Alan. We were at the hospital this AM and spoke with the trauma doctor. ***Her prognosis isn't good.*** She is in a very deep coma, and he doesn't expect any change for maybe 6–12 months. She isn't responding to any commands. ***Stable isn't good because there is no improvement.*** There was also talk of moving her to a nursing home for long-term care, but no decision has been made about this. Filters were put into her main arteries of her legs today to prevent blood clots from forming. We will keep you all informed, and thank you all so much for all the prayers and concern.

January 12, 2011 — Day 15

TO ALL THOSE WHO FAITHFULLY FOLLOW THIS BLOG

8:06 AM — From the beginning, perhaps unrealistically, I believed, and held out hope that Barb was on the verge of waking up. The Neuro on Sunday after her crash volunteered that he felt in 10-14 days she would *begin* to wake up. I knew when that happened, one day at a time, we would start to walk thru her recovery.

I am feeling somber and empty today… lost.

When Dr. Epstein, one of the trauma doctors, sat with our family his face was stoic, *"I have done this 25 years, and this never gets easy."*

He went on to explain — looking straight at me, *"Your daughter is in a deep coma. It is going to be 6-12 months before she awakes. You need to look for a nursing home. She is stable, but stable is not necessarily good. She can't go to rehab until she is responding and can cooperate. For you, as her mother, this had to be very hard to hear."*

I felt like I recoiled from his response, wincing in pain, as I remember clamoring for a response, ***"Dr. Stengel told me she would start to come out of this coma on about the 15th day. This is Day 13."***

His no-nonsense demeanor boomeranged off my ears when he refused to be diverted, returning to the point <of the meeting>. I remember his reply cutting through me like a knife through butter, ***"Neurologists tend to be optimists. Trauma surgeons are realists… Arrangements need to be made to move her…"***

I sat stunned and speechless as the color drained from my face. Sinking deeper into the chair, I felt my hope deflate. I looked at the faces of her siblings.

Was he telling our family he was giving up on Barb?

For a minute, I wanted to cry, *or maybe I needed to be angry* — not at him, but at *this unparalleled tragedy that seemed to be unfolding before my eyes – around my family.*

> It had taken on a life of its own ---
> A beast-like monstrosity, flailing its angry arms in all directions destroying everything in its path.

It didn't matter what I was feeling as her mother. *The facts were the facts and were not open for debate or discussion.* Dr. Epstein had made that infinitely clear. We had to deal with what this is (not what he hoped or preferred it would be) in a direct way. In the end, it all becomes quite civilized and logical — and *emotions had to be set aside.* Cooler heads needed to prevail.

He had called the meeting to ask for permission to do three additional procedures immediately, in preparation for moving her.

Those were:

(1) a Gunther Tulip Vena Cava Filter (IVC) to help prevent pulmonary embolism (blood clots in the lungs),

(2) a Tracheotomy in her neck (so she could breathe), and

(3) a gastric (feeding) tube.

Dr. Epstein's notes in my daughter's chart reflected this: *"Long discussion with family (mother, siblings) concerning her injuries. We discussed long-term outlook; current problems with temperature, check fractures, IVC filter."*

I am sure with him doing this type of discussion with families on a somewhat regular basis, making it part of his unenviable 'routine', and this was his impression... ***"long discussion with family..."***

My father had been a compassionate and caring doctor in family practice for 36 years, and there were many times when he had been in the same unenviable position to have "discussions" with families – and put on a brave and professional face.

Often, when dad was finally able to be alone, he had sat and cried at "the news" he had to bring to that family. It is one of the less coveted tasks assigned to "doctor" by virtue of his title and position.

Chapter 12

I wondered if Dr. Epstein had left our presence and found a lonely quiet corner so he could vent his frustration and regrets at relaying *this kind of news* to my family.

For me, it was very different. He sat with us for 15 minutes (a time that seemed entire too brief for me), and dropped **devastating news** in my lap that *I was not prepared to hear*. I doubt anyone is ever prepared to hear news like this.

Then he was gone.

I sat impaled by his words — attempting composure. I felt transfixed as my mind tried to grasp the "news" he had unveiled. The confidence and optimism I held tightly to, deflated like an over-filled balloon.

I recognized the words he had spoken, and my mind was struggling not to reject them. They had to free up a bed for Barb when she was admitted to Bayfront. I knew other people were (*unfortunately*) being admitted to Bayfront, and who needed a bed in Neuro ICU – just as she had needed the bed when she was initially admitted.

The problem?

I didn't know what the alternatives were.

꙳

Lord Jesus,
You held out a hand of mercy
so many who sought your help.
Take hold of my hand this day,
and see me through this time of trouble.
Grant me the strength to hope against hope,
and the courage to greet each new day.
Renew my faith in your healing touch,
and help me to put my trust entirely in you
in the days that lie ahead.
Keep me close to you,
That I may find comfort and peace
In the nearness of your unfailing love.
Amen.

꙳

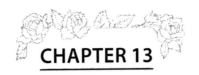

CHAPTER 13

Coming Out

Barb's temp is 104.2. MSSA Pneumonia continues.

Postoperative Diagnosis: Prolonged intubation

OPERATION: Bedside tracheostomy (the surgical formation of a temporary or permanent opening into the trachea)

6:54 PM — Bayfront Trauma Team have made a recommendation that HealthSouth RidgeLake Hospital in Sarasota (Fl.) is a correct placement for Barb. The social worker called me to explain that a proposal has been made for transfer to this facility as appropriate for her the next 30-60 days. They will provide many therapists and management of her case.

My son, a friend and I, drove there and took a tour guided by Mary, Nurse Manager. RidgeLake Hospital in Sarasota (Fl.) is a 4-year-old long-term hospital (LTCH – Long-Term Care Hospital). They were very kind to answer all our questions. I am feeling a bit relieved now that there is an answer.

The paperwork is now in process for her transfer from Bayfront to HealthSouth RidgeLake Hospital in Sarasota. All we are waiting for is Blue Cross Blue Shield to approve the transfer.

8:00 PM – I checked in on Barb in ICU. There is nothing in the blood cultures to show infection is present and causing her periodic spiking temperature. The doctors say when that happens it is probably a "neuro" cause. The brain does what is termed **storming**. Otherwise, her condition is stable but unchanged.

It is expected that Barb will be moved to Sarasota by ambulance, as soon as paperwork and approval can be accomplished – perhaps by week's end.

Today was a busy day because we were all in *"information gathering mode"*. Alan and Andrea went the legal route to gather information through Legal Aide on getting an Emergency Guardianship for Barb.

Janet (Barb's aunt*)*: Oh Betty, I was so sorry to hear the news that she wasn't getting better as I thought. I guess her movements and tears, don't mean much to the doctors if they are not asking it to happen??? I'm not giving up on her pulling out of the coma earlier than they say. So what is going to happen now? Nursing home? How? Will her insurance cover it? They are extremely expensive… Can't give up the hope and prayers.

Chapter 13

January 13, 2011 – Day 16 — Mark, Sonny (a friend), and I arrived at the hospital approx. 9:30 AM with no expectations. It's Barb's 15th day in a coma. We are holding on to hope that against (what appeared to be) all odds that by **God's Grace**, things would take a more hopeful turn.

One of the nurses approached me with a smile and remarked, *"Barb is responding! Bonnie, the Assessment Coordinator from RidgeLake, was here. She gave Barb command to open her eyes, and she did!"*

I checked twice to see if I was hearing her right. **"What do you mean??? How ???"**

"The lady from RidgeLake came to evaluate her for their facility, to make sure she is appropriate for placement in their facility. She was asked to squeeze her hand, and she did!"

"REALLY? She did?" I asked her again.

I could hardly believe my ears! I sprinted to the bedside and took Barb's hand.

"Barb, it's Mom. Open your eyes for me!"

Her eyes popped open very deliberately.

"Can you squeeze my hand?"

Again she responded appropriately.

WOW! I could hardly believe what I was seeing! She did! She did! I was in tears!

"Thank you, God! My daughter is finally waking up!"

"Your brother is here, Barb. He came all the way from Iraq to see you!"

I could see her trying to comprehend what I was saying. All three of us were laughing and crying. Barb blinked once, twice, and a third time for me, when I requested it.

Dr. Amy Kohler MD, one of the trauma doctors, came in. Dr. Kohler asked her to move her fingers, and she couldn't, but she **did** move her toes. *She is apparently trying to understand what is being said.*

We put in a call to Andrea in Bradenton she was at the hospital within the hour. She got the same response! We had to call people. They were crying! Shelley, Steve, Brandi and more… all thrilled.

Barb is being moved at 11 AM Friday (1/14/11) to Sarasota.

We found The Bloodmobile in the hospital parking lot and gave blood to replace the 2 units Barb was given. (Blood is $500 per unit when billed by the hospital. If you replace it the patient is not charged.)

"Barb it's Mom. Sweetie, can you open your eyes and look at me?"

She opened her eyes –for a bit and not very wide, but it was enough to tell she was hearing what I was saying.

"Thank you, God! My daughter is finally waking up!"

I will sleep well tonight knowing my Sleeping Beauty is waking up.

1:44 PM — Alan (my son-in-law) wrote on Facebook: **GREAT NEWS! BARB CAME OUT OF HER COMA. SHE OPENED HER EYES and SHE IS SQUEEZING HANDS. THANKS FOR ALL YOUR PRAYERS AND SUPPORT.** We will keep you updated.

Temperature 103.9

MSSA Pneumonia continues

3:22 PM — **Brandi:** *"That's my Barbalicious!!!..........."*

9:23 PM — I am sure they will get any cards and letters received to the right room. The capacity of the hospital is 40 patients. The hospital is asking that the first week, please keep visiting to a minimum. Too much information or stimulation is counter-productive. The danger is to "over-stimulate" her. One of two things can happen. She will become overly agitated or she will "cocoon" (withdraw).

People have been asking, *"What can we do?"* I don't currently have a printer. Photos are important in recovery. There are so many great pictures of her with friends and family. Could you guys photocopy some of the best ones, and send them to the hospital? It will help us to talk to her in identifying who everyone is, and we can also put them in her room. If you can help, I can replace the photo paper. I will be constructing a "Memory Book".

Those of you who love her have memories… touching, funny and memorable events you have shared with her. If you will send letters detailing those events I will put them in a Memory Book she will be able to review with therapists and family as we walk her through recovery. All this information (with photos) will help to bring her back. Sit down and write them down as though you were talking to her. I will compile them and make them available in her room for her to read thru and enjoy.

January 14, 2011 – Day 17 — 2:38 PM - **UPDATE:** Both hospitals have now confirmed that Barb was transported without incident and is in Room 113-B. Dr. Amy Kohler M.D. spoke to the receiving doctor at length this AM, and he was there at the time she arrived at the new hospital to access her entirely. I will be driving there later this afternoon after she is settled into her room and all procedures have been completed.

Her discharge summary read as follows:
Date of Admission: 12/29/10
Date of Discharge: 1/14/11

DIAGNOSES:
(1) Basilar skull fracture
(2) Right parietal skull fracture,
(3) Subarachnoid hemorrhage,
(4) Intercranial hemorrhage,
(5) Subdural hematoma
(6) Intraventricular hemorrhage
(7) Bilateral first rib fractures
(8) Right Clavicle fracture
(9) Methicillin-sensitive
Staphylococcus Areas Pneumonia
Staphylococcus bacteria
Hyperglycemia

PROCEDURES:
12/31/2010 — Right femoral triple lumen venous catheter
01/11/2011 — Insertion of inferior vena cava filter
01/11/2011 — Tracheotomy
01/12/2011 — Percutaneous gastrostomy tube

HOSPITAL COURSE: The patient remained on ventilator support throughout her hospitalization. She was seen by Dr. Stengel shortly after admission who places an ICP monitor on 12/29/2010. Tube feeding was initiated for nutritional support and well-tolerated. She was seen by Dr. Hamilton for her clavicle fracture. No surgical intervention was recommended. Her ICPs remained controlled. A PICC line was placed on 12/30/10, and the femoral line was removed...

She underwent tracheostomy and IVC filter placement on 01/11/14 and PEG tube. Placement on 1/12/11. The patient was gradually weaned off the ventilator but had difficult time tolerating CPAP due to low tidal volumes... *Her electrolytes are stable.*

Barb has been accepted into HealthSouth (RidgeLake LTAC). The case had been discussed by Dr. Koler with the receiving physician. The family is also aware of these plans. The patient is felt safe to transport at this time. She is day 11 of Vancomycin and day 4 of Levaquin. PEF tube feedings were initiated on 01/13/2011, and will be a goal. An IVC filter is in place for DVR prophylaxis.

11:22 PM - **UPDATE:** I drove south to the hospital today, and stayed approx. 1 hour. There were some procedures I needed to sign for.

Barb was able to open her eyes on command but *does not focus*. She listens to the sound of my voice. The plan is that Sunday, my son, a friend, and Brandi (Barb's friend) will be going to visit her.

Monday morning my son is flying out of Tampa, back to Ft. Hood, Texas, to his wife and back to his duty station. I promised him frequent updates and photos, so he is kept very much in the loop on Barb's progress and recovery.

Closed Head Injury

A closed head injury is any injury to the head that does not penetrate the skull. Closed head injuries are usually caused by blows to the head and frequently occur in traffic accidents, falls, and assaults. Closed head injury is also common in children who have suffered serious bicycle accidents.

There is a variety of risks associated with closed head injury. Sharp blows to the head can lead to complications such as brain swelling and intracranial pressure, which can permanently destroy delicate brain tissue and nerve cells, in turn leading to permanent brain damage.

Types of Closed Head Injury

The extent of a patient's brain damage depends on the severity of the injury. Closed head injuries range from mild skull injuries to traumatic brain injuries, which can lead to severe brain damage or even death. There are several different types of closed head injury, including concussion, brain contusion, diffuse axonal injury, and hematoma.

Concussion

Although definitions vary, the Mayo Clinic defines concussion as any head injury that temporarily affects normal brain functions. Most concussions are mild and do not cause loss of consciousness, but this is not always the case. Sports are a common cause of concussions in the United States. Almost half of the 600,000 total concussion cases reported each year are sports-related.

People suffering from a concussion can exhibit a number of immediate symptoms, including:

- Headache
- Dizziness
- Nausea
- Ringing in the ears
- Slurred speech
- Vomiting

Chapter 13

Concussion victims also may be confused, unable to concentrate or have difficulty balancing. In other cases, symptoms do not surface until hours or days after the incident.

These secondary symptoms include mood swings, sensitivity to light and noise, and changes in sleep patterns.

Brain Contusion

Brain contusions are bruises of the brain tissue that occur as a result of brain trauma. In some cases, brain contusions lead to hemorrhages which are absorbed into the brain tissue. If blood is absorbed into the cerebrospinal fluid, it can cause permanent neurological damage. Brain contusions are localized, a characteristic that distinguishes them from concussions, which are more diffuse (spread out).

Brain contusions are present in 20 to 30 percent of all severe head injuries. People suffering from brain injuries may feel weak and numb, lose coordination and struggle with memory or cognitive problems. Because brain contusions and other head injuries can increase intracranial pressure, it is important to seek immediate medical care after any head injury.

Diffuse Axonal Injury

One of the most debilitating traumatic brain injuries is a diffuse axonal injury. Frequently caused by high-speed transportation accidents — and sometimes associated with shaken baby syndrome — diffuse axonal injury causes permanent damage to nerves in the brain. As with other closed head injuries, the diffuse axonal injury may cause brain swelling and intracranial pressure. But unlike more minor closed head injuries, severe diffuse axonal injuries lead to vegetative states or comas in 90 percent of patients.

Intracranial hematoma

occurs when the brain is forced against the inside of the skull, resulting in a pool of blood outside the blood vessels of the brain or in between the skull and brain. The brain is not designed to drain this much fluid. As a result, an intracranial hematoma can compress brain tissue, requiring immediate medical attention. Blood that collects in the brain, or in between the brain and skull, may lead to unconsciousness, seizures and/or lethargy.

There are three types of intracranial hematoma: subdural, epidural and intraparenchymal.

Subdural hematoma occurs when a vein ruptures between the brain and the dura mater (the membranes surrounding the brain);

77

Epidural hematoma is caused by a rupture between the dura mater and the skull;

Intraparenchymal hematoma occurs when blood collects within the brain tissue.

Intracranial hematoma is a serious condition that often requires surgery and extensive recovery time.

Closed Head Injury Complications

A traumatic brain injury can put a patient at risk of developing a variety of complications, including intracranial pressure and swelling of the brain. Patients with severe closed head injuries may suffer from:

- Headache
- Dizziness
- Nausea
- Ringing in the ears
- Slurred speech
- Vomiting

Most patients suffering from mild closed head injury report headaches, dizziness, and short-term memory loss. A severe closed head injury can lead to death or cause a patient to remain in a permanent vegetative state.

Closed Head Injury Treatment

Traumatic brain injury treatment, such as for a closed head injury, depends on the severity of the injury. For patients with mild injuries, doctors recommend rest and over-the-counter pain relievers. Patients with severe closed head injuries require additional medical attention.

Doctors treating severe closed head injuries seek to prevent further brain damage from easing the intracranial pressure. This can usually be achieved with diuretics, anti-seizure medication or coma-inducing drugs. Patients with intracranial hematoma usually require surgery to drain clotted blood deposits. Surgeons also may open a "window in the skull" to accommodate brain swelling until it subsides.

Closed Head Injury Rehabilitation

Following surgery and medication, many patients with severe closed head injuries need therapy to regain basic motor and cognitive skills. Depending on what part of the brain was damaged, patients may struggle with walking, speaking or loss of memory.

Chapter 13

Closed head injury patients typically begin their therapy during their time in the hospital and continue it on an outpatient basis. A skilled team of neuropsychologists, physical therapists, and others works closely with patients to help them manage or regain their lost skills. The amount of traumatic brain injury rehabilitation required varies depending on the individual.

Closed head injury is a serious type of traumatic brain injury.

> We cannot choose our external circumstances, but we can always choose how we respond to them.
>
> Epictetus
>
> Sometimes we find ourselves in a situation that is not of our choosing. Our first reaction might be to complain. To feel hard done by. Maybe a better reaction would be to adapt.

The Blessing of Unanswered Prayers

I asked for strength that I might achieve;
I was made weak that I might learn humbly to obey.

I asked for health that I might do greater things;
I was given infirmity that I might do better things.

I asked for riches that I might be happy;
I was given poverty that I might be wise.

I asked for power that I might have
the praise of men;
I was given weakness that I might
feel the need for God.

I asked for all things that I might enjoy life;
I was given life that I might enjoy all things.

I got nothing that I had asked for,
but everything that I had hoped for.

Almost despite myself my
unspoken prayers were answered;
I am, among all men, most richly blessed.

Author:
Unknown Confederate soldier

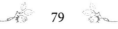

Traumatic Brain Injury Statistics

- *Emergency Department Visits: 1,365,000 (3,740 per day)*

- *Hospitalizations: 275,000 (753 per day)*

- *Deaths: 52,000 (142 per day)*

- *Nearly 1/3 of all injury-related deaths in the US involve a traumatic brain injury*

- *About 75% of TBIs that occur each year are concussions or other forms of mild traumatic brain injury*

- *Direct medical costs and indirect costs of TBI, such as lost productivity, totaled an estimated $60 billion in the United States in the year 2000*

- *Ages 0-4, 15-19 and 65+ are most likely to sustain a traumatic brain injury*

- *Traumatic brain injury rates are higher for males than for females*

- *Falls are the leading cause of traumatic brain injury*

- *Motor vehicle accidents are the leading cause of traumatic brain injury-related death*

Source: U.S. DEPARTMENT OF HEALTH
AND HUMAN SERVICES,
Centers for Disease Control and Prevention (2010)

CHAPTER 14

Who Can I Trust?

During her initial hospitalization, I would work 4 days a week from 8 - 4 PM. Then I would go to whatever facility she was in to check on her and any business I needed to take care of. There were times I was beyond exhausted, both physically and emotionally. However, I did not have the option to collapse, and take a vacation. I simply willed myself to keep moving forward. I am not a quitter, and Barb was depending on me.

January 16, 2011 – Day 19 — **Dawn:** (Barb's friend) I returned from RidgeLake Hospital (where I once worked) visiting Barbara. It is the first time I have seen her since her horrible accident. She has a trach and is on a ventilator, but she opened her eyes and followed commands (that is the nurse in me speaking). She moved her right side pretty good on her own! A bit weak on the left, but she is trying so hard! I asked her if she knew who Dawn was, and to squeeze my hand TWICE and SHE DID! We talked about the Bucs game, and how we missed her famous Buckeye candies this year! We praised her, and told her how much we all love her!

8:46 AM — We "worked" a bit with Barb last week. She was not squeezing our hands as much as she seemed to be pushing with it for days. She is doing the same with her right leg and foot. Her foot was reportedly trapped under the (gas or brake) pedal after her accident. Maybe she is re-enacting the accident over and over. We aren't sure what this is we are seeing. We have been advised to reassure her quietly,

"Barb, you were in a terrible car crash. You can come back to us now."

10:38 AM — Does anyone have a guestbook they could donate, so when everyone who visits can sign for a keepsake for Barb? Elizabeth Scott (Barb's Mom)

5:15 PM – **Shelley:** Tim and I visited Barb this afternoon. It was so nice to see her open her eyes in response to my voice. I know she had a long way to go, but Barb has always been determined and can succeed. A week ago the family was told Barb was in a very deep coma and may never wake up. Two days later Barb woke up and now is responding to simple commands. Keep up the good work Barb! God has a special plan for you. See you soon.

6:50 PM — We saw Barb today at 4 PM. They were happy to report she was more animated and held up 2 fingers *"just aren't there yet!"* My friends and

I will be going tomorrow (Sunday) to take some "home touches" to brighten up Barb's room. If you visit Barb, please update here (on FB). Everyone will see the same behavior from her and all of us want to share your experiences. PLEASE keep the cards, letters, and photos coming. They will be significant in her recovery.

8:40 PM I will speak to nursing staff tomorrow and find out what items she is (and is not) allowed to have in her room. I would think a stuffed animal would be okay, but 20 would be overwhelming. She has a lovely window sill by her bed. I will bring some playing cards, flash cards, and a few other small items so friends can work with her recovery. The company even when she can't (yet) participate, will help orient her. If I turn out to be wrong, I will let you know.

10:07 PM — **Paige:** I visited with Barbara this evening, and her nurse Isabelle, told me when I arrived that I had just missed her brother. I would have so liked to have met him! Isabelle also told me that the Occupational Therapist, Janet, had finished working with Barbara, and they were very pleased, with her progress! Isabelle told me that in caring for Barbara today, she had established a way to communicate with her throughout the day using a thumbs-up for "yes" and thrums-down for "no," using her right hand. Isabelle is an excellent nurse (I used to work with her), and she is awesome in taking care of patients with brain injuries.

She also shared with me that she will be Barbara's nurse for the next 3 days. This is very comforting. When I asked Barbara if she would like me to read some of her cards to her, she gave me thumbs up! I also asked Barb if she recalled Dawn and I am visiting the night before, and she gave me the thumbs up! I told her how all of us have been praying for her, and posting on her Facebook page, and that we all love and miss her so much. We know she can do this! In 24 hours, I am amazed at how she is more awake and alert and responding appropriately! I am confident with every day, she WILL continue to progress; we all know she can do it!

The hospital has given me a copy of ***Living With Brain Injury: A Guide For Families*** (2nd Edition) by Dr. Richard Senelick, MD with Karla Dougherty. The book tells of how people with brain injury are expected to make judgment calls that we might find peculiar, and we must understand their brains are not working "normally." ***One example***: One man, after going home, called 9-1-1 to report his cereal bowl was missing. It promises to be a fascinating read.

BARB IS THE BIGGEST "BUCS" FAN EVER as many of her friends can testify. Is there anyone who could make contact with them and get her a shirt/ball (something) they could sign to show their support for a fan that had supported them all these years? It would be huge for her, and mean more than anyone could imagine.

8:30 PM — **Brandi:** Hey woman. Sorry, I haven't made it there yet, but it sounds like you have had many visitors. I am watching the Golden Globes for you… I generally DO NOT watch, but for you, I will. I am not gonna remember who won what and for what show, movie or whatever like you do, but I will watch. I love you girl and will be there tomorrow to see you. We definitely need some one-on-one time. I have been lonely without you.

January 17, 2011 – Day 20 — 8:04 PM – **Andrea** (sister): I went to see Barb today, and she is progressing slowly. She is responding the same as the last few days, squeezing my hand on command, blinking twice for 'yes' and once for 'no.' I think she is doing a 'thumbs up' that's what it looks like anyway. It's better than she was Thursday. I was out of town for the weekend, so this was the first time had seen her since she woke up Thursday. We need to brush her hair out. It's pretty matted. I didn't have a whole lot of time today. I didn't have a brush. Otherwise, I would have brushed it. The next time I go to the hospital, I'm gonna take conditioner, brush, and a ponytail holder and braid her hair. She is moving a bit and left side not so much. She is very restless.

8:27 PM — Betty, please add Angela and Stacy to Barb's visitor list. We are going to visit her in the morning and perhaps we can work on her hair some more. Let me know when you plan to cut it. Before the accident, she told us she was planning to cut it and donate it to Locks of Love like she always does. Barb told me, Christmas Eve, she was planning to cut it. I went down today brushed out what I could. Hopefully, we can cut it this weekend. She has given her hair to Locks of Love and knew she would do that again.

9:00 PM — **UPDATE:** Dr. Prakash MD (Family Practice/Primary) visited with me this evening. Pupils are equal, and I was staying with Barb around 7 PM. He asked me details about the accident. We spoke in the hall, and he plans to begin weaning her from the trach in 2-3 weeks. He will keep me up-to-date as he reviews her progress.

11:35 PM — **Brandi:** I went today and spent some time with Barb. Also had a nice conversation with her nurse who seems very confident about her progress. I massaged and lotioned her feet and put socks on her. Those little piggies seemed cold. This is the most progress has been made since I last saw her at Bayfront. Baby steps but she is getting there. Keep up the good work Barb… luv ya.

January 18, 2011 – Day 21 — 11 AM – **Mark: (Barb's brother)** I had to leave back to Home Station, Ft. Hood, Texas. Since Barb's condition is gradually improving, I couldn't substantiate staying longer that I did. However, this is a good thing. All that matters is that my sister is getting better. We Love You Barb!!!

2:37 PM – **Tammy:** Went to see Barb today. They were getting ready to move her to another room. They told me they planned to take her off the trach today. Yesterday they had thought that is was going to be two weeks, but she is doing well, and they are planning on removing it today. She was kind of restless today.

The nurse and I worked on her hair some, while I was there and put some lotion on her hands. I also took her a pair of socks (she calls them 'sexy socks'!!) I was not able to put them on her because they were getting ready to move her. If the next person who visits her could do it for her, I would appreciate it.

When I mentioned Bodie (her dog), she got very agitated. I think she understands more and more each day. She squeezed my hand, and when I told her we missed her, a tear ran down her cheek. WE LOVE YOU BARB!!!!!

5:55 PM **_Thank you to everyone_** for visiting Barb and your comments on what you observed are helpful and allow each of us to participate in her recovery. I will be sitting down 11 AM with her case worker Lori RN, CRRN, CCM, to review the team evaluations that will be held on Wed. afternoon. Peggy, her case worker through Dept. of Health, Florida Brain, and Spinal Cord Injury Program will join me, and meet Barb, so she can access her as well. She will be following Barb's case until she returns to work. Barb's Mom

6:22 PM **Janet** (Barb's aunt): I sent a card off to Barb and then heard she is moving to a new room. I guess it will catch up with her. So very glad she is improving pretty fast, it seems to me. Love ya.

8:02 PM **Andrea:** We are going to talk to doctor tomorrow about Barb's case.

January 19, 2011 – Day 22 — 8:15 PM **UPDATE:** Apologies for not posting sooner. It has been a busy day. Andrea, Peggy and I met with Lori (hospital case manager). This was following a team meeting for all members of Barb's care team. There will be another meeting 11 AM on Feb. 3 for updates again.

I met with Dr. Diane Miller MD, the new psychiatrist today. She asked my permission to start Barb on a new medication "Geodon." She explained that this drug had been **very** successful in helping heal brains with Traumatic Brain Injury. Dr. Miller explained that Dr. Sears M.D. (a neuropsychologist – meaning she had a specialty in function of the brain) would partner with her in treating Barb. Also, Dr. Ancheta MD is the new Neurologist on her team. **Barb's Mom**

Chapter 14

UPDATE: Barb is being weaned from the vent, which is critical. Yesterday she was off the vent from 10 AM – 7:30 PM. Today, they are planning to leave her off all day and putting her on during the night, as tolerated. At the rate, she is going (hopefully) she will be entirely independent of the vent by next week!

Her ability to follow simple commands (thumbs 'up' and thumbs 'down') remains inconsistent. We feel this is due to the types of medications she is on. Her nurse says they will make an attempt to get her up in a chair Friday or Saturday. *Each day is a step forward.* **Barb's Mom**

January 21, 2011 — Day 24 — 2:26 PM - Saturday (1/22/11) at noon Andrea, Shelley and Angie will be going over to do "something" with Barb's hair. I am told that Moroccan Oil is amazing for getting mats out of hair. I have to go to work at 5 PM today and work through 5 PM Sunday. *Can someone help by bringing these products to her?* Maybe we can keep from having to shave her head. It would be a great help with this process. There is shampoo and a brush already there. And guys, please do not forget to sign her Guest Book! It will be there Sunday.

Someone I spoke to has suggested we may want to look into **Hyperbaric Oxygen Therapy** (HBOT) for Barb. I plan to research this subject. Does anyone have any feedback on HBOT with Traumatic Brain Injury?

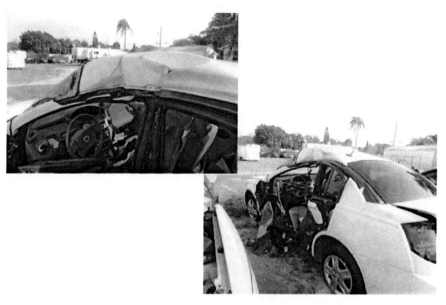

I posted the pictures of Barb's 2006 Saturn Ion here. It has now been established beyond a shadow of a doubt that she DID have her seatbelt on. Barb's Mom

Yankee 794 Trauma

January 22, 2011 – Day 25 — 3:53 PM - Angela: Barb now had an incredible short haircut thanks to Shelley and me. I even did two shampoo caps. Hopefully, this will help. The horrible mat of hair won the battle, so I had to cut it out. It was more of a dreadlock only round, lol. Her hair grows out, and Barb gets more strength to hold her head up, we can keep fixing it, so she has a fresh style. She did even put her arms on me as to hug me when I was done. Thanks Shelley for all your help. I couldn't have done it without you.

5:55 PM — **Shelley:** (Barb's supervisor at Pinnacle): Spent the afternoon with Barb today. She seemed a little restless in the bed, but once they got her in the chair, she seemed more comfortable. I can't imagine how her body feels, lying in bed all the time. Anyway, while she was in the chair I held Barb's head up while Angie cut her hair. After Angie was done, we washed her hair twice with a shampoo cap, and then dried her hair. Barb seemed to enjoy it. She still had a little residual conditioner build-up in her hair. A couple more shampoo caps should take care of that. Angie did a great job. She cut about 8 inches off Barb's hair, and it is going to donate it to "Wigs For Kids". Barb and Angie were planning to do this just before the accident. **Thank you to Angie for taking great care of Barb!**

6:36 PM **Andrea:** Thanks, Angie, and Shelley so much for doing her hair and spending time with Barb. Her hair looks a lot better, and we shouldn't have a problem again for a while.

6:57 PM Among Barb's things, I discovered a precious ponytail about 8 inches long she planned to donate some time ago. It is in gorgeous condition. Angie, can I meet up with you someplace and give it to you so it can be shipped with the rest? Betty (Barb's mom)

January 24, 2011 – Day 27 — I was with Barb yesterday noon. She was experiencing *Tachycardia*[1] (spiking a heartbeat of 135), and there was no answer for why this was occurring other than it is most likely "neuro". They gave her meds, and she was sleeping when I left. The staff did verify that she was restless before 11:30 AM.

I spoke to M.D. Stevens owner of *The Mikey Center for Hyperbaric Oxygen Therapy* in Lakewood Ranch. I will go there and visit tomorrow, so I can understand more about HBOT. I was told there *may not* be insurance

---

[1] Tachycardia — From Wikipedia, the free encyclopedia
Tachycardia, also called tachyarrhythmia, is a heart rate that exceeds the normal resting rate.[1]
In general, a resting heart rate over 100 beats per minute is accepted as tachycardia in adults.[1]
Heart rates above the resting rate may be normal (such as with exercise) or abnormal (such as with electrical problems within the heart).

money for this. It might be private pay. Barb has an excellent AFLAC (rehab/long-term disability) plan, and funds from that might be designated to pay for this therapy.

Brook: Barb – I just want you to know that I'm so glad the most recent profile picture you put up were or November trip to Shake Pit. That was a great afternoon, and it makes me smile to see you smiling... can't wait to sit on the Pit patio with you again, as soon as you are ready!

Brandi: Robert and I went to visit "Barbalicious" this afternoon. She was alert and seemed comfortable. I ask if she knew who I was and she responded 'yes' by squeezing my hand. I talked to her for a while, adjusting her left side and she helped by straightening her hand moving slightly. I made sure to tell her I love her and ask if she felt the same. She squeezed my hand tight. Love you girlie and you WILL be home soon!

January 25, 2011 - Day 28 — 10:02 AM Barb SMILED at me yesterday. Her eyes were fixated on me as I moved toward and away from her bedside. *My daughter SMILED at me Christmas Day in passing, and it almost went unnoticed. Yesterday it was a major triumph* of her finding her way back to us.

I took it to be a sign from God.

Shelley: Melanie and I visited with Barb yesterday. She was very alert and animated. She smiled as well as raising her eyebrows when we said something surprising. I ask Barb to do a "thumbs up" if she knew who Melanie was and she smiled and gave the thumbs-up sign. It is very nice to see Barb responding so well! This is the first time I have seen her so animated with her facial expressions. Keep up the good work, Barb. See you soon.

January 26, 2011 - Day 29 — 3:13 PM — A number of people have asked me to be placed on Barb's "visitors list." When she was at Bayfront, this was required, a limited number of people were only allowed in to see her if I put them on the list. This is no longer the case. RidgeLake, where she is currently, is open invitation 9-9 seven days a week. Anyone can visit her. Please keep the cards and letters coming.

January 28, 2011 — Day 31 — 8:33 PM — We went to see Barb at noon for an hour. She was up in a chair sound asleep. The nurse told me she had been "very active" this morning. I won't be here Sat. or Sunday. I will be in Tampa attending a medical class 8-5. I will see Barb again on Monday. I made an attempt to visit *The Mikey Center* (HBOT) today, however, I was unsuccessful. Please continue your prayers and visits.

January 30, 2011 – Day 33 — 3:52 PM — Andrea: Alan and I saw Barb today, and we could not get her to wake up. We hang out for a while. We talked to Barb's nurse, and she asked Barb to smile at her this morning, and the nurse said she did. Barb's nurses say she is doing really well. The nurse also said she was up all night and all day yesterday, so she probably wore herself out.

I went to RidgeLake this afternoon to see Barb. She was wide awake, but I noticed her pupils were extremely dilated. The nurse said she had *not* given her any medications that would cause this.

The case worker, Lori, came in and said the x-rays were excellent (meaning her lungs are healing well from all the bruising of the accident).

Dr. Simon, the psychiatrist (specializes in rehabilitation), was here to evaluate Barb this morning and was *"very pleased"* with the results of her evaluations she was given. They want to move her to HealthSouth rehab. (at the other side of the lake) by the weekend. Barb's mom

January 31, 2011 – Day 34 — 11:16 PM… Brandi: Robert and I went to see Barb this evening. WOW! What a change from last Thursday. She immediately smiled at us when we entered the room. She kept kicking that right leg like a ballerina… LOL! She was able to give me thumbs up, high five, and she touched her nose. When I would laugh, she smiled even bigger. It seemed like she wanted to giggle when I teased her about playing patty cake. It was very cute. As I was leaving, I was saying "goodbye" and hugged her and smiled. I waved, and she waved back! Today was a great day for her. These may be baby steps, but she is improving all the time. Love ya Barbalicious!

> *Dear Nurses,*
> *Thank you for guarding my heart.*
> *You were there during the most joyful*
> *moments in my life, when my children*
> *were born, and you were also right*
> *there during the most difficult,*
> *during heartbreak and when we*
> *soared. Thank you for what you do.*
>
> *Elizabeth A. Scott*

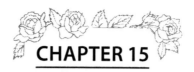

CHAPTER 15

Today I Received the Bill

February 2011

Today I received the bill from Bayfront for the 15 days Barb was in ICU-Neuro. It was a real eye-opener! At first, when I looked at the bill, I thought I saw things. Then, I thought I read it wrong, and had to look again! I realized I did not imagine the *$19 million dollars* at the bottom of the bill.

Nineteen million, seven hundred thirty-four thousand, three hundred and seventy-seven DOLLARS.

NOTE: The above figures are copied from the actual bill. Anyone who knows about hospital bills is aware that it is likely incorrect, and the agreement with insurance companies is that the hospital settles for less than the actual bill and writes off the remainder.

This bill did not include any EMS charges or Bayflite charges to the hospital. This was the first of what would end up being 4 months with 2 hospitals and 2 rehabs. She did not come home until early May 2011

When Barb was moved from Bayfront Medical Center in St. Petersburg, Fl., to RidgeLake Hospital, in Sarasota, Fl. I requested a copy of her total bill for 12/29/10–1/13/11. She had been in ER and Neuro-ICU the whole time. Because she had Progressive (Auto) Insurance and Blue Cross Blue Shield (Medical) she was covered. You might find it interesting. I did, when I saw it itemized.

They were amazing in their medical care, and they saved my daughter's life.

If someone neglecting to put her into a state computer system (for new TBI patients within hours because they were busy saving her life) and that was the worst that happened – then I think we were good!

There are not words in the English language to express how grateful my family is for the amazing and uplifting experience we had at Bayfront as she received the best care available beginning with a BIG thank you to:

Dr. Nicholas Price M.D. and Dr. Brian Hedrick D.O.

who were the trauma team that initially addressed my daughter's critical injuries. Without 9-1-1 first responders, Bayflite staff and the trauma team, there would be no book… *and no Barb.*

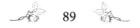

Yankee 794 Trauma

Description Service	Units	Total Charges
Intensive Care	3	$6,234.60
Intensive Care	13	28,637.70
Pharmacy	644	29,860.00
IV Solutions	8	120.30
Non-Sterile Supply	46	4,418.80
Sterile Supplied	40	3,824.60
Supplies/Implants	1	480.60
Laboratory	36	1,002.50
Lab Chemistry	169	16,333.00
Lab / Immunology	12	2,158.00
Lab / Hematology	20	13,364.00
Lab/Bacteria-Micro	31	6,464.00
Lab / Urology	3	239.00
Dx. X-Ray	3	965.20
Dx. X-Ray Chest	17	4,882.10
CT Scan	4	7,535.10
CT Scan / Head	3	3,809.00
CT Scan / Body	4	5,903.90
OR / Minor	2	4,081.90
Blood / Stor-Prod	2	707.20
Ultrasound	1	1,001.20
Respiratory SVC	17	23,150.10
Emergency Room	6	6,863.00
Pulmonary Function	84	14,701.94
MRI — Brain	1	2,498.30
MRI — Spine	1	2,498.30
Drugs / Detail Code	21	600.00
Trauma Response / Level II	1	8,009.70
Gastr – Ints SVS	1	2,200.13
Treatment Room	46	6,383.00
Peri Vascul Lab	1	420.20
Total Bill		$19,734,377.00

Initially, along with other issues of my daughter's untimely incapacitation her "legal needs" were not part of my consciousness. However, within days, it became apparent, that I needed to seek out help for a number of legal issues that needed to be addressed.

> The phrase "do not be afraid" is written in The Bible 365 times.
>
> That is a daily reminder from God to live everyday fearlessly.

I had been in the hospital only a couple of hours trying to absorb my daughter being in Neuro-ICU in a coma (and might be dying), when I was approached by the hospital's *"insurance lady"*. At the time, Dr. Stengel was drilling a hole in my daughter's already significantly battered and bruised head.

Initially, *"insurance lady"* was on a mission. She began to throw questions in my direction like The Coyote after The Road Runner.

All I wanted was to say was, **"My brain is full of mush lady! Please go away!"**

I think I must have stared at her in disbelief. She backed off. It may have been the expression on my face that clued her into the fact I was not receptive to speaking with her.

She turned out to be a wonderful lady that was initially assigned to find out about Barb's medical insurance. She was willing to "clue me in" on a lot of issues that I had yet to consider and turned out to be remarkably helpful.

Barb had been living away from (my) home for 20 years since she graduated high school and left for the Air Force in July 1990. Our "chit-chat" did not include information about any of her insurance. She took care of that at work.

I called Shelley, Barb's supervisor, at Pinnacle Medical. (Shelley was the 2nd call I received, that put up red flags, that my daughter was "nowhere to be found", before we knew she was gravely injured.) Shelley was to give Bayfront the information they were requesting, very quickly. I was grateful for that help.

What I discovered was that Barb's medical coverage from her auto insurance ($10,000.00) had been exhausted by Bayflite and the first hour in Bayfront ER. I was told the Bayflite helicopter ride from Bradenton to St. Petersburg (Fl.) one way was $6500.

I would later ask Barb about her ride in the helicopter,

"How was the view from up there?" I probed.

"I never got to ride in a helicopter until my accident, and now I don't even remember it!" came her reply a year later.

Thanks for help and advice, I was able to find out a lot about what direction my role as Barb's legal caregiver was to take. Being her mom *I was suddenly and unexpectedly thrust me into the unenviable role I had never expected.*

> I wanted to scream,
> "Our children are supposed to bury us, not the other way around!
> That is the Cycle of Life.
> You designed it God.
> Have you forgotten your plan?"

Then I remembered what I knew as a Mother – her Mother. This title **"Mother"** represents a position for which I would have responsibility for the remainder of both our lives – however long that turned out to be and whatever it brought our path.

I was responsible for another person, who I loved more than life itself. Now I had to make decisions not based on emotion, but based on common sense and balancing of facts. Now, more than ever, my brain had to be on top of its game – *or I would fail Barb*. **That was not an option.**

Making angry demands on God for answers to why, and placing blame, could have easily followed. Instead, I remember asking,

> **"Can I do this God? Can you please help me do this?
> I don't understand... Why Barb?"**

Being at the hospital created some moments I found ironic and (perhaps) amusing. Indeed, they made me stop and think.

I was handed a packet of general information on "Notice of Privacy Practices" and a sheet on "Patients Belongings and Valuables."

Along with a letter that read, *"Welcome to our family! Your choice of hospital is a wise one... You are the center of our family, the most important part of our organization's efforts. You will see this reflected in our mission to provide the best available healthcare to all..."*

"Welcome to our family"?

Somehow I think my feelings were very much like the guy who, in the 1960's got his draft notice from Uncle Sam, announcing *"Greeting."* when he knew that meant he was heading for Vietnam.

Neither my daughter nor I had "signed up" for this, and prior to 2:41 AM on 12/29/10, and we were not "eager" for their services. None-the-less, I will be forever grateful for their willingness to help us.

ॐ

I WILL...

I will start afresh each new day,
with pretty littleness freed;

I will cease to stand complaining,
of my ruthless neighbor's greed;

I will cease to sit repining,
while my duty's call is clear;

I will waste no moment whining,
and my heart shall know no fear.

I will not be swayed by envy,
when my rival's strength is shown;

I will not deny his merit,
but I'll try to prove my own;

I will try to see the beauty,
spread before me in rain or shine;

I will cease to preach your duty,
and be more concerned with mine.

Author Unknown

ॐ

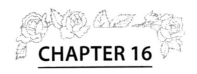

CHAPTER 16

The Legal and Financial Nightmare

Along with other issues of my daughter's untimely incapacity, her legal needs were not part of my consciousness. However, within days, it became apparent that I needed to seek out help for a number of issues that needed to be addressed.

While I was visiting RidgeLake Hospital in Sarasota, as the *next step* in this process, once she left Bayfront Medical Center, my daughter, Andrea, and her husband, Alan, began to pursue Legal Aid to see what help they might be able to obtain.

We discovered Barb qualified for assistance through Legal Aid. Once they were made aware of Barb's dire situation, Legal Aid immediately referred me to Neil Scott, Esq. an attorney in Sarasota, Florida, who specialized in civil law. I was informed I had 14 days to contact him, or they would drop us.

I called Neil Scott (no relation to our family) immediately, leaving him a message. Shortly thereafter, Neil called me regarding Legal Guardianship. He informed me that I needed him to represent me (as her mother and logical choice as her Legal Guardianship) and that Barb would have a *different* attorney, to represent her interests.

If I was legally representing my daughter's best interest, why did **she** need an attorney? She was in a coma. There was no way anyone could communicate with her. **Wasn't I representing her interests?**

However, he told me that was the law. Both would serve until discharged by the court, once appointed. No matter. Legal Aid was paying for this.

Mr. Scott's letter read:

Re: Barbara Suzanne Scott, Guardianship

Dear Mrs. Scott:

This letter is intended to confirm the matters we discussed by telephone, and email recently regarding this matter. You wish me to represent you as a person and property guardian for your daughter, Barbara. Once you are appointed a guardian, you would serve until you are discharged by the court.

I would represent you as guardian, by preparing and filing all legal documents needed to administer the guardianship, except for any tax returns, that may be needed (individual income, etc.). I suggest you find out who prepared your daughter's income tax returns, as you will be responsible for preparing and filing them. A good deal of my work will be in the beginning, getting you appointed and filing the reports due two months, afterward, and again each year when the annual report is due.

I understand your daughter was in an accident last month and is currently in a HealthSouth facility, here in Sarasota. You told me it was not clear how long her recovery will take, and how far she will progress, but you are optimistic. Depending how far she recovers, she may no longer need a guardian.I explained you must take a guardianship training course, within four months after you are appointed. The course is offered live in Sarasota three times a year. Incidentally, I will send you a copy of all correspondence, pleadings, etc., as we generate them. If this letter confirms your respective understanding of our agreement, please sign, date and return to me the enclosed copy of this letter with other original documents.

Thank you for your cooperation. I look forward to working with you. Please call or email me if you have any questions.

Sincerely,

Neil W. Scott

As I am reading the letter, I am overwhelmed with raw emotion, realizing this was all a far bigger picture than I had imagined.

(1) Initially I was at the hospital where my daughter was in a coma, and we have no clue if she would survive.

(2) I had to find temporary homes for her cat and dog because I was not able to be in three places at once. Then we are told she had to be moved to another location, **because she survived**, and the hospital needed the bed.

There was no way to gauge what the "short-term" (let alone long-term) circumstances were going to be. I was there every day, all day, dealing with her medical issues, as well as trying to hold down a job four days a week!

They were unsuccessfully attempting to wean Barb off her Life Support, and attempting rehabilitation when she couldn't talk to me – or anyone. How is that supposed to work? Now, this guy thinks I should be dealing with **her taxes** – somewhere in the future? **Was he serious?**

In all honesty, I must tell you *Neil W. Scott, Esq. turned out to be a gift from Heaven.* He is a wonderful Christian, a deacon in his Lutheran church, and **an**

all-around credit to his profession. This is a man who mentors young people, goes camping (which he calls 'vacation') and is knee-deep in charitable causes, including The Salvation Army, when asked. Many legal issues had to be dealt with, and I could only do it with **his** help and support.

I dealt with each one as it reared its unexpected or ugly head. Dealing with legal issues on my best day is not my favorite thing, and with Barb incapacitation, I had to choose the right path *each time, without failing her*.

There were meetings and reviews of legal issues and documents, over the next few months. Each time I found myself in Neil's office, it was with some sense of apprehension *about my ability to make the right choices*. There were times when we would go into his conference room, and all he had to do was asked, *"Mrs. Scott, how is your daughter?"*

As if on cue, I would dissolve into tears. He was always there to listen, *even if the issues were not legal ones*. He was never in a rush. This was remarkable and a real gift! He was kind, compassionate, and gave be a shoulder to cry on when I felt no one understood the path I was walking alone. He stayed on top of things when I couldn't, and he gently nudged me along, when he needed an answer, and I was too exhausted to think. Without Neil Scott at the helm of Barb's (and my) legal ship, I think it would have been scuttled more than once. I don't know how many times I stopped and **thanked God** for bringing him into our lives when we needed him most.

Mr. Scott's first order of business was to create the following documents for the court:

Order Appointing Examining Committee;
Petition To Determine Incapacity;
Petition To Appoint Plenary Guardian;
Notice of Petitions; and
Reports of Examining Committee

One of the first things Neil did was to request three medical people to form an Examining Committee to visit Barbara, in the facility, and evaluate her mental and physical state. Legally my daughter was deemed an "Alleged Incapacitated Person". There was only a short amount of time for the three of them to submit their findings/reports to the court for review. This list comprised three court-appointed health care workers: Dr. James L. Slocum M.D. psychiatrist, an R.N., MSN, and a social worker (MSW).

The Petition to Determine Incapacity alleges the person is incapable of exercising the following rights:

Chapter 16

To marry
To vote
To personally apply for government benefits
To have a driver's license
To travel
To contract
To sue and defend lawsuits
To manage property or to make any gifts or disposition of property
To determine his or her residence.
To consent to medical or mental health treatment.

The Examining Committee is charged with determining whether the *"alleged incapacitated person"* has the ability to exercise those rights which the petitioner has requested be removed in the petition to determine incapacity.

February 20, 2011 — Day 54 — Report by Diane S., RN, MSN

"The patient is s/p motor accident in December 2010. She fell asleep at the wheel and crashed her car. She had three head injuries and multiple broken bones. She had a trach which was removed last week, but she still cannot speak. She has respiratory issues, and she is fed by feeding tube. She is wheelchair bound.

At this point, the patient's physical prognosis is fair. She has made good progress in rehab. According to her mother, the doctors state that "only time will tell." Cognitively, theoretically, she could continue to "clear her head" and regain full cognitive function. However, that is not the case right now. The patient should remain in rehab.

The patient cannot speak. She nods that she knows her name. She does not know the day, date, or time. She has no idea how long she had been hospitalized. She is clearly frustrated at not being able to communicate. She cannot write. She appears to comprehend some of what is said to her. However, it is very difficult to validate this as there is no clear response from her. There is no evidence of critical thinking, sequencing of thought, or abstract thought. The patient is entirely dependent on others for all activities of daily living."

February 22, 2011 – Day 56 — Report by Anne O. LCSM

"This young woman was involved in an auto accident leaving her with traumatic brain injury. In an acute phase, she is being treated for a skull fracture, hemorrhages, subdural hematoma, rib fractures, hip fractures, hemorrhages, spinal cord, and phenomena. She had a tracheotomy and Peg tube. She had been weaned off the ventilator, but still had a feeding tube. Difficult to assess because of brain recovers over an extended period of time. She will always have cognitive deficits due to brain injury. She needs a plenary guardian. Hopefully, she will

continue to receive physical rehabilitation for the purpose of getting to her highest level of function.

She is alert but quite agitated and restless. She had no speech, but could respond to simple questions with a nod or lifting a finger. Recent psych reports indicate she has a history of depression and is being treated with psychotropic medications for depression and agitation. She is full care. She cannot ambulate, nor do self-care. She could not communicate verbally, although she could follow a simple command: hold up your hand. She is receiving comprehensive inpatient rehabilitation, at this time, but it is too early to know her outcome."

"She will always have cognitive deficits due to brain injury."

The next legal step was to:

Petition to Appoint Plenary Guardian — *who was me.* There was an office: Letter of Plenary Person and Property Guardianship, who was me. Then there was an: Amended Notice of Petitions to Determine Incapacity and to Appoint Guardians for March 4, 2011, at 10:00 AM to go to Judge Williams.

That alone was a court fee of $631.00 (for the filing fee), and court costs of $725.00 (for the examiners who evaluated her.) Another hearing was held on May 3, 2011.

A Verified Inventory — was required by the court. This was a list of all Barb's bank accounts, cash assets, possessions, and real property and holdings. Once I had the officially signed document from the court, I was able to move forward with matters of business I had postponed.

Early in her hospital stay, I was informed that Barb had taken AFLAC insurance at work. I got in touch with the insurance agent who knew her well.

She had three policies with AFLAC

(1) Personal Disability Income Protector
(2) Personal Accident Indemnity Plan
(3) Hospital Protection

This was in addition to her auto insurance, and her Blue Cross Blue Shield Medical Coverage, which paid most of her hospital/rehab bills. She also had GAP Insurance that paid off her (now demolished) car, a 2006 white Saturn Ion.

Sometime in mid-February AFLAC paid the 3 first claims.
There were three checks that came on February, 2011…

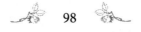

Chapter 16

$ 4035.00
$ 2,548.00
$22,965.00
_____

$29,548.00

From that point on each month, I submitted a claim to AFLAC, and they paid approx. $1,820 per month (through December 2011)… 80% of her salary. Her HCA COBRA Continuing Coverage Medical Insurance premium was $8,841.76 for 16 mo. of coverage.

It was essential when her Blue Cross Blue Shield ran out March 1, 2011, because *Pinnacle* (her employer) *had sold.* This kicked in when her Blue Cross Blue Shield covered lapsed.

I also opted for
Dental coverage…..$439.53
Vision coverage….. $106.08

Her COBRA kicked in March 1, 2011, and was a significant investment with major rewards.

The wonderful people at Pinnacle Medical, where she worked, took up a collection, and they paid her rent for February – then I began to pack and move her, and letting the apartment go back for rent.

By then, it was entirely clear to everyone she could not live alone – and I would have to move out of my apartment and combine our households, whenever she was able to come home. This meant I needed to find the two of us a place to live.

February 24, 2011 - Day 57

I have scheduled a meeting with Jennie, the case worker at 2 PM to discuss a number of critical issues with rehab regarding Barb's safety, day and night.

Dr. Simon has agreed to write an order on her chart for a sitter, so that when the family/staff (therapists) can't be present, there will be someone with her 24/7. The reason? *Barb won't stay in bed, and legally they can't restrain her.* She keeps scooting out of bed and chairs!! This is agitation from her TBI referred to as "neuro", but also, it is a desperate need for attention; more than the staff can supply, even with a staff-patient ratio of 6:1. We are being required to go at this from another angle, to try to get her the protection that *everyone agrees she requires* currently.

My concern and that of the staff went up a new level when Barb discovered that she had a new 'play toy' – *her seatbelt!* She seems to think it is a game to unbuckle it. *Two days ago she unbuckled it and lunged – going over head first, followed by her chair!*

By the time the nursing staff realized she could unbuckle it, it was too late! *Eleven staff members* were at the nurse's station and *watched in horror as she took a header onto the floor.*

This happened because I told them, *"Barb hates being in this room alone. She is a nurse. She wants to be out at the nurse's station where the action is."*

Her bed is now as low as it is possible to get it. Gym mattresses cover the floor in her room. **She refuses to remain in bed.** No matter what hour I arrive, I am likely to find she has made her way out into the middle of the room. She can't walk, but that never stopped someone as determined as she seems to be.

I told her she reminds me of a "slug" once, a year later, and she grinned ear to ear. Sometimes I think it is those moments where we can laugh at ourselves that are keeping us sane. I can't stay all night and work all day.

February 25, 2011 - Day 59 — The guardianship hearing in Sarasota County (her current address) is now scheduled for March 4 at 10 AM. Today at 1 PM, I went to Social Security Administration to follow-up on Barb's SS Disability. The process was begun 6 days after she entered Bayfront, but I had to provide updated medical records to them. I have been keeping 3-ring binders of everything. The lady picked what she needed and copied them. Hopefully, this will satisfy them.

February 27, 2011 — Day 61 — Barb has a really glorious day Saturday (yesterday) according to her nurse. However, as it describes in the book on TBI that I am reading, *the emotional roller coaster she is currently riding is extreme.* I was called this morning at 8 AM. She was crying and calling for me.

Part of her "recovery" is that she is starting to realize that she is away from home and her animals, Lily and Bodie. She has been having crying episodes since last week for no "apparent" reason.

We learned the term ***"storming"*** at the hospital is a description of the brain after traumatic brain injury (TBI), and how it functions.

She is awake for long periods now and becoming increasingly aware of her surroundings. She knows movement, especially standing and taking steps is a tentative matter. I am sure she feels **a prisoner of her circumstances** though I am not sure to what extent she realizes the details.

Barb is still not wanting to use her voice through Speech Therapy is encouraging her to do so. It has been 2 weeks since the trach was removed. She speaks coherently – in a whisper. She is trying to use her good (right) hand to write notes... much of it starts out somewhat legible, but then becomes scribble due to her current lack of coordination. This infuriates me.

One of the nurses asked Barb about Lily. *"What color is your cat?"* she was asked. Barb's response was to hold up 3 fingers. Lily is a Tortoiseshell Persian (black, red and cream) so 3 fingers were correct.

There was one note she wrote that we finally were able to decipher. It said, **"I do not feel safe here!"** I immediately spoke with the Director of Nursing about this concern.

A lady came in to visit her husband with their dog. Barb needs and wants to see Bodie (her Pomeranian) and the sight and interaction with the dog, a black Poodle, overjoyed and upset her. Her emotional outbursts come without warning.

She keeps writing us notes, **"I want to go home!"**

My response is as follows: **"Barb, if you went home now, could you take care of yourself?"**

She always acknowledges that what I am telling her is correct. This has to be very frustrating for her.

I have tried a million times to imagine what she is processing, and what it must be like to lay there in that bed, unable to walk or talk audibly, and trying to piece together what happening to her.

We have not yet told her a lot of the details because we were warned that telling her "too much" (who knows what that is???) will confuse her. We hold her and reassure her, and *we tell her that we will be there for her no matter what happens. Isn't that what a family is about?*

The family is defined as those who LOVE her... so all those who are following this blog are included.

March 1, 2011 – Day 63

A month ago the doctor said he *didn't* believe that Barb would walk again. Today she "pivoted" from her wheelchair (w/c) to her bed with minimal help! She can now place 3 events into the sequence, and she is counting to 10. Dr. Miller says she is making "wonderful progress." We are very encouraged.

Now if she could swallow, so she could get off the peg tube (tube feeding) and on to real food. It is a goal that will come with time.

I explained to her today that she will (probably) be moved next week, and she seemed to understand. Two places are recommended for her next destination.

(1) Jupiter, Florida, which we have heard, has a wonderful program for TBI. The downside? It is 3 and ½ hours away.

(2) Heartland here in Sarasota. Dr. Simon could follow her there. Andrea and I can visit Heartland, as can her friends.

All things being equal, sending her to Jupiter (where none of her friends or family could often visit) would be counter-productive to her emotional state of mind, and we feel her therapy would suffer.

Anything she might stand to gain from going to Jupiter (Fl.) would be offset by the isolation she would experience if we move her there.

We are voting for Heartland.

Riding Out the Storm:
Sympathetic Storming after Traumatic Brain Injury
Denise M. Lemke

Following multiple acute traumas, hypothalamic stimulation of the sympathetic nervous system and adrenal glands causes an increase in circulating corticoids and catecholamines, or a stress response. In individuals with severe traumatic brain injury or a Glasgow Coma Scale score of 3-8, this response can be exaggerated and episodic. A term commonly used by nurses caring for these individuals to describe this phenomenon is *storming*.

Symptoms can include alterations in level of consciousness, increased posturing, dystonia, hypertension, hyperthermia, tachycardia, tachypnea, diaphoresis, and agitation. These individuals generally are at a low level of neurological activity with minimal alertness, minimal awareness, and reflexive motor response to stimulation and the storming can take a seemingly peaceful individual into a state of chaos.

Diagnosis is commonly made solely on clinical assessment, and treatment is aimed at controlling the duration and severity of the symptoms and preventing additional brain injury.

Storming can pose a challenge for the nurse, from providing daily care for the individual in the height of the *storming* episode and treating the symptoms, to educating the family. Careful assessment of the individual leads the nurse to the diagnosis and places the nurse in the role of moderator of the *storming* episode, including providing treatment and evaluating outcomes.

After acute trauma, an immediate sympathetic surge provides the needed rapid response to compensate for the effects of the injury (Keller & Williams, 1993; Neil-Dwyer, Cruickshank, & Doshi, 1990; Stanford, 1994). The outward expressions of this surge are hypertension (HTN), hyperthermia, pupillary dilatation, tachycardia, cardiac arrhythmias, profuse sweating, an increased release of glucose, and an increased basal metabolic rate (Cartlidge & Shaw, 1981; Stanford).

Some individuals suffering severe traumatic brain injury (TBI) have demonstrated a spontaneous episodic exaggerated stress response, or *storming* (Baguley, Nicholls, Felmingham, Crooks, Gurka, & Wade, 1999)

Sympathetic storming tends to be associated with the lower neurological functional level and can be caused by injury or pressure created by tumors, hydrocephalus, or *subarachnoid hemorrhage* though it is most commonly seen in the TBI population.

"Trusting yourself means living out what you already know to be true."

Cheryl Strayed

"Creativity is straddling the tension, leaning into the discomfort and finding your way through the dark."

Dr. Brene Brown Ph.D

CHAPTER 17

Weathering the Storm

or

PBA: You Can't Make Sense Out of Nonsense

February 1, 2011 – Day 35 —4:06 PM - I went to the SS Admin Office today to make sure where Barb is in the process of her disability approval.

The paperwork for Barb's Social Security Disability that was submitted by Bayfront Medical Center on January 6th. Social Security has no record of any submission in Barb's name, even though I filled out the paperwork and Bayfront promised (insisted) they mailed it. Interesting… sigh. The best Social Security could do was to give me a phone appointment for Feb. 16 at 8:30 AM. Sigh (again)!! *That means the whole process is held up 6 weeks.* I am not a happy camper. Could you guess?

Margaret "Peggy" Giaramita, Barb's case manager with Brain and Spinal Cord Injury Association, helped me fill out paperwork to get Barb approved for Medicaid. It is a process that has to be submitted, because of issues with her insurance that may be coming up after the beginning of March. She gave me a 3-ring binder to keep all the paperwork.

Neil Scott, my attorney, has filed for Guardianship Monday morning. This process will allow me to manage Barb's legal affairs if that is needed in the future. She may not need this. However, it is a 6-8 week process. It is best to get it going. We can always rescind the need for this in the future.

Moving Barb to the adjacent facility, we are told, is now appropriate, and will probably occur before the weekend. This will most likely occur Friday, February 4.

February 2, 2011 – Day 36 — We went to Tampa this evening to recertify CPR Class. Last weekend we spent 16 hours in class on Saturday and Sunday recertifying medical updates. This is to prepare for when Barb is finally discharged home.

Chapter 17

I am only now being told that he ER bill for 12/29/10 at Bayfront was $118,899.00 (This is only a partial bill.) There is a $10,000 fee that had to be paid *before* her insurance kicks in. I am wading through the details and struggling to understand.

Barb began daily physical rehabilitation, following her move from RidgeLake Hospital to HealthSouth Rehabilitation. The first thing that happened was that the doctor ordered her indwelling catheter *removed*. I was concerned because I knew there would be skin breakdown. This **could** turn into a radical situation **if** she did not quickly learn to retrain herself to bowel and bladder habits. The floor help frequently does not get there *"in time"*, even when they do bed checks every two hours. This situation will remedy itself given time.

The therapists suggested that I come and watch them work with her in rehab. Monday, I arrived and went with her to Physical Therapy. She was wheeled down to the end of the hall, and they began to work with her. **She started crying uncontrollably.** (I would come to understand this was **PBA** — **Pseudobulbar Affect**.) At this point in time, I had no idea what it was or how to react.

> Pseudobulbar Affect
> I have no idea what it is or how to react.
> I remember feeling perplexed, bewildered and mystified.
> I am struggling "to make sense of nonsense."

How do I advocate for her when she isn't capable of communicating with me? My daughter was incapable of talking to me! My heart breaks for both of us. When she had these uncontrollable crying spells, I didn't know what is triggering them.

Did she not want me there?

Was she glad I was there and couldn't express it?

I could not tell why these outbursts were happening. Barb couldn't talk to me at that point, but she certainly was trying to give me some sort of message. *Should I leave – or stay?* I, of course, related them to her attempting to communicate with me.

This was my first encounter with PBA — Pseudobulbar Affect – a part of her TBI. It was not until months later that "Dr. T" (more about him to come soon) explained to me what PBA is, and I began to read about it on the internet.

I would observe her react by sobbing uncontrollably more and more frequently, as she gradually became increasingly aware of her surroundings.

Her actions and reactions did not seem logical to me. I struggled to understand. I remember feeling perplexed, bewildered and mystified because (I later learned) *I was struggling "to make sense of nonsense."* That day did not bring any answers.

February 3, 2011 - Day 37

When I arrived at RidgeLake today, I discovered Barb was out in the hall in a chair! She also had 7 nursing students that visited. The case worker, Lori, said that yesterday (Feb. 2) they took Barb outside, and she seemed to enjoy that.

Barb spiked a temperature, and they are doing blood cultures on her. We held our collective breath, hoping it was *not* Pneumonia (with her lungs so bruised). Her pupils were normal size, and she was wide awake.

I plan to request the nursing staff to have The Super Bowl on for Barb Sunday. We all know, she is a real fan, and certainly won't want to miss the commercials... huh?

Storming in TBI (Traumatic Brain Injury): *the brain is confused, and sometimes it will send out the wrong "symptoms"* (temp. and shivering) *because it is unstable.*

February 4, 2011 - Day 38

I am currently reading the book ***Successfully Surviving A Brain Injury: A Family Guidebook From Emergency Room to Selecting A Rehabilitation Facility***. Author Gary Prowe – 2010.

I am highlighting statements in the book, and will share those with you. I hope no one will feel I am breaking any copyright laws. I believe we can all benefit from my sharing portions of what I am learning. Note that I am referring to the stages Barb is in.

Please allow me to explain.

"Rancho Los Amigos Scale of Cognitive Functioning" is commonly used in describing the condition of a brain injury patient. It begins with Level 3 and ranges upwards.

Barb came into the ER with a #3 which is the lowest possible and still sustain life. For everyone who loves and cherishes her, this will be a learning experience for all of us together.

Level III - Localized Response: Total Assistance

- Demonstrates withdrawal or vocalization to painful stimuli.
- Turns toward or away from auditory stimuli.
- Blinks when strong light crosses the visual field.

- Follows moving object passed within the visual field.
- Responds to discomfort by pulling tubes or restraints.
- Responds inconsistently to simple commands.
- Responses directly related to the type of stimulus.
- May respond to some persons (especially family and friends) but not to others.

February 5, 2011 - Day 39 — The liaison has visited Barb today from Heartland and believes she is *"appropriate"* for their facility. I am assuming they will be moving her soon – certainly by next week, from what they are telling me. I am told there are negotiations between Heartland and Blue Cross Blue Shield.

Barb seems restless today, thrashing about in bed and only semi-responsive to me. I am told all this movement is "neuro." I sat in her room for an hour, reading my book on brain injury and trying to get *"enlightened."*

I kept watching her, and for me, it can be overwhelming. Confusion, panic, fatigue, and grief are my constant companions every hour of every day now. I guess reality is setting in. I have been running on adrenalin.

I work, I come to the hospital, and then I am alone with my thoughts and fears. People tell me I have to rest.

What happens when your mind won't shut down?

Refusing to go to those "dark places" does not keep my mind quieted. Those places can be like nightmares – and yet I know we can't predict the future. Every fiber of my being is willing me to have a meltdown. Yet, there is a spark— a continuously flickering ember that smolders, and from time-to-time that ember erupts into a Flame of Hope. I give in to it, and for a time, I can sense things will get better.

There are excerpts from the book:

Successfully Surviving a Brain Injury: A Family Guidebook: From Emergency Room to Selecting a Rehabilitation Facility
by Garry Prowe

"Traumatic brain injury statistics in the United States are staggering: 1.4 million people sustain an injury each year: 50,000 people die... ushering an onslaught of neurologic and neuro-endocrine disorders: bowel, bladder... and sometimes psychiatric disorders. Just as every individual is different, every brain injury is different. This could be likened to fingerprints or snowflakes.

Every injury affects the entire family (and friends). Understanding brain injury is the first step in regaining control over many challenges brain injured presents. Understanding brain injury is also critical to becoming an effective caregiver and advocate."

Andrea and I have decided this weekend not to keep Barb's duplex. She has long months (or possibly years) of rehabilitation ahead of her. We will be moving her.

A few weeks ago, I could not comprehend making such a decision. That having been said, *my daughter should not be alive with the injuries she sustained, and so I am grateful for her still being with us.* I have no clue at this point exactly what that means, however with the help of God we will deal with every new day as it comes.

My prayer is that God will smile on her and show me the way.

Every fiber of my being is willing me to have a meltdown.
Yet, there is a spark — a continuously flickering ember that smolders,
And from time-to-time that ember erupts into a Flame of Hope.

February 6, 2011 – Day 40 — **Shelley:** "...Barb has begun speaking. They have a voice valve on her trach and are actually encouraging her to talk. Right now, her voice is just a whisper, and her speech is minimal. She said 'yes' and 'bye.' They are encouraging Barb to speak as much as possible, or at least try to mouth the words. She started yawning. I asked her if she was tired. She shook her head 'yes'. I told her I would go, so she could rest. She waved goodbye and closed her eyes. Get some sleep Barb. See you again soon.

February 7, 2011 – Day 41 — 4:48 PM Andrea: Alan and I went to see Barb today and had a excellent visit. She gave me a hug. She told me she wants to go home now by pointing at herself and pointing at the door, then pointing at me and out the door. She asked me about her phone, and when I told her I had her phone at my house, she gave me a 'thumbs up.' She tried to write something on a piece of paper, but I couldn't make it out. She moved her left leg for me, but she still couldn't move her left arm. She is getting better every day.

8:05 PM Barb complained of having a headache this morning. They called to ask to take her for a CT scan...

She has been having a tremendous amount of agitation the past few days, causing the doctors to increase her medication. We are not sure if this agitation is because she is starting to wake up and realize her surroundings and circumstances, or some other reason including *storming.*

Heartland sent a liaison. She did not feel it was advisable to move Barb for another week and wait to see if the agitation subsides. The plan is to reevaluate her in a few days. I had asked for a consultation with the doctor for an update and progress from when she arrived 3 weeks ago.

I find myself wondering what I am missing. What is right here in front of me, and I am too ignorant <of the facts of TBI> to recognize what other, who work with TBI patients, would observe and note as significant. It frustrates me, yet if I overload myself with too much information too quickly, I will end up with even more overwhelmed than I already am.

How am I failing Barb? The fear is continuous with me. What more is there for me to do and pay attention to? We are following all the guidelines, rules, and guidance offered. **Conventional medicine has its benefits. However, it is bound to the guidelines of what insurance companies choose to allow and will pay for.**

Frankly, I think a lot about dad when I am alone with my thoughts — a general practitioner for 36 years, he "ran by the seat of his pants." He was a country doctor, who made house calls, and he led with his heart. He made things happen for his patients. He had a personal and interactive partnership with them. *They knew he cared.*

I sometimes shudder to think what his reaction would be if he saw the medical system *now.* I think he would be hard pressed to recognize or make sense of the institution he took such pride in 40 years ago, in which insurance (not the doctor) determines care given to any person in medical care.

Sadly, that is far removed from the experience many people now have. *My soul cries out for my daughter's welfare* in this ever-evolving medical establishment.

My father retired in 1977, *without ever having paid a penny in malpractice insurance.* Yes! You read that right! Remarkable, huh? There were mutual trust and respect between doctor and patient. If you told that to a physician now, many would look at you in disbelief.

People have forgotten about the established bond that used to occur as you saw the same doctor year after year. That doctor delivered the new members of the family, cared for women and children and saw to it that the men's health issues were addressed. He was there when they celebrated births, and when they mourned the passing of loved ones. He became an appreciated extended branch of the family tree, *grafted there out of necessity.* He saw families almost like a marriage vow – *"in sickness and in health, forsaking all others, as long as we both shall live."*

When I was growing up, the doctors who operated on me, and later, delivered my babies, were friends of the family. It was a very personal relationship. It took leadership, perseverance, loyalty and dedication. In a nutshell, that was who my father was. Those are the values I grew up with. It was not for quitters. You remained steadfast in the face of adversity. You did what was required, no matter the cost or sacrifice, and you did it for as long as it took. There was no time limit on loyalty. You did it until…

Self-examination haunts me. The limitations of my knowledge bind me to reality. At times, my brain is jumbled and bewildered – scrambling to find answers. The lines of conformation become blurred.

There is more than the conventional medical constraints here. This is why I am seeking information about HBOT (Hyperbaric Oxygen Therapy) to assist in Barb's overall recovery.

The first thing God gives you when you are born — oxygen.
The last thing God takes away when you breathe your last — oxygen.
Without oxygen you die.

Such a simple concept —perhaps we sometimes
make things too complicated.

Can concentrated amounts of oxygen at 95%, help heal Barb's brain? I feel I am compelled to seek out more information on this.

The Guardianship hearing (for me to become a court-appointed legal guardian for Barb) is in Sarasota and scheduled for March 9, 2011.

11:15 PM **Brandi:** WOW! is the only word I can think of using to explain my visit with Barb. When I went into her room, she immediately started crying, and her heart rate shot up to 157! The nurse came in and gave her meds to slow that down. It took a few minutes, but she calmed down. She tried so hard to communicate with me. I asked her many questions to find out what she was attempting to tell me. She kept pointing outside then pointed at me, then Robert, then to herself. I finally ask if she wanted to go home and she nodded *'yes'* as if to say *'right now.'* I giggled and made sure she knew she would be going home soon. She also kept writing letters and numbers in the air with her finger. The therapist tells me they had her standing today. I ask if it hurt, and she said *'no.'* I asked if it felt good and she nodded *'yes'* and smiled. When saying *'goodbye'* she waved for me to come closer, and she hugged me. Wrapped her right arm around me and squeezed. It truly was a wonderful visit today!!! *Today was a milestone of improvement in just a week.*

February 8, 2011 - Day 42 — 5:50 - Ryan and I were at RidgeLake to see Barb at noon. She was in a chair out in the hall when we arrived. Her eyes brightened with recognition when she saw us. She communicated to me that she was ready to go back to her room. (Ry is the one she was on her way to see the night of the accident.)

Ry asked *her "Do you remember anything that happened the night of the accident?"*

She signed, *"No"*, which I would expect.

The trauma doctors at Bayfront told me that *90% of TBI (traumatic brain injury)* patients have *no memory* of what happened when they start to wake up from a coma.

Both the Occupational and Physical Therapists came over and gave big grins of encouragement – saying she was actually making progress following every command they give her – approaching Stage 5 on the *Glasgow Coma Scale.* They feel that next week she will be Stage 5-6, which is what she needs to be moved to the next facility. This is encouraging news!!

My daughter was in a coma. Look how far she had come! When I spoke to her doctor later in the day, and told him that two therapists, today, said she might be a Stage 5, his response was, *"Yes, and she could be higher than that, I think."* He feels she will be ready to graduate from RidgeLake shortly.

February 9, 2011 – Day 43 — 7: 32 PM - **Jenn**: I wanted to let you know that I received an **autographed Bucs football** from the Bucs organization! We are all aware Barb is their biggest fan! I wanted to find out what was a good time to get it to you? I had them send it directly to me, because, I wasn't sure when Barb was being moved to another facility before she got it… and wanted to make sure it did not get lost. Honestly, I didn't think they would get it here that quickly! Let me know what works for you. Talk to you soon.

An Epidemic of Disconnection

8:43 PM — In this world there is an *"epidemic of disconnection"* with people. This blog on Facebook is a testimony to the fact that when people love someone, they can and will connect and step up for a person. Everyone has continued to keep up with Barb in your thoughts and prayer. I believe that those prayers are what is bringing her back to us now. *I thank you from the depths of my heart, for all you have done, and all you will continue to do for my daughter. The support system we have here will be critical to supporting her after she returns home.* (During this time friends stepped up to care for Barb's dog and cat.)

LOVE AND PRAYERS CAN MOVE MOUNTAINS

February 10, 2011 - Day 44 — 9:46 AM - A lot of people, including the guardianship attorney, Neil Scott, and Lori, Barb's case worker at RidgeLake, have been concerned that I take care of my health. They have reminded me that if I do not pay attention to my health, I can't take care of Barb later. So today, I am seeing my doctor to bring my health issues up to date, and see what "game plan" we need to follow.

5:53 PM - Barb seemed very alert today. This is her 2nd day with her Trach capped. After the 3rd day of success, it can be removed. She did not pass the "swallowing test" but most people do not pass on their first try. It is not a big deal. I believe she is ready for the next step in her recovery, and so does her medical team.

She seems to be understanding most of what is happening around her now, and is trying to talk to me – but *I just can't understand her.* Once the trach is out, she will be able to speak to us, and we will understand her better.

7:30 PM - I went over to *The Mikey Center for Hyperbaric Oxygen Treatments* today to get more information. I spoke to the director, M.D. Stevens. The center is named after Mikey, her son.

There have been *significantly positive outcomes with TBI* (Traumatic Brain Injury) patients in receiving HBOT. 20 treatments of 1-2 hours will be $1400 as opposed to other commercial centers closest to where we live (Largo and Venice, Fl.) which charge $9000. One hundred percent oxygen can explode, and is therefore not recommended. However, the 95% oxygen treatments are widely accepted now and have no explosive characteristics.

I will continue to gain education on HBOT for Barb, so we can pursue this when she is finished with other therapies.

February 11, 2011 - Day 45 — 3:13 PM — The therapist concurs that in the past 2 weeks Barb has made incredible progress and is now ready for her next transition —- to another facility. This is where the real work on her recovery begins.

She had been downsized to a #4 trach, the last step before she had her trach removed. We are waiting for approval from Blue Cross Blue Shield, as I write this, to accomplish this next big step.

Barb (finally) had a shower this morning – her first since her accident. They took her on a water-proof gurney and promised they will shampoo her hair.

Once she is moved to the new facility, she will have to meet the requirement of 3 hours of therapy (physical, occupational, psych) per day. She is also going to be required to dress each day (with help).

Chapter 17

February 12, 2011 – Day 46 — 7:30 PM — My son rushed home from Iraq in light of my daughter's grave condition. For 17 days, we kept vigil at her bedside in Neuro-ICU. She had *six* separate traumatic brain injuries. *Realistically, any one of them could have killed her.* No one can explain why she is alive.

Prior to this event, my daughter was charge nurse at the largest state-of-the-art walk-in, subacute care medical center in our county.

She is 38 years old, the middle child, and the peace maker. The one who is close to both her sister, 4 years older, and her brother, 6 years younger. Their father died in April 1978, of a brain aneurysm at age 30. When *this* happened to my daughter, four days after Christmas, the entire family was blind-sided. I have been posting on Facebook during the entire painful and slow recovery (a description more appropriate to her family's experience than hers) process.

> *It is amazing to be part of such a wonderful network of friends who are stepping up with offers of help, support, and unconditional love, returning what she had given.*

She has just reached a milestone: Stage 5-6 on the Glasgow Coma Scale. We are encouraged. Her family will be here every step of her recovery.

February 13, 2011 – Day 47 — I went to the hospital today at noon. Barb was out at the nurse's station (where else would she be? Ha!). Isabelle, her nurse, says she hates being in her room alone now that she is awake much of the time. We spent 30 minutes pushing her up and down the halls in her wheelchair. Every time I sat down to talk, she wanted to keep moving. I wanted to get a photo to send to Mark so he could see how good she is doing and she allowed that.

Then I asked, *"Do you mind if I put it on Facebook for your friends?"* She said, *"Yes, it's okay to do that!"*

Another big milestone: Her trach came out today.

Feb. 14, 2011 – Day 48 — This morning for the first time, I discovered there are some issues with Blue Cross Blue Shield. Primarily that of the 21 days they allow for intense rehabilitation. Can you imagine putting a limit on that – if the person needs it? Insurance – bah humbug.

AFLAC is moving ahead with processing Barb's claims, and soon we will know more information. She needs to go to the most aggressive rehabilitation available. We are looking at a day-to-day prospectus.

She is restless and agitated because her brain is *storming* and she has BPA.

She needs more stimulation and interaction. HealthSouth can provide this, and we are having her approved for admission in the next couple of days.

A grateful *"Thank You"* and acknowledgment to the generosity of the employees at Pinnacle Medical. The employees took up a collection and paid her rent through February.

Now we need to move ahead with packing up her things and getting them moved to a safe and secure place. I live on a fixed income. I have a small one bedroom apartment to maintain. I cannot access her bank account until after March 9 when her Guardianship Hearing is scheduled. As her mom, it falls to me to be her legal "Next-Of-Kin" and the court will appoint me to handle her affairs, until she can do that again.

February 15, 2011 – Day 49 — At 3 PM Barb was moved to HealthSouth (on the opposite side of the lake from where we are now at RidgeLake). She will be here for 21 days (or perhaps longer) before we investigate the next move. I am told therapy is 8:30 – 3 PM – but they are pretty liberal. She is to dress each day. **I asked God to help us** so we can manage this since my feeble mind can't begin to comprehend how we are going to do that – but some way we will "get 'er done."

February 16, 2011 – Day 50 — Shhhhhhhhh… Barb is the biggest Bucs fan ever! Barb is not aware that The Buccaneers Football team in Tampa, Florida, has sent one of Barb's friends, Jenn, a football that had been autographed by her favorite player ever — #40 Mike Alstott ("A-Train"). This football was one that was used in the Super Bowl!

Monday noon Jenn is coming to HealthSouth to present the football to Barb with this *super surprise*. If anyone would like to join Jenn and me, you are welcome. Jenn got a display case for this unique football. We know this will be one of *Barb's prize possessions.*

Barb now had 3 hours a day of therapy. It is obvious to everyone she understands everything being said. She responds appropriately, although I still have no clue if she knows what happened to her. I ask her if the first day of therapy wore her out. She shook her head *"No."*

She tends to be restless, and it is hard to tell when she is restless and when she is agitated (which is a Neuro-generated condition *"storming"*).

I spoke to the new case worker today, Jennie (MSW) and she encouraged us to bring Barb's dog, Bodie, for a visit. This is a "pet-friendly" facility.

February 18, 2011 — Day 52 — It was suggested that I spend a day going to therapy with Barb. That will help me to understand, more in-depth about

Chapter 17

her experience, and what they are trying to set goals for her development and progress. I will do this on Monday, Feb. 21. I plan to ask a ton of questions. I see a terrific opportunity presented to me and will take it as such.

Meetings with therapists, Dr. Simon (physical medicine/therapy doctor), Dr. Miller (her psychiatrist) and her social worker, Jennie. We had an absorbing and informative conversation that I feel was valuable for each of us in understanding more about how to treat Barb. She has admitted to depression in the past, which is expected. There is a unanimous consensus among the doctors and therapists *"Barb is making progress!"* However, on the **Glasgow Coma Scale (GCS)** of minimum, moderate or severe, Barb is currently "severe".

I spoke to Dr. Simon about her personal experience and information she might share on HBOT. *She was incredibly encouraging about the positive effects seen when adding HBOT for TBI patients.* She spoke of **The Mikey Center** locally, and also told me of the center in Palm Harbor. Dr. Simon just put Barb on a new medication that is supposed to help her regain her speech and some vitamins that are known to help with healing the brain with TBI. **Dr. Simon stated that she saw high potential for recovery over time for Barb.** She agreed that there is currently a "communication issue" that is causing frustration (hers and mine). She feels this will pass soon. Barb's indwelling catheter was removed Tuesday. Bowel/bladder training is being done every 2-3 hours. Visits are now encouraged and are more important than ever after therapy – 3 PM.

February 21, 2011 – Day 55 — I spent the day with Barb going to her different therapies. (Occupational, Speech, and Physical). Andrea was here for a couple of hours. I also spoke to Jennie, the case worker. She will gather all the resources and options that are available to review for more care and rehabilitation when the current stay at HealthSouth is completed approx. March 8. I will have a meeting with Jennie, Feb. 24 to go over possible options, and for us to consider so far as Barb's progress.

February 23, 2011 – Day 57 — Hey "MHS Peeps". (MHS = Manatee High School class '90 and the "peeps" were Barb's classmates) It is time to get together and have a cyber "group hug". She needs everyone soon and often. HealthSouth is asking for volunteers to come and stay with Barb for a while 24/7. She is very agitated and restless. This is a temporary situation due to her "re-awakening" from her coma. *The staff is asking me to put out a call for HELP with her nights, days, weekends, so someone will be with her all the time.* **It is obvious she is lonely and needs company.** The rehab will put a bed in her room for someone who can stay the night. She can and will respond *"yes"* and *"no"* to questions. Her trach is healing, and soon she will be audible. If you can go for just a few hours or a night, please let me know.

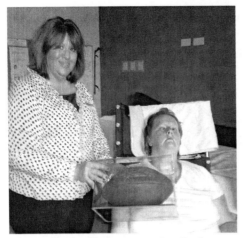

Jennifer Tratz presenting Barb with her Buccaneer football.

February 24, 2011 — Day 58 — Jenn presented the Bucs football to Barb today at 3 PM. It is one from The Superbowl XXXVII Official Wilson football signed by #40 Mike Alstott ("A-Train") with a case to protect it. Barb was really excited to get it and smiled as big as I have seen her smile lately. Sadly, not one of the photos of her "big smiles" was worth putting on FB. That was disappointing. (Actually when I asked her later, she did not remember this. However, it is now one of her prized possessions. She keeps it on a shelf in her room.)

❧

Don't let what you can't do
stop you from doing what you can do.
John Wooden (1910-2010)

❧

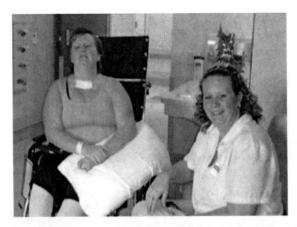

Andrea visiting with Barb in her room at HealthSouth.

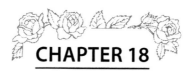

CHAPTER 18

"Forget the Person You Knew..."

March 2011

I have just gotten an $8900 cashier's check and sent payment overnight by FEDEX to Colorado to ensure Barb would be covered by Cobra Insurance, as soon as Blue Cross Blue Shield ran out. It is a big chunk of her AFLAC money. I was simply thankful that the money was there to ensure her continuing care with the situation so up in the air. This had to be done now, because Pinnacle had been sold, prior to her accident. . The change of ownership was to occur March 1, 2011. I was confident that I had kept ahead of them. The wheels were already moving forward for her to be transferred to the next (and last) rehab, prior to her coming home.

The lady from COBRA had even called personally, that day while I was at work, to assure me that the check had arrived, and my daughter had been put into their system – and she was covered immediately.

I arrived at HealthSouth after work, confident that the move would go off seamlessly the following day.

4:30 PM - Jennie, Barb's case worker, approached me. She looked worried.

"Mrs. Scott? There is a problem," she informed me.

"Problem? What kind of problem?" I queried.

"Your daughter has no insurance. We can't find her in the system anywhere."

I stared at her in disbelief. I had just spent days getting all our ducks-in-a-row, so Barb would not fall off the grid for insurance coverage. Barb was scheduled to transfer to Heartland the following morning, however **without confirmation** by the system, *that she was covered by insurance, they could do nothing but send her home!* At that time we had no place for her to go!

Jennie and I put our heads together and went to work to try and find a way to rectify the erroneous information being received by their office. *It did not matter what I knew.* Unless they could find *proof that Barb was insured* (and her bill was covered) *what I knew did not count.* I spent a sleepless night trying to understand what was happening.

I had previously had one encounter with *"The Insurance Liaison"* while I was attempting to get information on Barb's insurance in early January. I had used determination and guile to locate him. He was beyond the stacks in the medical records department, and deep into one corner in an office that appeared to be **not** much more than a large utility closet. I finally managed to locate him and appeared in his doorway, looking a bit exasperated and frazzled, not to mention feeling perplexed and determined.

He seemed shocked to see me materialize. For some unknown reason, I had felt that he should have, as part of his job description, been prepared to meet the public, and have **insightful information** to impart to them. *Imagine me, expecting that! What a fool I was!*

The first thing I noted was *the lack of a chair* in which anyone could sit. I tried to be pleasant, once I uncovered his "secret" whereabouts, but by now I was feeling really frustrated. I kept reminding myself that a person is more likely to respond in a positive manner. Something about "a bee to honey" came to mind.

The guy did an excellent imitation of a "deer in headlights," and seemed at a loss when I appeared. All I could see on his bewildered face,

Obviously he had never had an encounter with a mother Grizzly, trying to shield her cub!

"Lady, how did you find me? I thought I was buried so deep you would have to pipe in the sunshine."

I introduced myself and ignored his obvious frustration at my uninvited presence. The fact that I had been so thoughtless as not to call for an appointment (so he could tell me he was not available), before appearing in his office /utility closet, was obviously an affront to his sensibilities.

I began pummeling this oaf with a list of questions on a slip of paper in my hand. He hemmed and hawed — totally at a loss with any useful information. He seemed unable to apologize even for his distinct and complete incompetence.

He had kept himself hidden, hoping he did not have to encounter the public during his days "working." He was not only devoid of information about anything useful, but his social skills were woefully inadequate.

He struggled to keep up with my conversation and I became less than sympathetic to his "social disability". The longer I tried to wrench information out of this "Insurance Liaison" the more frustrated I became. *I felt like Alice, who had just fallen down The Rabbit Hole into Wonderland.*

Finally with nothing to show for my efforts, except frustration, I moved on, leaving him to his illogical and uninspired existence. I wondered how he managed to find his way to work. That is when I concluded that *"Insurance Liaison"* was a buzz term for *"Idiot-In-Residence."*

I spent most of the morning e-mailing back and forth to various people, trying to get information on what to do. It didn't seem as if I were making any headway, and Barb's rehab hung in the balance. Time was evaporating. *If I failed, it would not matter how hard I had tried. I would still have failed.* They would release her even though they admitted she was not ready to come home — to a place that no longer existed!

While I was dealing with the process of problem-solving, I got a call from HealthSouth. It was explained to me that there had been *"an incident"* with Barb.

She had been taken in a wheelchair to rehab downstairs for the first time. While she was sitting and waiting, for the therapist, another person had an incident of choking. She had observed this, and it had upset her. I knew immediately what had happened. Barb had become frustrated and overstimulated because she still could not walk and could not help! Her training and orientation as a nurse created a need in her to help. She became overwhelmed because she was helpless. She became so upset that she had a panic attack, and that caused her PBA to go into overdrive. She ended up having to be removed from therapy and taken back to her room to be suctioned because she hyperventilated. Basically, Barb had a meltdown! She had ended up having to be suctioned of phlegm that had clogged her throat.

Dr. Simon had decided to postpone her transfer to Heartland until the end of the week, in order to give Barb time to recover from what she had witnessed.

I later realized that **God had intervened once again.** He had created a situation that would *allow me extra time* to work out the details of the insurance issue I was faced with. (Of course then, I did not see that message as clearly as I do now.)

By afternoon, I was feeling as if I were sitting on a powder keg. I had to do *something* before time ran out, and they called to tell me that I had to move Barb from HealthSouth *due to lack of insurance*, when I knew that was not the case.

At 2:15 PM I headed to Pinnacle Medical. *Something* told me that I needed to go there. I was on my way to see the "head honcho" at Pinnacle. I had never met her, but I was determined I would find a way to see her, avoiding "The Insurance Liaison" at all costs, no matter how long I had to boycott the waiting room.

Yankee 794 Trauma

As I headed down the road driving to Pinnacle and passing a gas station, I actually had a daydream. It's funny what frustration and fear will drive a person's mind to imagine. I had this clear visual image – picturing myself sitting cross-legged in the parking lot of Pinnacle, pouring gasoline on myself and lighting a match – *turning myself into a human torch*! As brief and desperate as that daydream was – I found it interesting in a macabre sort of way. *That certainly would have gotten their attention! It might have actually made the news! The headline might have read "Desperate Mom Lights Up Issues Regarding Daughter's Health Care."*

I parked the car, dismissing the daydream as demonic and *said a prayer for strength*.

I marched into the side-entrance waiting room at Pinnacle, and up to the desk. There was an elderly volunteer attending the desk. Her eyes met mine. I quietly and calmly spoke to her in a low, slow and determined voice, *"Is Janice here? I'd like to see her. Please tell her that Elizabeth Scott is here. I need to speak to her regarding my daughter Barbara's situation."*

I am not sure what I must have looked like, but that volunteer jumped up like she had seen a ghost. She motioned for me to wait, and then disappeared into the back.

It was not long before Janice, the administrator of Pinnacle, arrived. She introduced herself and asked me to follow her. I complied. I could tell she did not want a public scene in the waiting room.

She showed me into a conference room and closed the door. Showing me to my seat she sat down directly across the conference table from me. By this time I was beyond furious, and *fixated on purpose* that was *fueled by fear*.

I collected my thoughts, took a deep breath, and began to explain the situation step-by-step. There was no way I planned to look like a raving lunatic to my daughter's employer, by ranting and raving about Pinnacle dropping my daughter's insurance right in the middle of her stay in rehab. I waited for it – *the question*.

"What can I do for you, Mrs. Scott?"

There it was. The question.

Hearing *that question* opened the floodgates, and my thoughts poured out like an avalanche tumbling down a mountain.

I did not raise my voice and tried to be logical in the way I explained things I recognized appearing hysterical was counterproductive. To get this one done,

Chapter 18

I needed to possess a clear head and organizational skills. What I was requesting was not unreasonable and (I knew) it was within my grasp.

"Barb has been fighting so hard to come back after almost dying. How fortunate we are, that she did not die… and now I have to fight every day to try and help with her recovery when I have no idea what the future holds. If you could only see how hard Barb is trying to come back to us, it would make everyone so proud. Pinnacle is Barb's employer, and my daughter has been a good and faithful employee. Not once have you been to see for yourself what is going on with my daughter's recovery. I tried to get information early on from the insurance guy, who appears to be lost somewhere behind medical records. I got her COBRA (insurance) check sent by overnight Fed Ex, and they called me and said Barb had insurance. Now the rehab has cut us off at the knees, because of Pinnacle canceling her insurance. I have been trying to do everything the right way. I am her Mom and all she has. Don't you understand they have dropped my daughter's lifeline to recovery?…"

I went on and on.

I finally wore myself out, running out of anything persuasive to say, and stopped talking. I took a breath, and I looked at her. She sat quietly for several minutes, never taking her eyes off of me. (I suspect she wondered if I was going to lunge across the conference table at her though I never indicated that was my intention.) She never once interrupted me. (It was nice to know someone seemed to be listening.)

She began, *"Mrs. Scott, from the bottom of my heart you have my deepest apology for what has happened. It should never have happened. I was concerned about the insurance issues that might occur with Barbara, considering the change in ownership of Pinnacle on March 1, and took my concerns to the board 6 weeks ago, hoping we could get ahead of the problem. Apparently, I did not do enough. I promise you that before this day is out, the issues with your insurance will be fixed. I will take care of this right now. I will send you an e-mail confirmation later today and information on how to proceed."*

There was nothing more to be said. I quickly deflated.

I was initially skeptical of what she told me, yet it seemed sincere. Her words, *"I promise you that before the day is out, the issues with your insurance will be fixed."*

The statement reverberated in my head. It was all I had wanted.

I wanted to believe her… and it certainly wouldn't take long for me to find out if she was going to follow through.

By 5:30 PM I had an e-mail from Janice attending to **the situation**. She did exactly what she promised she would do.

What I still don't know is what would have happened if I had not gone there and this matter had not been rectified!

By Friday, the way was cleared for Barb to be moved to Heartland and our journey to healing continued while everyone breathed a collective sigh of relief.

March 1, 2011 — Day 63— 11:41 AM

INFORMATION: On March 8 Barb will have been at HealthSouth Rehab Hospital for the 21 days allotted to her by her insurance policy with Blue Cross Blue Shield. We are now reviewing what *the next step* is to be in this process.

UPDATE: – 7:06 PM

I arrived at the hospital at 1 PM. Barb was in good spirits. She went to therapy, and that is making excellent progress. We picked up Bodie, her dog, and at 2:30 brought him to see Barb. She was overjoyed!

March 3, 2011 — **Day 65 - 08:58 PM - Day 66**

UPDATE: I was at the hospital from 2-5 PM today. Barb is a real unhappy camper. I have spoken to Dr. Miller, her psychiatrist, who keeps reminding me that her crying spells are the result of her brain trauma and are not to be taken personally. (I wish she had taken the time to help me understand PBA then!)

Because of her impulsive nature (again, due to Brain Trauma from "storming" and PBA) we have to "keep her safe" because she can't understand right now. This means when she moves to Heartland they require us to have 24/7 supervision with her for an unknown period of time.

Unlike the hospital setting, Heartland will not be allowed to have any type of restraint on her either in her wheelchair or bed.

Last week she unbuckled her seat belt and took a header (chair and all) in front of the nurse's station, to the astonishment of eleven members of the nursing the staff, including the Director of Nursing.

There will be **no seat belt allowed at Heartland by law** for 60 days. The family is now trying to find a way to accomplish this.

March 4, 2011 – Day 66

Elizabeth A. Scott 08:23 PM

UPDATE: Today was unlike any other. At 10 AM with the attorney, Neil Scott, I appeared in Sarasota County court. It felt like a nightmare, but it was real. It made me feel sad due to the circumstances that brought us to court

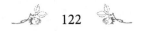

Chapter 18

today. Actually, it was a very simple process. The judge granted me Legal Guardianship so I could manage Barb's affairs.

Barb has been one of the most independent, delightful, funny and socially outgoing people I know. She has a heart as big as all outdoors, and her laugh is contagious. I would like to feel perhaps I had something to do with that.

> A DECLARATION OF LOVE MEANS NOTHING WITHOUT THE ACTIONS TO BACK IT UP.

March 6, 2011 — 06:47 PM — Day 68

I arrived at the rehab today at noon. My friend Ray came after church, and we visited with Barb for a while. She is still not verbal, and communication is minimal at best. It was a perfect Florida day; temperature hovering around 80 degrees and the sky was a perfectly gorgeous shade of azure.

I thought she would enjoy the fresh air. I longed for a conversation with her, no matter how brief, but it was unlikely that would happen. For now we would manage to be optimistic with God's perfect day. We wheeled her out to the patio to sit. Ray and I would visit a bit.

Barb immediately pointed to her temple and uttered,

"Better now!" and she smiled at me.

I looked at her in amazement and queried,

"What did you say Barb?"

She smiled and focused on me, "Better now!" pointing to her head.

I glanced at Ray to see if I saw things. He smiled and nodded in acknowledgment. I turned again to look at Barb and gave her an approving smile.

"Do you mean you are understanding more now?"

"Yes," She replied.

"Do you feel like you are coming out of a fog?"

She shook her head *"yes."*

"When was your accident?" I asked.

"Dec. 29," she replied.

"What day is it today?" I asked.

"March 6th," she responded.

She was communicating! My attention to her reactions was heightened. I

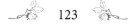

wondered if it would last or if, soon, she would fade again. **I felt hope restoring itself, if only for a minute.**

She appeared to be in exceedingly robust spirits today, and really enjoyed having company! Two of her friends from work arrived, along with the "Art Therapist".

We all went to the waiting room to do "art stuff." The Art Therapist rolled out a long, white sheet of paper and gave everyone crayons.

Then she said, "Draw whatever you would like."

Barb's eyes twinkled like "a kid in a candy store". She picked up a crayon and started writing, ***"Hospitals Suck!"***

We all started laughing as we could certainly sympathize with her opinion. Then she continued to doodle. The two girls who could see what she was writing thought she was writing "nonsense."

What she actually wrote was: ***"Snicklefritz!"***

She looked at me and there it was – that mysterious grin – a hallmark of who my daughter was! I took a second look and YES! *there it was reminiscent of who she had been under all this damage. A sense of comfort and tranquility fell over me.*

Not being able to see her doodle, I asked the others what she had written. Then I got up and looked.

"Snicklefritz"

I looked at her. There was that twinkle of mischief in her eye that I had missed for so long, and ***that grin*** was still there as well.

I started to laugh, and everyone looked puzzled. I knew what it meant, and she knew what that meant.

"Snicklefritz" was her Grandpa Moore's <my dad> pet name for her when she was a little girl. No one else could have known that but she knew Mom would get it. ***She is coming back!!!!!!!!***

Snicklefritz – From Wikipedia, the free encyclopedia

Snicklefritz or **Schnickelfritz** is a Pennsylvania Dutch term of affection usually for young, mischievous or talkative children.

March 9, 2011 — Day 71 - I met with Nurse Corp to do an intake this morning in preparation for moving Barb tomorrow. They are the ones who have been hired when we move Barb to Heartland. I was explaining to the intake supervisor her history and specifically why they were needed.

We then drove over to Heartland so she could meet Barb and assess the situation. As we were walking off the elevator toward Barb's room, I was explaining that I had entered Barb's room a number of times and witnessed the CNA's attempting to move her from bed to wheelchair or vice versa, and because her legs won't hold her weight, they have dropped her to the floor. With the gym mats on the floor, no injury ever resulted.

As we entered her room, we witnessed *three* CNA's in the bathroom with her. They were attempting to pivot her from the wheelchair to the toilet when she shifted, and they dropped her to the floor like a ragdoll – where there were no gym mats. Startled, we both just stood and watched the fiasco.

HealthSouth is a really nice place – clean, well lit, beautifully appointed, and staffed with a 6:1 ratio of staff to patient. I do not know that she could have been in a better place anywhere! Luckily, Barb was not hurt, but it is disturbing when such incidents happen — and are witnessed by family!

March 10, 2011 — Day 72 — 09:29 PM — UPDATE: This afternoon Barb was moved to Heartland HCR Manor in Sarasota, Florida. The length of stay is unknown at this time (perhaps 60 days). She was in good spirits today. I was at HealthSouth before they transported her at 4:00 PM and followed them over to Heartland to get her settled in. For the first week or two she will have 24/7 Nurse Core staff with her. This is a pet-friendly facility, providing regulations are followed.

We are seeking a laptop for Barb since she is not using her voice much, and her handwriting is uncoordinated. We feel (and Dr. Simon concurs) a laptop would be a great help for her to communicate her needs to family and staff. She is right-handed, and it is her left side that has the weakness. Barb believes she could type. That being said, a lock would be required to keep it at the rehab in her room. We would also need someone to set it up on Heartland's WIFI.

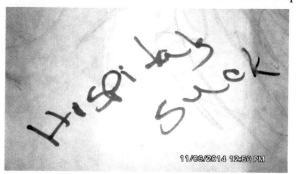

March 13, 2011 — 03:42 PM – Day 75

Barb scribbled: ***"Hospitals Suck."***

She wrote last Sunday. Apparently she has not altered her opinion in a week!

We ask her... so you think "Hospitals suck?" to which she wrote:

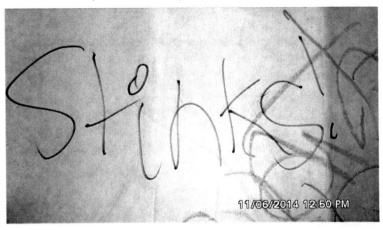

05:26 PM — Barb is watching Mom's Facebook account until Brandi can set up a new password on hers. We tried, but could not find the right one <the one she had been using> last night. It appears my statement about Barb being able to read your posts, but (possibly) not posting for a while was premature... but that is my tenacious daughter for you!

I ask Barb, and she believes she could type with her right hand. It is her left hand that is (temporarily) paralyzed. That being said, a lock would be required to keep it at the rehab in her room. Also, we would need someone to set up on their WIFI.

Elizabeth A. Scott - 07:12 PM — Hey MHS peeps – Barbara Scott is online! Thanks to Jennifer Ford-Cote! She hasn't remembered her passwords yet, so for the time being she's using her Mom's account. You can post to her page, and **she will answer as "Elizabeth Scott." WOO HOO!**

March 14, 2011 — 08:58 AM – Day 76

Everything about my daughter's mind is intact! She is with us. (Thank you, Lord!) We just had to realize what it would take to

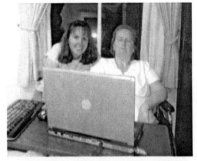

Jennifer Ford-Cote brought Barb a computer at Heartland.

allow her to talk with us. Obstacles are no match for Barb and her tenacity. The computer arrived, and when we got her on Facebook, she began to read the messages.

I said *"Barb, can you read this?"*

She looked up at me and beamed, nodding, *"YES!"*

The computer opened a door for her to communicate once again with her world and her family. At first just glimpses of her began emerging, and then more and more of her disposition and personality were evident.

"She is in there." I kept thinking.

09:04 AM – Gary Prowe's book on Traumatic Brain Injury told me, *"Forget the person you knew. Whoever is coming back to you will be someone different from the person you knew before."*

I had been trying to adjust to loving someone I had not known before, through this unimaginable struggle. Then, a couple of weeks ago, we started to see her sense of humor come shining through.

Sharon, the CNA from Nurse Corp, was talking to me last Thursday, following moving Barb to Heartland. She had her back to Barb when I saw her jump. The look on her face was priceless.

"Barb! Did you just goose me?" she exclaimed!

Barb was grinning from ear-to-ear. Sharon started laughing, as Barb knew she would. I suppose that is one way for nurses to communicate. HA!

CHAPTER 19

Incredible Breakthrough

March 13, 2011 - Day 75

Barb is using Mom's Facebook account until Brandi can help her set up a new password on hers. We tried, but could not hit the right one last night. She wrote last Sunday "Hospital Sucks!" Apparently she has not altered her opinion in a week!

It appears my statement about Barb being able to read your post, but (possibly) not posting for a while was premature... but this is my tenacious daughter for you!

"... this sux ... hospitals are horrible ! " she soon wrote.

Hey MHS peeps - Barbara Scott is online thanks to Jennifer!!! She hasn't remembered her passwords yet, so for the time being she's using her mom's account. You can post to her page, and she will answer as "Elizabeth Scott." WOO HOO!

She is with us. We just have to realize what it will take to allow her to talk to us. Obstacles are no match for Barb and her tenacity. The computer arrived, and when we got her on Facebook, she began to read the messages.

Everything about my daughter's mind is intact.

The computer that Jennifer so generously volunteered to donate has opened a door for her to communicate once again with her world and her family.

At first we just had glimpses of her, but more and more her disposition and personality began to shine through.

"She is in there." I kept thinking.

The books on Traumatic Brain Injury told me: *"Forget the person you knew. Whoever is coming back to you will be someone different from the person you knew before."*

I had been trying to adjust to loving someone I had not known before — through this almost unimaginable struggle. Then, a couple of weeks ago we started to see her sense of humor come shining through.

Chapter 19

March 16, 2011, Sunday — Day 78

When I got home from work, I received a call from Mark.

He asked me, *"Mom? Is Barb posting on Facebook?!?"*

"I don't think so son. Jennifer put a laptop in her room at the new place yesterday, so she could see the posts on Facebook, but I don't know if she can post yet."

He replied, *"I think you better go and look because it looks like she is posting!"*

I got off the phone, and I logged on to Facebook to see what he was referring to. I thought maybe someone had hacked into her account.

That is when I saw her post and realized the floodgates had opened!

I sat there reading the posts coming in from people who had been following her page all along, but had never posted anything.

It looked as if I was posting, — *but I wasn't.*

I began to scream and jump up and down. I would have given someone a big hug – but, no one was there.

I just sat there with tears streaming down my face, in utter disbelief and *astonished at the miracle everyone was collectively witnessing.*

(Barb typing) 12:50 PM (posting as Elizabeth Scott)

"hi, guys."

Barb sent a text by Facebook!

"hi, all!!!!"

Kelly: Hi Barb! I miss you like crazy! I am so impressed with how well you are doing! But I'm not all that surprised since it's you we are talking about! I've always admired you! You are a true fighter!!

Barbara S Scott:

trying … miss you too Kelly

Kelly: I'm going to come and see you on my next days off! Can't wait!

Barbara S Scott: ok

Kelly: I have to get ready for work… I hate it when I'm late :) Have a great night!

Barbara S Scott: u2

Tammy W: Hey Barb! How are you today? Good to see you again today.

Oh, Barb... it's soo great to see you again... YOU have been truly missed.

Cassandra: Hey Barb, I'm glad to hear about u r progress. I miss and love u dearly. Keep up the great work!

Tonya: Hello barb. its great to see your progress in all this, but you have always been our go-to girl. Keep up the good work. Hope to see you soon.

Melanie: BARBARA SUE!!!!! I MISS YOU!! Kiya says hi, and she misses you too!!

Susan: Hi Barb!!!!! How exciting to see you on here!!!!! Nothing less than a miracle! I hope you got my card. I'd love to come visit you one day :):)

Inda: We love you and pray for you every day.

Andrea (sister): Hey sis I poked you back

Casey: Hi, Barb!!

Rich: HI!!! Barb glad to see you back in action, so happy to see you're doing better stay positive we'll see you soon

Richardo: (uncle): Hello glad to see you back. Mom and Sharon also say hi. We hope to keep seeing you progress.

Elizabeth A. Scott: Look carefully – Barb is sending messages to her friends.

I think she likes Heartland better than HealthSouth for a number of reasons. I was at rehab yesterday and again today. Tomorrow I worked. She was in good spirits and thanks to Jenn, she is really enjoying her laptop !!!

Cindy: Hey Barb... am thinking about you every day and sending you prayers!! God speed on your recovery! Look forward to working with you again. I know you are going to heal... I can just feel it! Anything you need... just ask!

March 17, 2011 – Day 79 — I saw my daughter take 100 steps today, in three spurts this afternoon with assistance. She is doing so well. Lots of "issues" with her neck that have created problems with her swallowing and talking.

It's been a month since the trach came out, and we discussed this with Speech Therapy. They are asking for a consultation with a throat doctor to see if there is *something* we are not aware of. Barb agrees we need to look into this.

When Blue Cross Blue Shield had her insurance coverage, they approved 60 days at Heartland. United Healthcare is a new provider, and they have just told Heartland. *"No limit on rehab, as long as she is making progress."* This is great news.

Barb continues to do well, and we are encouraged by her progress. *She is really enjoying being back on Facebook. She likes reading the comments and encouraging notes. Keep them up!*

March 19, 2011 – Day 81 — Barb loves seeing her friends. Please understand she tires quickly, but not seeing everyone would be worse. So if you have not seen her for a while, this weekend would be great — anytime is great. If she is in therapy, just hang around. She will be back soon!

Tammy W: 08:31 AM — Barb, I am so glad that I got to spend some time with you yesterday. I know this "sucks" but just remember you are getting better every day!!! Love your girlie! If you need anything, just let me know!

Now, more than before, she needs to keep in touch.

> "We do not think ourselves into new ways of living. We live ourselves into new ways of thinking."
>
> Richard Rohr

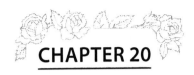

CHAPTER 20

Hyperbaric Oxygen Therapy (HBOT)

The first thing God gives you when you are born – Oxygen.
The last thing God takes away when you breathe your last – Oxygen.
Without Oxygen you died.
Such a simple concept –
Perhaps we sometimes make things too complicated.

Within days of Barb being grievously injured, my instincts told me to find out about Hyperbaric Oxygen Therapy (HBOT). I began doing research within a week.

Initially, I was told the closest commercial facilities were in Largo and Venice (Florida). They charge approximately $9000 for 20 hours. That was cost-prohibitive for us, no insurance company would cover the cost for TBI (traumatic brain injury). They tell us "There is no verifiable research that it works."

Newsflash!

We don't need "valid research"! We have been able to see with our own eyes; it works in many cases where no other medical help has done the job. Traumatic Brain Injury (TBI) is one of those success stories.

꒰

"The person who says something is impossible
should not interrupt the person who is doing it."

Chinese Proverb

꒰

Something told me to keep looking. The more I read, the more I was convinced that Barb needed HBOT to help her brain heal, as well as the rest of her body.

HBOT was the key to maximizing her recovery.

One of the doctors with whom she had worked at Pinnacle Medical, Dr.

Chapter 20

James W. Raniolo, D.O., was certified in emergency medicine. He also had a master's degree in Nutrition and had taken a 3-month residency beside the doctor who had pioneered HBOT for medical purposes. Dr. Raniolo reviewed her MRI and other medical records, and was *absolutely convinced* that the type of TBI Barbara had sustained, would reap *enormous benefits for her recovery.*

I approached several of her doctors to see what they knew about HBOT and although they admitted knowing little about it, they all seemed to be in agreement *it could not hurt.*

In fact, her doctors had seen nothing but good results from patients who they knew had benefited, when they sought out HBOT.

Dr. Simon, her physiatrist (rehab doctor who specializes in physical medicine) told me that in the patients who she had followed that had independently sought out HBOT she had observed *significant improvement in a shorter amount of time.*

Those patient's families had sought out more information as they investigated further. The result was that, like us, the families was so convinced of its benefits, that they used alternative resources to pay for it.

> HBOT may help hasten her improvement and recovery.

One evening, while on the internet, *The Mikey Center for Hyperbaric Therapy* popped up. It is a unique and innovative center that offers the latest technology and advancements at reasonable rates. A private business owned by M.D. Stevens, and dedicated to the memory of her son, Mikey, who had died when he was 5 years old. After talking to M.D., I understood that this facility was a labor of love.

The Mikey Center offers Hyperbaric Oxygen Therapy to infants, children, adolescents, and adults for a broad range of conditions and symptoms such as aging, autism, infections, Cerebral Palsy, diabetes, fatigue, dementia, injuries (such as sports-related), ADD/ADHD and many more.

The Hyperbaric chambers are the most advanced and spacious in their class of chambers. It's designed for individual use for the ultimate privacy and relaxation during the Hyperbaric Treatment. It is spacious and roomy enough to accommodate a parent and child for dual treatments.

The Mikey Center was located in Lakewood Ranch, Florida, half way between Bradenton (where I lived) and Sarasota, FL (where Barb was in rehabilitation). Approximately 10 miles in either direction. (As of January 2016 it is now in Osprey, FL.)

There was only one Hyperbaric Oxygen Chamber in her office since each chamber if purchased privately, costs approx. $25,000. The miracles that were radiating out of The Mikey Center were undeniable. ***The Mikey Center*** offers Hyperbaric Oxygen treatments 6 days a week. Call 941-724-1861 to schedule an appointment, or for information.

It seemed as though M.D. Stevens was there endlessly, accommodating schedules of people who needed her services. Many nights she worked so late that she wouldn't go home. Instead, she would climb into her own chamber and sleep. I had never seen anyone so driven to "do the right thing" for people she didn't know, but who needed her services. It's about COMPASSION.

By now, I was no longer saying Barb's disabilities were a tragedy, but rather an opportunity. There was no alternative but to try. There were naysayers, but I looked at my daughter and thought, that without the attempt, there was no possible result.

In March 2011, when Barb finally got to Heartland Rehabilitation in Sarasota, I was able to arrange for HBOT. I had spent a lot of time studying the benefits of this alternate therapy. I was convinced that this was going to help in her recovery. The cost would be $1400 for 20 one-hour treatments.

***"Take the first step in faith.
You don't have to see the whole staircase,
just take the first step."***

***Martin Luthur King, Jr.
(1929-1968)***

As determined as I was for Barb to have these treatments, I was equally determined not to interrupt her rehab schedule during the day. M.D. agreed that when Barb finished at the rehab, we would transport her to *The Mikey Center*, arriving at 5:00 PM. She would remain in the chamber until 7:00 PM, *giving her two uninterrupted hours each visit.*

M.D. had Wifi at The Mikey Center, so I ran down to Best Buy to try and find one of the new I-PADS. This would allow her to watch a movie each time she was in the chamber.

My heart sank, as I was told the store was sold out, having just hit the market that week. However, I said a prayer right there in the store that in some mysterious way God would make a way to get one for Barb. While I was chatting with the salesperson about back ordering one, and how long the projected delay would be (perhaps a month or more), a store clerk walked up with one that had just been returned — unopened.

"Do you want this one?" she inquired. It was a though she knew why I had come.

"Oh yes! Thank you so much!" I exclaimed. "This truly is a miracle. You just don't know!"

It felt as if God had opened another door, furnishing us with something that seemed out of reach. This gave Barb an opportunity to watch a movie each time she was immobile in HBOT for those two hours. The fact is that more often than not the patient sleeps through most of their treatment.

As time moved forward, and Barb began to adjust gradually dealing with her disabilities, I was reminded that whatever lies ahead of us is always in **God's Hands**. He had given me Hope!

My main concern was finding out if Barb was claustrophobic. I am. I don't remember being that way as a young person, but it seems to have developed as a bi-product of my aging. Prior to us going, I asked Barb, *"Are you claustrophobic?"* Her answer was *"No."*

When we arrived at The Mikey Center, she was unable to walk. M.D. Stevens provided a Hoyer Lift to get Barb into and out of the hyperbaric chamber.

Barb said the first couple of sessions she got the distinct impression she could not breathe and felt trapped and unable to get out, but that feeling did pass. She also was concerned about being zipped into the chamber. What would happen if she needed anything? Would anyone hear her? She needn't have worried. M.D. gave Barb a bell, which she still has, so she could ring it if she needed anything.

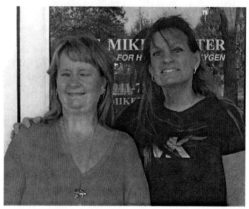

As each obstacle occurred, the answer to overcoming it also came. It was not long until, with her I-Pad and her movie, Barb could spend two hours in the chamber, and feel good about it.

When our money began to run low, M.D. gifted Barb with her birthday month (July 2011).

Barbara with M.D. Stevens at the Mikey Center — Nov. 2014.

In total, Barb ended up having 47 hours of HBOT.

For veterans with PTSD:
US Army Medical Dept.
Dwight D. Eisenhower Army Medical Center

Exceptional Family Member Program
Location: Family Medicine Clinic
300 Hospital Road
Fort Gordon, GA 30905
Phone Number:
(706) 787-9300/9310
Hours: Monday-Friday 0700-1530 hrs
If you have any questions for the local EFMP staff,
please send to DDEAMC EFMP
For more information, please visit the AMEDD EFMP Web site.

Our program is currently the only clinical hyperbaric medicine service in the U.S. Army. The hyperbaric medicine service is managed and supervised by a physician who is trained in hyperbaric medicine. The service is also staffed by a nurse and technicians trained in the medical, physical, and mechanical aspects of hyperbaric medicine.

Outpatient and Inpatient Care
Accepted Indications: Approved Uses

Air or gas embolism, carbon monoxide poisoning , clostridial myonecrosis (gas gangrene), crush injury, compartment syndrome, and other acute traumatic ischemias, decompression sickness (The Bends), enhancement of healing in selected problem wounds,exceptional blood loss (anemia), intracranial abscess, necrotizing soft tissue infections (subcutaneous tissue, muscle, fascia) Osteomyelitis (refractory), radiation tissue damage (radionecrosis), skin grafts and flaps (compromised), thermal burns.

"Whatever happens to you belongs to you. Make it yours. Feed it to yourelf even if it feels impossible to swallow. Let it nurture you, because it will."

Cheryl Strayed

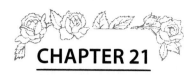

CHAPTER 21

Every Brain Injury is Unique and Unpredictable

Successfully Surviving A Brain Injury
Author: Gary Prowe:
Chapter 8 "How to Succeed as a Caregiver:
Focus on What You Can Control."

"While you are unable to predict how well your survivor is going to recover, there are two things you can say with certainty:

(1) She is facing the challenge of her life;

(2) She will need your undying support to succeed."

"When a patient emerges from her coma, she will need you to comfort her through her bewilderment and agitation.

In rehabilitation, she will need your encouragement as she is pushed to the limits of her ability. When she returns home, she will need your support in countless ways. Through all this, your loved one will rely on your patience, guidance, creativity, stamina, selflessness and love. In other words, your survivor is going to demand every minute and every ounce of energy you can muster for a long time. It is time to get ready for that demanding job."

"Preparing physically, intellectually and spiritually – to be an excellent caregiver is the challenge. Caring for a person with brain injury leaves you vulnerable to stress-related illnesses…

(1) Get some sleep;

(2) Eat well;

(3) Exercise;

Helplessness is a hallmark of brain injury.

(4) Have some fun.

Focus on the future and not the past. *Much of what will happen in your patient's recovery is beyond your control. Helpless can be maddening. Most important, it can be lethargic.* **Fatigue inevitably leads to illness, and an ailing caregiver is a poor caregiver."**

"Use it or lose it" applies well to brain injury. A survivor who had lived an active, challenging and full pre-injury life, has conditioned her brain to be

*well-prepared for the rigorous reworking necessary to recover well... **every brain injury is unique and unpredictable...**" How unique and how unpredictable?*

Keep the humor in mind.
Humor can help with anything.

When Barb started rehabilitation, after moving to Heartland, one day I brought her a gift of four T-shirts I had hand-picked. Each had one large, legible phrase. They were designed for wearing to therapy, as well as an example of the humor that kept us going, in the face of the uncertain adversity through which we were moving.

The Blue one had white letters and said:
"Just pretend I'm not here. That's what I'm doing."

The second one was bright Yellow with black letters and read,
"Are you trying to piss me off?"

The dark Mauve one announced in big white letters,
"I live in my own little world. But it's okay... they know I am here."

The Turquoise one with black letters read:
"Remember my name. You'll be screaming it later!"

"All we have is all we need. All we need is the awareness of how blessed we really are."

Sarah Ban Breathnach

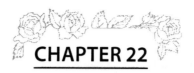

CHAPTER 22

Shake, Shake, Shake

March 2011

One Sunday I decided to take Barb something which I thought would be a treat. She was eating "institutional food," which we jokingly remarked was difficult to identify.

The food was pureed, and I had joked that the secret kitchen was where secret dieticians "pre-chewed" the food for the residents before it was served! Their "pizza" was something completely unrecognizable; a sort of a red lump that Barb referred to as "a hockey puck."

None-the-less, while I tried not to watch, Barb would sit there, and she would eat whatever they brought to her room, like a trooper. I joked that she had an admirable fortitude and her trademark tenacity.

Later she explained that she had been told, "If you don't eat, we can't remove your feeding tube." So she decided no matter how distasteful the food looked, she would eat it, one way or another.

So on that day, I decided that she would surely enjoy a shake. I stopped by Dairy Queen and ordered a chocolate/marshmallow shake – my favorite – for her. I was excited. I thought I had actually favored her with something special.

She spent the next couple of hours S-L-O-W-L-Y slurping up the shake and ended up leaving half of it in the cup. I thought that was odd, but maybe she just wasn't hungry. Finally, I "asked" her if it had been okay, and she gave me an approving smile and put her stamp of approval on my good deed.

A few days later Paige, one of her friends, asked me if there was anything special she could bring Barb since she was planning to see her. I suggested a chocolate/marshmallow shake from Dairy Queen, and Paige followed my instructions. She showed up with the shake in hand to surprise Barb — and Barb took the drink, slowly sucking it through the straw — gratefully acknowledging Paige's thoughtfulness.

Months later, after we were settled in at home, I would look for activities to get us out of the house. I would take her for a walk to The John Ringling Bridge in Sarasota, or to the mall, or the sidewalk on Anna Maria Island, so she could get her practice walking. The more walking, the better. For many months whenever I left the house, Barb was my constant companion.

One day I was looking for an outing and suggested we go to Dairy Queen for two chocolate/marshmallow shakes. Barb scrunched up her nose, and shook her head, "No." Then she informed me that she wanted a chocolate/peanut butter shake. It turned out Barb hates marshmallow – in any form, a fact that had totally eluded me... apparently.

March 20, 2011 — **Day 82**

My 64th birthday was spent at Heartland Rehab in Sarasota, Florida.

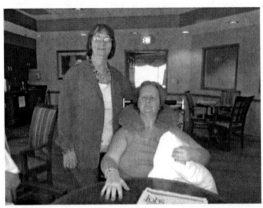

Barb with me on my birthday, March 20, 2011 at Heartland.

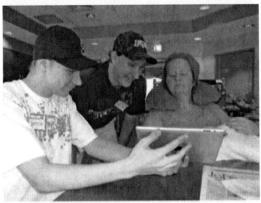

Ryan Simmonds and Matthew (son) trying out her new I-Pad.
Barb was on her way to Ryan's the night the accident happened.

March 21, 2011 — Day 83 — 08:15 PM

Paige: Well, hello my friend! I have been gone for 3 1/2 weeks, and look at what I come back to: You are truly amazing! It is so wonderful to read about all of your progress, and I can't wait to see ya in person! I will be coming to see you soon now that I am home! I miss and love you!

Andrea and I transported Barb to see Dr. John C. Shelton, M.D. He is a board-certified ear, nose and throat doctor whom she had seen in 2004.

Barb did well pivoting from wheelchair to back seat and from the back seat of a wheelchair. He has ordered an MRI for her head and neck, which have been creating a lot of pain.

He scoped her throat and told us *her vocal cords are not opening and closing properly.* This explains the difficulty of her projecting her voice and swallowing.

He feels that *her brain injury is contributing to her inability to speak.* Again, for those who have not seen her, Barb is talking quite frequently and coherently, but she is not able to project her voice. She speaks in a whisper.

We are also making an appointment with a Neuro-Ophthalmologist about her left eye. Once those three "pieces of this puzzle" are in place, we will know much more about how to proceed with her recovery.

March 23, 2011 — Day 85 – Dr. Shelton's office is now cleared thru insurance for Barb to have an MRI on Thursday, March 24. Andrea will transport, and Donna (CNA) will accompany her.

A report on the MRI of head, neck, and lumbar is to be sent to Dr. Shelton's office, and we will go for a review of the report Monday, March 28.

March 24, 2011 — Day 86 – Reports from the CNA's at Nurse Corp confirm *neck pain is worsening.* The past two weeks the CNA's have been with her 24/7. They report how bad she is feeling. She's having an MRI at 10 AM, to try and discover why her neck pain (back to the left side and more recently back of neck to right side) is increasing.

Barb is complaining of pain and not sleeping. My daughter is not a complainer. If she says she is having neck pain at a 9 out of 10, then I want her pain to be lessened. Pain meds are obviously not adequate to make her comfortable so that she can do therapies or sleep. I called last night to request more powerful pain meds be used. I think it might be time for HBOT to begin soon but she needs pain meds for that to be effective.

9:58 PM – **UPDATE:** Barb had an MRI this morning. On Monday, the doctor will give us the news of what it reveals. Pain issues may have been dealt with – we shall see. They have doubled her pain medications plus gotten an order for Soma (a muscle relaxer.) That, in conjunction with pain med, may improve effectiveness.

I will call in AM to see what kind of night she has had. This morning her good right arm went numb and became useless with tingling. It sounds like a pinched nerve. Barb needs a good nights sleep to work well in therapy. She explained to me her left eye was not tracking correctly.

10:11 PM - I had a busy day taking care of legal issues. Finally got the court document to direct Progressive to pay off her car. I went to the bank and got two cashier's checks for 16 months of coverage:

(1) COBRA/HCR Met Life Dental insurance

(2) COBRA/HCA-Vision Insurance.

I put them in the mail. Then I went by to the Progressive Insurance office in Lakewood Ranch to sign papers to pay off her car.

Following that, I went to where her MRI was done and paid a co-pay. Next, I met with Neil Scott, my attorney, to review documents the court requires. I feel as if I have been chasing my tail all day! I am not sure how many miles I put on my car while running all over town. I did not make it to rehab until 6:20 PM. I am tired but I have accomplished a lot.

March 25, 2011 – Day 87 - 6:35 AM — Renee, CNA on the night shift, reports Barb had a better night and did sleep for intervals. The pain level was not as bad with the increased medication plus Soma. Today we are cutting back on private duty nursing from 24/7 for the last two weeks, to 12 hours this coming week. Both Donna (days) and Sharon (evenings) from Nurse Corp have agreed to do a 9-3 and 3-9 shifts for a week. We will see how that goes.

March 26, 2011 - Day 88 — 9:25 AM — Her pain level at 4:00 AM was a 6-7 even with doubling the OxyContin plus Soma. She also had Percocet ordered between the OxyContin. It is a battle right now to keep her pain at a level where she can tolerate therapy. That pain is counter-productive to her reason for being at Heartland Rehabilitation.

The week before her move to Heartland, to everyone's astonishment, Barb was sitting in a wheelchair at the Nurses Station. She was going through a very impulsive stage with her brain injury. She unbuckled her seatbelt and took a "header" (chair and all) *hitting her head on the left side, hyper-extending her neck.*

At first it was reported that she did not "hurt" herself. She even confirmed not hurting herself. However, her neck pain is now causing increasing anxiety about additional (or possibly new) damage to her neck.

The MRI was overdue, because of her move from HealthSouth to Heartland. I have now obtained a CD of the MRI, and we are scheduled to see Dr. Shelton,

Chapter 22

ENT / swallowing specialist, on Monday, 3/28/11 to read the MRI of head / neck / lumbar.

My fear is that Barb may have herniated or bulging discs in her neck, not related to the car accident on Dec. 29 2010. The pain is interfering with her therapy and her sleep, as well as making her miserable.

Barb is asking to see an ophthalmologist because her left eye is not tracking properly. I am going to be making that appointment now that we have the current MRI.

(Two years later Barb told me that sitting out by the Nurses Station that day was the first time since her accident that she actually became aware of her surroundings. Not aware of her accident, she thought she was at a facility to see a patient, and so she tried to get up, not realizing the circumstances.)

I arrived at 4:00 PM at Heartland. Barb is again feeling miserable. The pain is so severe that she can't get comfortable, no matter what she tries or anyone else tries. *The pain is steadily increasing,* even with increased pain meds. It will be Monday afternoon before the MRI is read by the doctor, and we know how to proceed. I feel so badly for her.

6:52 PM — I was at Heartland from 12:30 - 4:30 PM. Barb seemed to be having a better day. She has been so miserable that it had to get better. I now have the name of a neurologist in Bradenton that is being recommended to us for Barb's consult, Dr. Frank Loh MD, whom I will call in the AM to make their first available appointment.

March 28, 2011 - Day 90 - 04:25 AM

We are cutting back on Nurse Corp now — simply a financial issue. Nurse Corp is charging $19 an hour, and this is our 3rd week 24/7 with them. The cost has been near $10,000. Her money is running low. New appointments are now set: Dr. Frank Loh MD - Neurology - April 5 at 2:30 PM., Dr. Eric Berman MD - Ophthalmology - April 19th at 2:00 PM

5:31 PM — **UPDATE:** — Good news and bad news. Barb, Andrea and I were at Dr. John Shelton's office at 3:15 PM. He is the ENT (throat and swallowing specialist). He reviewed the MRI from last Thursday. The mystery deepens.

There are no bulging or herniated discs in Barb's neck as far as they can tell. That is unexpected, but fantastic news. *So from where is all this pain coming?* No answer yet. Dr. Shelton is referring Barb to a Dr. Vincent who is a Throat Specialist in Tampa, for a second opinion. He did discuss some possible procedures that could be considered later. He will consult with the other specialist and together they will try to find what will come next.

March 29, 2011 — Day 91 — 06:23 PM—

UPDATE: Alan, Andrea and I attended a staffing meeting at Heartland with Barb. It was good to have her there to contribute to her own care. She says her pain was less today, which I was happy to hear. One day at a time, we are moving forward.

March 30, 2011 — Day 92 — 07:36 AM (Facebook)

Good Morning Barb.
Remember I am working today.
My phone will be on. What is your pain level this AM?

March 31, 2011 — Day 93 — 08:25 PM

Barb's pain seems to have lessened. We're not sure why. I have spoken to Dr. Simon's office and asked for a letter to state that HBOT may help to hasten her improvement and recovery. We need documentation to give permission for her to leave Hearland Rehabilitation. I talked to M.D. Stevens, who runs **The Mikey Center** in Lakewood Ranch. She can take Barb for 6 weeks between 5:00 and 7:00 PM Monday, Wednesday, Friday as soon as I get the letter, which Dr. Simon had agreed to furnish, clearing the way.

I have put together a whole 3-ring binder on HBOT, and it is amazing what is being discovered. We can start almost immediately. Going to HBOT treatments at 5 PM will prevent any interference with her current therapies at Heartland.

Her first HBOT treatment will be one hour to see how she tolerates it. After that, if everything seems right, she will be in the chamber between 90 and 120 minutes each time for 20 treatments. Then we will evaluate to see how she is doing.

I was there for three hours this afternoon and went to Physical Therapy. She is walking with someone balancing on each side of her, but *step-by-step she is making progress.*

> "Vulnerability
> is our most accurate
> measurement of Courage."
>
> Brene Brown

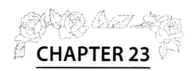

CHAPTER 23

A Gift More Precious than Gold

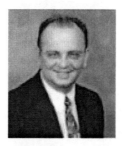

Dr. Craig Trigueiro, M.D.

> I choose to see God's world as full of miracles.
> It was that hope and faith, when I did not know if Barb would live or die, that kept me moving forward one-day-at-a-time.

Among the most surprising and unexpected miracles in our life was "Dr. T."

Dr. Craig A. Trigueiro M.D. had been Barb's employer from the time she graduated nursing school in April 1996, until April 2004, when she left his employ to go to Pinnacle Medical. He specialized in the field of Family Practice for 30+ years, and he had both a walk-in-clinic, as well as a by-appointment general practice.

His office was the perfect fertile ground for Barb's experience, being fresh out of school. He trained her to do all sorts of nursing skills: triage, drawing blood, running his lab, stocking supplies, inventory, filing, drug screens, breath alcohol testing, to merely carrying out doctor's orders. Eventually, she did the training of new employees and managed his back office.

Betty, who was to become his wife, was his office manager, and she and Barb became friends.

Dr. T saw patients of all ages and treated a wide range of ailments and conditions, usually acting as the first line of defense and contact. He then referring patients to a specialist, if necessary. This is also known as a Primary Care Provider (PCP).

Dr. T has a gift for taking a medical puzzle (a lot of seemingly unrelated issues or symptoms) and putting the pieces into some semblance of order, so they made sense. He knew his associates in the local medical community, and the top people in their specialties. Perhaps just as important, *he knew which ones to steer clear of.*

When Barb left his employ, it was on good terms, following eight years of employment. There was only so much he could teach her, and the offer of more money and better benefits eventually lured her to greener pastures. He simply was not in a position to provide what the competition was offering.

When I began to post day-to-day updates on Facebook the day following Barb's accident, Dr. T's wife, Betty, began reading my posts. She gave Dr. T updates on Barb's condition and any other news I had posted. Even though I was unaware of it, through his wife, he was keeping tabs on Barb's condition, progress, and recovery.

In March 2011, following her move to Heartland Rehabilitation in Sarasota, Betty posted a note to me, requesting that she and Dr. T come to visit Barb on Sunday, following their church services.

I placed Barb's newest MRI into her laptop so that Dr. T could take a look when they arrived at 2:00 PM. Barb was elated to see both of them. He took a look at her MRI, and then they visited a bit. It was as if no time at all had passed between them.

The staff came in and announced that we needed to retreat to the visitor's lounge for a bit while some things were done in Barb's room. So we walked down the hall and sat down at a table. I looked at Dr. T and smiled, *"Why haven't you been here before?"* I quietly asked.

He lowered his head, and with tears in his eyes he said, *"I couldn't see her like this. I just couldn't."* shaking his head.

Then he took a long, deep breath and said something I will never forget. *"What can I do to help?"*

They were six simple, uncomplicated words. It was only later that I reflected on that moment and the gift he had just handed me for my daughter. **I thank God every day for this man, and what he brought to us with those words. It was a gift of immeasurable value.**

"You could walk us through the maze of medical specialists that Barb is going to need," I pleaded.

From that day to December 2014, he was the guiding light to every aspect of Barb's medical care.

First he referred us to Dr. Berman, the Ophthalmologist, who spent two hours on Barb's first visit, evaluating her optic concerns, and determining the extent of her sight issues. Dr. Berman confirmed her diagnosis of 6th Nerve Palsy.

**His cherished affection and devotion to my daughter,
and her care has been the Shining Star
that has guided every aspect of her recovery.**

They were six simple uncomplicated words. It was only later that I reflected on that moment and the gift he had just handed my daughter.

What Is Sixth Nerve Palsy?

Sixth Nerve Palsy is a disorder affecting the sixth nerve, which supplies the lateral rectus muscle. This ocular muscle is responsible for turning the eyeball outward, away from the nose. When a person has Sixth nerve palsy, the eye begins to point inward toward the nose, often resulting in double vision. This condition is sometimes known as Abducens nerve palsy, or Cranial Nerve VI Palsy.

His second referral was to Dr. Frank Loh, MD, whom he told me was the most brilliant neurologist he had met in all his years of practice. There were a number of issues we needed to address. Dr. Lowe's first encounter with Barb was for the pain she was having in her neck and left shoulder. He was able to diagnose *Frozen Shoulder Syndrome*, and start appropriate treatment for that.

FROZEN SHOULDER SYNDROME

Frozen shoulder, also known as adhesive capsulitis, is a condition characterized by stiffness and pain in your shoulder joint. Signs and symptoms typically begin gradually, worsen over time and then resolve, usually within one to three years.

Your risk of developing frozen shoulder increases if you're recovering from a medical condition or procedure that prevents you from moving your arms — such as a stroke or a mastectomy.

Treatment for frozen shoulder involves range-of-motion exercises and, sometimes, corticosteroids and numbing medications injected into the joint capsule. In a small percentage of cases, arthroscopic surgery may be indicated to loosen the joint capsule so that it can move more freely. By Mayo Clinic Staff

Yankee 794 Trauma

For three weeks, Barb had been complaining of pain in her neck and left shoulder that measured an 8 or 9, which the pain medication would not touch. She was miserable, and I had been at a loss to know what to do for her. Fearing a disc had been ruptured in her neck, due to a recent fall, an MRI was performed and found to be negative for damage of any type. It was a relief, but if not a ruptured disc in her neck, what could be causing so much pain?

It turned out that her clavicle on her right side had been comminuted (shattered) during her auto accident, and there are vital blood vessels in that area. The physical therapist had probably been hesitant to exercise her arm. But by now, she was healing nicely. With some persuasion and a report from Dr. Loh, we got her on a regiment of exercise that relieved the intense pain she had been experiencing, and slowly she began to report less pain and overall improvement.

> "For everyone of us that succeeds,
> it's because there's somebody there
> to show you the way out. The *LIGHT*
> doesn't always necessarlily have
> to be in your family."
>
> Oprah Winfry

Yankee 794 Trauma

For three weeks, Barb had been complaining of pain in her neck and left shoulder that measured an 8 or 9, which the pain medication would not touch. She was miserable, and I had been at a loss to know what to do for her. Fearing a disc had been ruptured in her neck, due to a recent fall, an MRI was performed and found to be negative for damage of any type. It was a relief, but if not a ruptured disc in her neck, what could be causing so much pain?

It turned out that her clavicle on her right side had been comminuted (shattered) during her auto accident, and there are vital blood vessels in that area. The physical therapist had probably been hesitant to exercise her arm. But by now, she was healing nicely. With some persuasion and a report from Dr. Loh, we got her on a regiment of exercise that relieved the intense pain she had been experiencing, and slowly she began to report less pain and overall improvement.

> "For everyone of us that succeeds,
> it's because there's somebody there
> to show you the way out. The *LIGHT*
> doesn't always necessarlily have
> to be in your family."
>
> Oprah Winfry

CHAPTER 24

I Wrapped My Butterfly Wings Around My Injured Chrysalis

Barb is finally coming home.

For two weeks, beginning mid-April, I started fighting to keep Barb in rehab. It was a stalling tactic. Nearly every day the social worker, and rehab therapists, were writing reports to stall the insurance company from discharging her. For one more day, she would be getting the intense rehab that she desperately needed, and I felt she was entitled to under COBRA insurance.

I was not at all sure she was ready to come home, and I was even less sure that I was prepared to deal with whatever her coming home meant. I was still arranging to get our households consolidated to a new duplex when I was told by the social worker that she would be released "soon," although we had no date.

I hurriedly arranged to move from my apartment, and for her things to be moved out of the duplex she had occupied for 10 years. My daughter was a pack rat, and that proved to be a monumental undertaking. I had been packing and sorting her place for a while, knowing this was inevitable. The move was quite a feat. A church in town agreed to move both of us for "a donation."

Saturday the movers arrived at my apartment with a large truck at 9:00 AM. Four burly and polite guys had my apartment emptied and neatly arranged in the back of the truck, in little more than 90 minutes. We then drove over to Barb's place and loaded up. By 3:00 PM, they had unloaded all the boxes, and furniture into our new place. I stood watching their efficiency with amazement.

Sunday I remained home to start unpacking. I was up to my eyeballs in boxes when I returned to Heartland on Monday.

I was immediately hustled into the social worker's office with the news that Barb was being released Thursday. I took a deep breath. Facing a deadline I could no longer avoid, I went home that afternoon and did the only thing that made any sense. I organized the bedrooms, so we had somewhere peaceful to land and sleep, and I tried to organize the kitchen. The rest of what seemed like hundreds of boxes were piled three deep and high in the living room and third bedroom. I would get to them as time allowed.

I bought a new washer/dryer and a new freezer. They were delivered just prior to moving. There was no way I could think about going to the laundromat – and Barb's old W/D were shot. She was still wearing Depends, and the laundry/bedding was going to be huge for a while.

Peggy, Barb's case worker from The Florida Brain Injury Assoc. persuaded me that when we got home, we needed to call for the intake to Suncoast Center for Independent Living (SCIL) whose primary focus is resources for all types of traumatic brain injury (TBI). Almost immediately after Barb left rehab, I called them for an intake appointment.

May 5, 2011—Day 128 — COMING HOME

On the day she was released from Heartland Rehabilitation, we went straight to Dr. T's office. I had been handed a huge grocery bag filled with drugs. I carefully laid each of the drugs out on a table in his office. When he entered the room, and carefully examined all the medication she was on, he just shook his head.

"There must be $2000 worth of medication here!" he remarked.

He was not even close to accurate. It turned out, because of the cost of some of the medications she was being prescribed, I had the pharmacy calculate what each medication would have cost, *if we had not had insurance.* There was more like $4,500⁰⁰ worth of medication in that bag.

When we got home that evening, and I sifted through the many medications, and realized that I had no clue when or how to dispense these drugs, and *Barb's life depended on me being accurate!*

Befuddled by this prospect, I high-tailed it up to Walgreens Pharmacy on the corner. The pharmacist was not busy, to my amazement. I arrived overwhelmed and nearly in tears. I explained my dilemma.

"Not to worry," he reassured me smiling. *"Bring them in and leave them with me for an hour. I will figure out what and when, and write you a computerized med sheet. That way you will know what you need to give her, and what time to give it."*

I drove home and retrieved the bag of drugs, delivering them into his capable hands. One hour later we had the magic formula for which pill or liquid we needed to give her — and when. The drug sheet he prepared had a place for me to note when I gave the medication, very much like I had been accustomed to doing when I worked. I felt like he had saved the day — *and my sanity!*

In a nutshell, Dr. T's goal was to reduce slowly and methodically and then stop **all** of the meds. He sent her to see Dr. Loh again to be sure every single medication dosage was *reduced correctly.*

Over a period of the next 6 months, Dr. Loh gradually and systematically weaned her from all medications. From time-to-time, something would be tried and added.

Here is a list of the medications on May 5, 2011

Chlorhexidine 0.12%	(A mouthwash for keeping her from getting mouth ulcers)
Temazepam (Restoril) 15 mg	(for sleep) at HS (Nightly) 1 tab at bedtime (HS)
Lorazepam Intensol (Ativan) 2 mg./ml	every 6 hours for anxiety
Metoprolol Tartrate (Lopressor) 50 mg.	(forTachycardia/Hypertension) 1 tab twice daily
Exelon Patch 4.6 mg	(Memory) Apply 1 daily
Geodon 20 mg.	IM every 4-6 hours as needed (Agitation associated with dementia)
Amantadine 50 mg./5ml	(Dyskinesia prevention) 5ml twice daily
Ibuprofen (Motrin) 600mg.	Take 1 tab. Every 6 hours as needed for mild pain.
Donepezil (Aricept) 5 mg.	(for memory) Take 1 tablet by mouth every day
Parlodel 5 mg.	daily
Ultram 100 mg.	daily
Oxycodone 5 mg	1 tab. 3 x a day PRN as needed for moderate pain
Carisoprodol (Soma) 350 mg.	PRN Take 1 tab. 3x a day as needed for pain
Pantoprazole (Protonix) 40 mg.	Take 1 tablet by mouth daily GERD/Acid Reflux Prevention
Sertraline (Zoloft) 20 mg.	Take 7.5 ml. By mouth daily for Depression
Namenda 10 mg.	Take 1 tablet by mouth twice daily for Memory
Acidophilus Florastor Folate	(Folic Acid)

May 10, 2011 – Day 132

We arrived at Suncoast Center for Independent Living (SCIL) and were greeted and made welcome by clients and employees.

Tim, the Intake Coordinator, interviewed both of us, trying to determine what services would fit Barb's needs most accurately. Barb cried through much of the interview. Tim later admitted he felt baffled by her behavior, wondering if he had said or done something to upset her. It was the first time he had done an intake interview with a client with severe PBA (Pseudobulbar Affect). It was a perfect example of how the PBA affected her and those around her.

SCIL turned out to be a major player in Barb's recovery, offering support groups, classes, activities, evaluations, and help.

One of the services they offer free to clients is wheelchair ramps and various handicapped bars in their bathrooms, for example. Eventually, SCIL became a place she could feel at home and at ease.

In 2016, Barb still volunteers to this day there each Friday from 10:00 – 2:30 PM. This allows each of us a time for a breather each week. It also opened up avenues for new friendships, as (inevitably and unavoidably) many of the old friends, who had been so close watching her Facebook page, fell away and went on with their lives. She would hear from them infrequently, however as with life, for everyone the shift in Barb's life was *undeniably and permanently altered.*

Prior to Barb being released from rehab, a number of concerned friends had suggested we make an appointment to see **Dr. James McGovern, Ph.D.** He is a psychologist specializing in the brain and how it functions. It was he who could do the testing on her to determine long-term effects, if any, that Barb has suffered, directly the result of her near-fatal accident and T.B.I. Armed with her test results and personal interviews, he could determine the long-term prognosis for Barb's future and what we could reasonably expect.

One thing that was already apparent, slow as it seemed, Barb was making progress daily.

Our faith in God had taught us to have hope.

The first two years in recovery from TBI are the most startling and significant in terms of the amount of progress that is easily seen and readily apparent. However, we should expect progress for the rest of her life. People who suffer TBI will recover and improve for years after they are injured. People in Barb's TBI circle were telling us that *significant numbers of TBI patients report improvement for 20+ years.*

Chapter 24

Simply stated, the fact is that much of an individual's brain is "on vacation." When a significant part of the brain is injured and/or dies, parts of the brain that were not really being used are called to work. The brain begins to rewire itself slowly so that the previously "on vacation" part of the brain kicks in. The more rehabilitation the person has given, the faster the recovery.

Therapy teaches us that repetition is the key; *movements repeated over and over to "retrain the brain." so that it creates new neuro-pathways to become proficient at the skills that were lost. Over an extended period of time, another area of brain learns to master this lost skill.*

Conclusion: The earlier rehab is started, and the longer it lasts, the faster the brain will retrain itself.

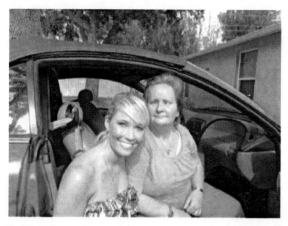

Barb's friend Natalie Briggs taking Barb to lunch on a visit.

Little Things — So Many Little Things – And Simple Solutions

MAY – JUNE 2011

So many "little things" began to come up after Barb came home.

"Little things" seemed to be a struggle.

"Little things" that didn't occur to me, because I was busy dealing with the big things.

She had not lived at my home for twenty years. There were many things about her personal habits I was simply unaware of – even though we would see each other often.

One example was *shampoo*. It should have been a simple thing – but because she could not talk to me it turned out not to be. It had been years since my orientation was to have a baby in the house. It never occurred to me that Barb kept getting shampoo in her eyes – and she could not tell me.

One day, while I was washing Barb's hair, I noticed she got shampoo in her eyes. She began to panic. I hadn't thought about it, but I should have.

There were many things in the beginning; she could not tell me. She only had one functioning (right) arm and hand. After that, I got Johnson & Johnson Baby Shampoo. That turned out to have a simple solution.

We found lowering shelves helped her reach things. The therapists told her about a battery-powered can opener that worked with one hand, along with a knife and utensils that were designed for use with one hand.

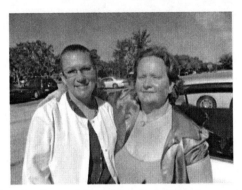

Shelley Anglin and Barb reunited after she came home.

Barb's most challenging feat to overcome was her left leg. She could see it. However, **she could not feel it!** She described her leg as a "phantom". When she tried to walk the physical therapist, Robert, had to put gait belts on her consistently and reassure her that if she lost her balance, he would be there to steady her. She could will her legs to go through the motions of walking, but **she could not comprehend her foot impacting the floor!** It frightened her, and *that* scared me. There were times when I stood back, fighting tears and knots in my stomach, biting my lip, willing her progress, silently watching her struggling to keep her balance. She would put one foot in front of the other, with the gentle encouragement of her physical therapist. She could will her legs to walk, but she couldn't will her leg to *feel* what the left side was doing! Just imagine walking when you can't feel it! It was inconceivable to me.

When her physical therapist suggested she try to walk outside, she panicked.

Chapter 24

In Barb, fear plus PBA (Pseudobulbar Affect) makes for an ugly cry. In the first couple of years, she did not really have "control" of her emotions.

We were out at the mall walking, and ran into a friend, Tammy, she had not seen since her accident. Barb began to sob uncontrollably. Tammy did not understand what she was seeing, and more than once asked, *"Did I say something wrong?"*

Once I had a grasp of what PBA was, and how it affected her, I realized that all I needed to say was, *"Nope. It's part of her brain injury. She is just happy to see you!"* Barb would stand there sobbing uncontrollably and shaking her head in agreement.

June 2011

The step up or down (even as elementary as one step) was frightening. Then the thought of trying to walk on uneven ground terrified her. It took some coaxing, and the promise that Robert would not let her fall, but slowly and gradually, she began to conquer her fear.

The left leg was "bone chilling" cold from the knee down. She frequently described it as feeling like it was sitting in a bucket of ice. Putting blankets on it did not relieve the problem. It is due to nerve damage, which is neuropathy that is centered in her brain. In other words part of her TBI. To this day, she has this issue. I suspect it is permanent.

For months, while she was having issues relearning to walk, I had not fully grasp the fact that she could not feel her left leg! *Learning to walk was far more complex than I could have imagined.*

Each day Barb and I would go out. We made many trips to The John Ringling Bridge in Sarasota, FL where it was safe for us to walk. This meant one mile over the bridge and one mile back to where we had parked the car. Because it was easier for her to walk uphill rather than downhill (because of gravity), we would take her GoGo Scooter, and she would walk as far as she could, uphill, while I followed on the scooter. When she got tired, we would shift "modes of transportation." I would then continue to walk to the bridge and back again. It was a good exercise for the both of us and the more she walked, the better her gait became.

Sometimes we would go out to Anna Maria Island and walk the sidewalks at the beach, as well as up and down the ramps and stairs, which give us a change of scenery. Occasionally, we would make a trip to the mall. It was not uncommon for me to be approached by strangers who would quietly ask me, *"Why did you stay?"*

To make things more complicated, she had **vertigo** (defined as a feeling of spinning) when she got to her feet every time she moved her head. Again, it was nearly a year, before she was able to voice this to me, and so I had not fully grasped the challenge she faced. I had been utterly clueless. Barb described it as *"an flawed perception of her surroundings."*

In truth, the room was spinning. She described it as feeling like she was in a centrifuge. As long as she held her head straight she was fine. The minute she turned her head, the whole place was spinning. Usually, when this happens, the eyes are darting back and forth – almost like the person is watching something move rapidly back and forth. This is occasionally one (of several) symptom the doctors look for to achieve a diagnosis.

HYPERACUSIS

Another thing that happened was that as she got into recovery, she became **hyper-sensitive to sounds of human voices**. I would be speaking in (what I thought was) a normal voice, and she would motion for me to turn down the volume. Sometimes she would put her fingers in her ears.

Hypersensitivity to many things, the rest of us pay no attention to, is common in people with TBI. Barb's friend, Jeff, is a victim of electrocution. His is a very different type of TBI. However, he also had this issue with hypersensitive to sound and perfume – things as subtle as baby powder made her breathing labored and noticably distressed.

Hyperacusis is a condition that arises from a problem in the way the brain's central auditory processing center perceives noise. It can often lead to pain and discomfort.

Individuals with hyperacusis have difficulty tolerating sounds which do not seem loud to others, such as the noise from running faucet water, riding in a car, walking on leaves, dishwasher, fan on the refrigerator, shuffling papers. Although all sounds may be perceived as too loud, high-frequency sounds may be particularly troublesome.

As one might suspect, the quality of life for individuals with hyperacusis can be significantly compromised. For those with a severe intolerance to sound, it is difficult and sometimes impossible to function in an everyday environment with all its ambient noise.

Hyperacusis can contribute to social isolation, phonophobia (fear of natural sounds), and depression.

Chapter 24

What is Neuropathy?

Neuropathy is a condition in which nerve damage has occurred in the peripheral nervous system often due to an underlying disease. Many people refer to this condition as peripheral neuropathy, and it usually results from infections, traumatic injuries, metabolic disorders, exposure to toxins, or, most commonly, diabetes.

The motor nerves and sensory nerves are often affected in a person who suffers from neuropathy. Symptoms of some types of neuropathy may mimic others, and treatments for neuropathy differ based on the cause.

What is Vestibular Disorder?

The vestibular system includes the parts of the inner ear and brain that process the sensory information involved with controlling balance and eye movements. If disease or injury damages these processing areas, vestibular disorders can result. Vestibular disorders can also result from or be worsened by genetic or environmental conditions, or occur for unknown reasons.

The first two years in recovery from TBI are the most startling and significant in terms of the amount of progress that is easily seen and readily apparent... Neuro-pathways become proficient at the skills that were lost. Over an extended period of time, another area of the brain learns to master this lost skill.

In Barb's case, the neurological cause of vertigo she was experiencing was considered a secondary issue, in lieu of other, more significant and medical findings. Consequently, it was overlooked for a time, in favor of more pressing issues. The problem with this was that it was interfering with her overall recovery until it was addressed.

CHAPTER 25

"Why Did I Stay?"

July 2011

Depending on your perspective, you may find it surprising that I asked that question, *"Why did you stay?"* frequently. It came from strangers when I would take Barb out in public to the mall. Anyone with half a brain could see how grievously she had been injured.

"Why did you stay?"

Four simple words that became a perplexing puzzle. I did not understand the question or what response I needed to give, in the beginning. To me, it was incredibly and fundamentally obvious. I was a nurse and caregiver by nature. It fit the mold of the motto my parents had raised me to believe, *"The only value you have is the value you have in serving others."*

> My gut response was resentful of the nature of question and suspicious of anyone who would ask such a thing.

> The very humanity of my staying came from my core values and beliefs and made it implausible for me consider otherwise.
> It was a haunting question, and one that was to fly in the face of "the right thing to do".

Yet it kept coming. It was a daunting question, and one that was to fly in the face of "the right thing to do".

I was her mom. Why wouldn't I stay?

For me, the only response was obvious. One time I recoiled by responding, "If you knew my daughter you could not possibly ask me that!"

The problem was the question kept coming. The question came from strangers, and I knew they were not gathering to target Barb or me.

When I sat down and began writing this book, it was never my intention to write an autobiography. Although, through the years, a number of people who knew my story, had remarked that I should write a book on my 3-year-search for my birth family, I blew the idea off. Who would care about my adoption or my search for my birth family, I wondered?

I had heard that many authors start a book for one reason and finish it for another; It was not until I began the mission of writing this book that I realized and understood *I needed to know why I stayed.*

Just being Barb's mom and a caregiver was not enough. I needed specifics — better and more plausible answers to why I stayed when others did not. That is how my second book *The Search for Judith Ann* (2016) came to be.

In the beginning, it was only my intention to write a chapter for this book. It turned out to be a prequel to this book and held the answers I needed. What began as a project to write one chapter in this book, ended up being another whole book! No one was more surprised than I was, when this development occurred.

I wrote most of the second book while writing the first book in ten months. I have been told that is remarkable. **Remarkable?** I never saw that at all. I was simply on a mission – and these books are the outcome of finishing what I started. I'd say it was simple — but I would be lying. It was a struggle — writing — but beyond everything it was probably the most rewarding thing I have ever done.

When we began to seek out the help of specialists in the private sector, Dr. T recommended Dr. David Tsai MD to guide her Physical Therapy and Speech Therapy, and Dr. Frank Loh MD (her neurologist). Both suggested Barb see Dr. James McGovern. PsyD. a neuro-psychologists. His specialty is in understanding the human brain and its function. Dr. McGovern does not prescribe medications.

I called Dr. McGovern's office to make an appointment in early May. It took 8 weeks for her to get in to get an appointment, because, between his private practice and his court-mediated practice, he is in high demand – because he is so expert and proficient, as well as, is highly regarded. We soon discovered this might have been an understatement.

We arrived at Dr. McGovern's office with some anticipation and a lot of apprehensions. He appeared in the waiting room at the appropriate time and greeted us with a welcoming smile and introduction. We were invited into the office, where he motioned me to bring Barb front-and-center in her wheelchair. I sit in a chair in "the peanut gallery" to the left of Barb. He then deliberately pulled up a chair directly in front of her and sat down.

He took a new and entirely different approach to addressing Barb's recovery. It was obvious immediately this was going to be a whole different type of interview. With most of the specialists, I had been interviewed, with Barb sitting as the audience. Then they would proceed to examine Barb and continue interviewing me.

I had become her mouthpiece.

Her speech was halting and difficult to understand, because of diminished lung capacity, and because her vocal chords had fused. (This was due to the trach being in for such an extended period.) Most of the time she just let me do the talking. I knew this frustrated her, but you have a limited amount of time with doctors, and I wanted us to get the most beneficial results of the time we had with her specialists. I was more able to understand what she was saying. Daylight was burning, and the professionals needed to get the greatest amount of information they could, in a limited time allowed for an appointment.

Her inability to express herself inhibited her communication with people. Instead, questions were directed to me as her legal guardian and mom. I was the person who had been there with her, every step of the way, through this journey. They felt I had the answers to their questions.

The way Dr. McGovern approached this situation was a departure from what we had been dealing with. I got the impression that I was not there in my capacity as Barb's Legal Guardian or her "mouthpiece", but mainly as her chauffeur.

I was there in case he asked her a question, and the answer was unclear, or he could not understand her. If that were to occur, I would assist his ability to map a strategy for how he fit into her on-going recovery as her Neuro-Psychologist.

Gently, in a non-aggressive, pleasant, determined, professional manner, he began to ask questions — and *she began to respond with appropriate answers.* That was to help him understand what she knew and didn't know, about her background, the past few month's events, and her recovery. Twice, during the hour, he looked over at me for confirmation of timeline of facts he would write down. Then he would ask more questions, and write down additional facts as she responded to his inquiries.

He managed to put both of us at ease. Never once did either Barb or I feel the least bit uncomfortable with this approach. At the end of the hour, he had gleaned a wealth of information, and masterfully developed a concise timeline of facts & figures about her accident, and what she knew. He asked to set her up for testing immediately. I explained to him that Barb's physical stamina was still severely lacking. He assured me that if she became too fatigued, the parts of the 4-hour test she did not complete could be scheduled for another day. Reluctantly, I left the office with the promise that I would be called when she showed signs of fatigue.

Chapter 25

It was the first time I had handed her over to anyone since she had gotten out of rehab. I remember feeling like I had the first day Barb went to Kindergarten.

I was to go home and come back.

I had wrapped my butterfly wings
around my injured chrysalis, protecting
her from anyone who would try to invade her space,
until she was (again) ready to spread her wings and fly.

To my amazement, Barb's tenacity took her through the entire test, and she finished early! To say I was astonished and relieved would have been an understatement.

Her first comment to me was, *"Mom! I like Dr. McGovern!"*

I smiled. I had liked Dr. McGovern's approach to my daughter as well. However, initially I was a bit surprised at her reaction. It was because *I had been paying attention to the wrong things.*

Barb finally explained to me that she kept wondering why "everyone" kept asking *me* all the questions when she was sitting right there. It annoyed her, but she remained silent, because, from the time she started becoming aware of her surroundings, she had followed their lead and done what she was told. In rehab no one asked for her opinion. They only *informed* her of what came next.

She said she didn't realize she had the right to say "No!"

Dr. McGovern's approach, which was for me to sit "in the peanut gallery", turned out to be *the right one* — different from all the other medical professionals.

"Mama! He talked to me! He asked me the questions! All this time, the doctors asked you, and I am sitting right here. I couldn't understand why, when I was in the room, they all talked to like I'm not there. They just didn't ask me – __but it is all about me!__"

I was preoccupied with advocating for her, and achieving excellent medical care. I was trying, perhaps too hard. I *was* her Legal Guardian. Because her return to consciousness was very gradual, I had lost sight of the fact that my daughter was now trying to advocate for herself! I felt terrible that she felt this way.

From that point on, I tried very hard to make everyone aware that if they had questions about what and how Barb was feeling, they needed to address these to her, rather than to me.

Barb helped me realize that although no one had intended to hurt or overlook her feelings or insult her intelligence, she felt slighted. *She stated that she had felt people were discounting her opinion in favor of mine!*

I was told that in two weeks, Dr. McGovern would have us return. By that time, the test results would be scored, and he would review and explain them.

In order to do an accurate examination Dr. McGovern's associate had to administer a series of twenty-two tests, lasting four hours, which included, but were not limited determining her levels of function in **nine (9) major areas**.

(1) Intelligential findings
(2) Global functioning
(3) Attention/ Information processing
(4) Sensory-motor function.
(5) Sensory-Perceptual functioning
(6) Spatial/Perceptual function
(7) Language function
(8) Executive function
(9) Memory function.

Two weeks later we returned to meet with Dr. McGovern for the results of all tests. He was the first doctor to explain

"The fact that Barbara has a skull fracture was a really good thing!"

I gave him a look of surprise — and then curiosity.

"Please explain that one to me." I inquired.

When he finished explaining, it all made sense.

The fact that Barb's brain was sloshing around (like Shaken Baby Syndrome) resulting in bruising, tearing of tissue and blood vessels, for a period which caused, among many issues, the Right Temporal Lobe bleed. *This action caused her to build up lots of energy inside her skull.*

The skull fracture occurring during her hitting her head, allowed that 'energy' to escape and her brain to swell — decreasing the amount of her TBI (traumatic brain injury) that resulted. This was significant to her recovery.

The fact that the right side of the brain controls the left side of the body and vice versa explained why Barb appears like a CVA (stroke) patient. Her left side was virtually useless — and the challenge was to relearn to use that side again.

The upside?

She was right-handed and working on her computer was a piece of cake.

Chapter 25

Her "coming back to us phase" remained painfully slow and tedious (even five years out she continues to make slow and steady progress). Barb was acutely aware of this and did not like talking to strangers when she did try to express herself. She would text.

Dr. McGovern's report read (in part): *"Ms. Scott is a 38-year-old, right-handed, single Caucasian female who is seen in neuropsychology evaluation at the behest of her physiatrist, Dr. David Tsai, for the purpose of determining whether she suffers from any cognitive and/or emotional sequelae secondary to a traumatic brain injury sustained during a motor vehicle accident in December 2010. She was reportedly rendered unconscious and was airlifted to Bayfront Hospital for a 15-day stay. She remained in a coma for 15 days. She estimates that posttraumatic amnesia lasted approximately 60 days and that retrograde amnesia covered two days. She suffered a basilar skull fracture, left-sided fracture and parietal bleed, and a right-sided countrecoup injury involving a temporal tear. Also involved was a subarachnoid hemorrhage.*

She is hemiparetic on her left and reportedly has sixth nerve palsy that continues to produce left–facial paresis. She also continues to experience diplopia, apparently due to CN VI damage, but she states that her visual fields are full. She denies anosmia (loss of smell). She was rehabilitated at HealthSouth for about a month, and she spent about another month in a facility named Heartland.

Post-concussive irritability (*) has reportedly improved. She was placed on Geodon, but she is currently weaned from this medication. She is being followed neurologically by Dr. Frank Loh. He wrote in his last note that post-concussive dizziness and fatigue have improved. He also reports that the results of a vocal cord assessment that reveal the next.

Ms. Scott also describes a post-traumatic sleep disturbance that is alleviated with medication. She denies all other mental health symptoms, but on one of our office registration forms, many concerns were endorsed having to do with issues related to self-esteem, loneliness, helplessness, and trepidation about what the future will bring...

Simple attention and working memory were found to be relatively spared, as was visual discrimination. Because she is contending with so many stressors, she had developed adjustment problems, characterized by depression and anxiety.

I will be recommending to her that this feature of her profile be addressed both psycho-pharmacologically and via psychological therapy aimed at helping her develop and enhance her adaptive capacities. It is to her great advantage that she had already been in contact with the Brain and Spinal Injury Program."

It was also Dr. McGovern that explained to me why I kept hearing the question, *"Why did you stay?"* from strangers.

To my surprise folks would come up to me when I would take Barb out in public to walk. I tried not to stay too close to her as if smothering her. I decided to stay just far enough back so that if she fell or had a major problem, I was there to address the issues as they immediately arose.

These were people who I did not know and did not know Barb. Yet I *repeatedly* experienced the same strange question "Why did you stay?"

Frankly, when I first heard the question, I was blindsided. I had no idea how to answer that question – and initially dismissed it. However, the question kept coming, and could not be ignored.

Finally, one day, I posed this issue to Dr. McGovern. *"Why did you stay?" "Can you please explain to me why I keep hearing this question?"* I ask him. *"I keep hearing it, and I don't understand why I keep being asked this."*

"Yes." he answered, *"I can explain it to you."*

"Specifically, in cases of auto accidents with TBI, the statistic is that 75% of them are young men between18 – 25. They come from dysfunctional families. These families were never really functional to start with, and the kids have been allowed to follow the example set by the adults in their world — taking (illegal) drugs and/or drinking and then driving. When these young men get a driver's license, they tend to follow the example.

When they end up in an auto accident, and are diagnosed with TBI, the family finds getting resources and services to be very challenging and overwhelming, as you have now discovered.

Those families say they plan to stick with the young men initially. After a time, the family becomes so overwhelmed by the obstacles they encounter that they throw up their hands — abandoned their family member to the system — and walking away."

I looked at him and protested, *"Barb and I don't fit in that category!"*

"No, you don't," he confirmed. *"But that is the answer to your question."*

I have thanked God every day for bringing Dr. McGovern into our lives, at a time when we needed to make sense of things. He was there to encourage and to unscramble and process a lot of vital information in a way that made sense.

He also helped us to come to terms with facts we were struggling to understand the mechanics of how Barbara's injuries would affect her.

༅

Dr. James McGovern was truly "A Gift from God."

༅

Dr. James M. McGovern's Profile

Dr. McGovern received his undergraduate degree from Northern Illinois University and his Masters' and Doctoral degrees from the Florida Institute of Technology. Dr. McGovern is a Licensed Clinical Psychologist, who is Board Certified in Clinical Neuropsychology by the American Board of Professional Psychology, the oldest and largest organization of its kind. As such, he has expertise in understanding how behavior and skills are related to brain structures and systems.

Practicing in Manatee County since 1988, much of his work has focused on evaluating and treating individuals with suspected or documented diseases and injuries of the brain. As such, he helps patients and their families maximize their abilities to adapt to the changes imposed upon them by neurologic and other medical conditions.

Dr. McGovern has a strong background in traumatic brain injury and stroke rehabilitation, and he served on the Board of Directors of the Florida Brain Injury Association from 1995 to 1998. He was also a Clinical Assistant Professor of Neurology at the School of Medicine at the University of South Florida from 1998 to 2001. He has hospital privileges at Blake Medical Center and Manatee Memorial Hospital.

Dr. McGovern has been qualified as an expert witness by the courts on many occasions. In both the state and federal courts, the cases he has consulted on have addressed many different issues including disability, decision-making capacity, guardianship, the ability to stand trial, and legal sanity.

> "The more you believe in your own ability to succeed the more likely it is that you will."
> Shawn Acher

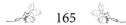

CHAPTER 26

Happy 39ᵗʰ Birthday Bash!

We decided since so many people had been keeping up with our FB page since Barb's accident, it was time for a celebration of life. What better day that to celebrate on her birthday, July 27ᵗʰ?

Sonny, a friend, of ours, managed a bar and grill in a central location, and so he offered to have her birthday celebration there. We made the big announcement on Facebook, and that night 50 friends showed up. Many were people who had not seen her since her accident. Everyone ordered their own food, and we served Tarimusu for dessert. I bought her a new computer.

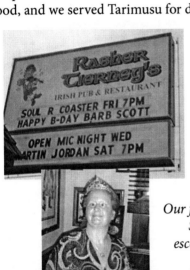

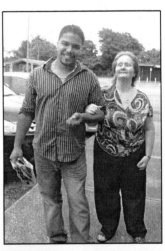

Our friend Sonny escorting Barb

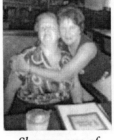

Sharon, one of Barb's CNA's at Heartland

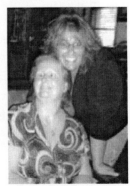

Andrea with Barb

Brandi

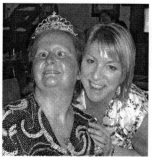

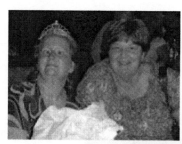

Barb with Katy

Barb with Paige

Barb with Heather and Joe

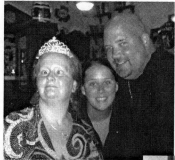

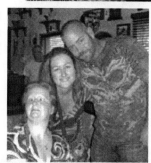

Barb with Tammy and Kaitlyn

Barb with Dawn and Todd

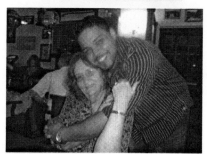

Shelley, Barb, Melanie

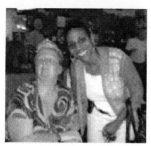

Sonny with me at Barb's 39th birthday party. Sonny and Mark on 4 months apart. I call him "My son by another mother."

Dr. Mowett

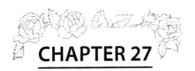

CHAPTER 27

If God Brought Us This Far

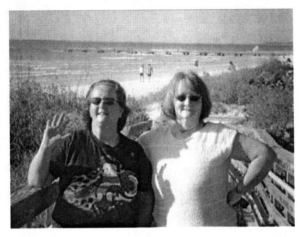

Barb and me out at Anna Maria Island for a walk.

September 2011

With the assistance of Dr. Loh and Dr. T, Barb had gradually been weaned off all her medications. We felt that this was a significant step forward.

One day while on a visit to his office, I mentioned to Dr. T my uneasiness with how I viewed other people's reactions to Barb's emotional outbursts (PBA). She was aware and uncomfortable with what she was experiencing, and I could not help her.

He addressed my concerns by again mentioning a new medication called Neudexta. He said we had no way of predicting if it would assist the uncontrollable outbursts of laughing and crying (PBA).

He warned us that it might also be cost-prohibitive. I suggested he give me the prescription and let me present it to the pharmacy. We would see what her insurance had to say about cost.

To our relief, it only cost $35 a month, with the insurance. Without insurance, the cost would have been $600! She began to take this daily.

I had been told, that along the journey through Barb's recovery, ten (10) months after TBI is often a significant time for "awakenings," following a TBI injury.

Chapter 27

I don't think that any of us will ever know if it was the medication that woke up her brain, or if it was just time for her brain to start functioning at "a different level." All I know is that a month after she began taking Nudexta, she began to realize and understand, on a much deeper level, what had happened to her.

October 2011

One day mid-October, when I entered her room I noticed Barb seemed more pessimistic than she ordinarily was. She was now faced with repressive limitations that prior to her accident, would have been unimaginable. In this minute, I wanted to wilt. I sat down next to her. She looked up at me and made a statement I will never forget,

"Mama, no one should have to live like this. Why don't you just put me in a nursing home?"

She began to cry. I looked at her and took a deep breath.

"Barbara, this is temporary. It isn't going to last forever. Besides, we don't have the money to put you in a nursing home. So I guess you are just going to do the best you can, and keep moving forward. You will see. It is going to get better! God didn't keep you alive, to have you give up! There is something He wants you to do. We have to find out what that is."

> I wondered what her future held but we just kept moving forward one day at a time.
> Realistically that is all we could do.
> I am a perputal optimist, and Life goes on.
> That is the message, isn't it?

> Optimism is like a muscle.
> The more you use it, the stronger it becomes.

We had climbed so many mountains since her accident, and met challenges that other people could not imagine. There was no way we were giving up now. There was not one doubt in my mind that in time she would put this behind her, as well, with the determination and tenacity I knew she possessed.

Both my daughter, in her recovery, and me along for the ride, had understood, that God had plans, yet unfilled.

I would take her out to walk. It was obvious to anyone (who was not blind) how horrible her injuries were – and how far she was going to have to go if she hoped to have any resemblance to a meaningful life. People, whom I had never met, and who I knew did not know each other, continued to approach me and simply and quietly asked me, "Why did you stay?"

Steve Harvey once said to Oprah Winfrey in a TV interview:

"The two most important days in your life are,
the day you are born,
and the day you find out why you were born."

I have a friend who had attended The United States Air Force Academy. He had been a Red Beret in the medical corps three tours in Vietnam. He told me that one of his professors had given the class an assignment to wrote a paper for half the semester grade. The subject: Define Death and explain what it is.

The students had two weeks to prepare a paper. When it came time to hand in his paper, my friend observed his classmates handing in pages and pages of work in a futile attempt to define Death.

He handed in 1 page.

When the papers were handed back, he got an "A".

The page had one word on it — INEVITABLE.

Comparing our situation?

The alternative was— UNTHINKABLE.

> Yes, there were times when
> I got angry with God.
> It's okay to get angry – He can take it.
> Eventually I got over my anger.
> After a time, I found that
> I processed things differently.
> I was in for the long haul –
> whatever that took.

After all –

*The alternative had been **unthinkable**.*

Chapter 27

&

We Thought We Were Alone
By Debbie Wilson

We thought we were alone.
We did not know how to contact a fellow survivor on the phone.

We noticed many family and friends seemed to care no longer.
We saw from the very beginning this brain injury wasn't fair.

We have since learned we are not alone.
We have heard many others also lose, moan and groan.
We are learning to be thankful we don't each have a headstone.

We are learning how to go forward with our brain repair.
We are working hard not to give in to frustration or despair.

We were all thrown into a very scary world of the unknown.
We all felt like we were hit by a very destructive cyclone.

We realize we don't have to live alone in solitaire.
We realize there are survivors everywhere.

We only thought we were alone

&

Dec. 31, 2011 (FB post) One year ago I spent New Year's Eve and New Year's Day at Bayfront Medical Center in ICU-Neuro with my daughter, Barb, who was in a near-fatal auto accident 12-29-10. I don't really remember being aware it was New Years. The only good thing was that my son, Mark, came home from Iraq for two weeks immediately following. Barb has no memory of the first 60 days after her accident. We are now on the way to recovery. She and I live together now, and she is being encouraged by all the great therapy and recovery. We are quietly home tonight enjoying TV, cheesecake and eggnog.

Happy 2012 to Everyone!!

𝒬

The Farmer & The Donkey

One day a farmer's donkey fell down into a well. The animal cried piteously for hours as the farmer tried to figure out what to do. Finally, he decided the animal was old, and the well needed to be covered up anyway; it just wasn't worth it to retrieve the donkey.

He invited all his neighbors to come over and help him. They all grabbed a shovel and began to shovel dirt into the well. At first, the donkey realized what was happening and cried horribly. Then, to everyone's amazement he quieted down.

A few shovel loads later, the farmer finally looked down the well. He was astonished at what he saw. With each shovel of dirt that hit his back, the donkey was doing something amazing. He would shake it off and take a step up.

As the farmer's neighbors continued to shovel dirt on top of the animal, he would shake it off and take a step up. Pretty soon, everyone was amazed as the donkey stepped up over the edge of the well and happily trotted off!

MORAL:

Life is going to shovel dirt on you, all kinds of dirt. The trick to getting out of the well is to shake it off and take a step up.
Each of our troubles is a stepping stone. We can get out of the deepest wells just by not stopping, never giving up!

Shake it off and take a step up.

BARB DID!!! YOU CAN TOO!!!

𝒬

Chapter 27

ঽ

<u>Five Simple Rules For Happiness:</u>

1. Free your heart from hatred –
Forgive.

2. Free your mind from worries
Most never happens.

3. Live simply and appreciate what you have.

4. Give more.

5. Expect less from people — but more from yourself.

You have two choices...
smile and close this page,
or pass this along to someone else to share the lesson.

ঽ

ℒ

<u>To my daughter Barb</u>

December 29, 2010,
was a date that altered everything for both of us.

Look how far you have come back from "The Brink"!
There is not one mother alive on Earth
prouder than you make me.
I am so proud of you!

The prognosis for your recovery was
initially catastrophic and now look at you!

When you are depressed,
because you can't accomplish something immediately
that used to be so easy,
just think what the alternative could have been.

Remember:
Life is a Gift from God.
Always seek out His purpose for you.
Cherish Life
Embrace Life.
Sit in the wonder of Life.

Love you "Snicklefritz",
Mom

ℒ

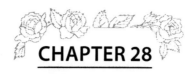

CHAPTER 28

Double Vision

January 2012

When my daughter, Barb, was nearly killed, the obstacles we had to overcome seemed insurmountable. It took all the strength I could muster to spend those hours, days, weeks and months, guiding her medical care and watching someone I loved so much learning to do all the same things, she had learned as an infant. She had to relearn the most rudimentary skills – swallowing, talking, walking – and eventually processing what had happened to her. These came with big challenges, and we met them one-by-one, as they resulted in "the ugly cry" for Barb. Her eyes were crossed due to "6th Nerve Paralysis," causing her brain to process differently than before. She was literally "seeing double" in the beginning. It was difficult for her to know which image was real and which was not. We used to joke that one was the good twin, and the other was the evil twin. Evidentially she learned to ignore the second ghost-like image.

For someone with Traumatic Brain Injury (TBI), this has to be frightening. I am sure she felt *she could not trust what she was seeing.* She did not feel safe for many reasons. She was ***finally*** able to express that *she saw two images.* There was the one that was clear, and then there was the one that looked like a ghost. She knew it was not real.

The ophthalmologist hinted this might be correctable – either naturally over time or with surgery. The double vision created a problem with her perception shortly after she came home. When she tried to guide her Go-Go battery-powered scooter, park benches and other objects seemed to jump out in front of her! Although her brain told her this was not real, her vision was also told her that they were real and not an illusion! She was overwhelmed with confusion. At first she would get upset and cry because her PBA ran rampant. Then we stepped back and calmed down. She had to think how to deal with what she was seeing, yet knew was not real.

Sixth Nerve Palsy

From Wikipedia, the free encyclopedia

Sixth nerve palsy, or abducens nerve palsy, is a disorder associated with dysfunction of cranial nerve VI (the abducens nerve), which is responsible for contracting the lateral rectus muscle to abduct (i.e., turn out) the eye. The inability of an eye to turning outward results in a convergent strabismus or esotropia of which the primary symptom is double vision or diplopia in which the two images appear side-by-side. The condition is commonly unilateral but can also occur bilaterally. The unilateral abducens nerve palsy is the most common of the isolated ocular motor nerve palsies.

Characteristics

Limitation of the abduction of the right eye. This individual tries to look to his right, but the right eye fails to turn to the side. The patient sometimes adopts a face turn towards the side of the affected eye, moving the eye away from the field of action of the affected lateral rectus muscle, with the aim of controlling diplopia and maintaining binocular vision.

While this is a positive adaptation in the short term, in the long term it can lead to a lack of appropriate development of the visual cortex giving rise to a permanent visual loss in the suppressed eye; a condition known as amblyopia.

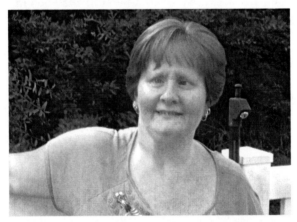

This photo was taken May 2011, shortly have Barb came home from rehab. Notice how her right eye does not line up with her left eye.

For two years and with every visit, the ophthalmologist held hope that, at some point, this might be surgically corrected. However, he explained that she had to get to a particular stage in her recovery before that would be possible. Then, following her two-year examination, we were told he felt it was not progressing to the point they had hoped. *Surgical intervention was not recommended.*

Initially, it was disappointing. However, like everything else, the upside to this whole potentially sad outcome, was that *the brain is amazingly adaptable.*

Her brain had retrained itself resulting in blocking the second image out. Unless someone talked about it in conversation, Barb forgot it was there! She had no problem focusing on TV or anything else. *We felt that was a miracle!*

Her most grievous and long-lasting brain injury is a ***Right Temporal Lobe bleed***.

The temporal lobes of your brain control the opposite side of your body and how it functions. In other words, Barb's right temporal lobe of her brain controlled the left side of her body and vice versa.

For a year, while she was having issues relearning to walk, I had not fully grasped that *she could not feel her left leg!* Learning to walk was far more complex than I could have imagined. The effect was very much like someone who had a CVA (stroke). At first, her left side was useless. Even though she went through the motions of walking her left side was unable to function, and there was no guarantee she would ever fully regain use of it.

The upside was that she was right handed, and so she was able to access and use her computer. I shudder to think what we would have faced, if it was her left temporal lobe that had been injured, affecting her right side.

Temporal Lobes

"Kolb & Wishaw (1990) have identified eight principle symptoms of temporal lobe damage:

1) disturbance of auditory sensation and perception,

2) disturbance of selective attention of auditory and visual input, 3) disorders of visual perception,

4) impaired organization and categorization of verbal material,

5) disturbance of language comprehension,

6) impaired long-term memory,

7) altered personality and affective behavior,

8) altered sexual behavior."

Selective attention to visual or auditory input is common with damage to the temporal lobes (Milner, 1968). Left side lesions result in decreased recall of verbal and visual content, including speech perception. Right side lesions result in decreased recognition of tonal sequences and many musical abilities. Right side lesions can also affect recognition of visual content (e.g. recall of faces).

The temporal lobes are involved in the primary organization of sensory input (Read, 1981). Individuals with temporal lobe lesions have difficulty placing words or pictures into categories.

Language can be affected by temporal lobe damage. Left temporal lesions disturb recognition of words. Right temporal damage can cause a loss of inhibition of talking. The temporal lobes are highly associated with *memory skills*. Left temporal lesions result in impaired memory for verbal material. Right side lesions lead to the recall of non-verbal material, such as music and drawings.

Seizures of the temporal lobe can have dramatic effects on an individual's personality. Temporal lobe epilepsy can cause preservative *speech, paranoia, and aggressive rages.*

Barb did not have her first (and only) seizure until January 2013 a full twenty-five months after she was injured. This took me totally off guard and was very frightening. It came out of the blue. As odd as it sounds to me looking back, I am not one to borrow trouble, and prior to this happening, not one doctor had mentioned to me that Barb might have a seizure disorder! It had not once occurred to me this might happen!

Additionally, in Barb's case, the neurological cause of *vertigo* she was experiencing was considered a secondary issue, in lieu of other, more significant medical findings. Consequently, it was overlooked for a time in favor of more pressing issues. The problem with this was that it was interfering with her overall recovery. Finally in Feb. 2012, when she enrolled in Blake Medical Center's Outpatient Rehabilitation, she started to have vertigo issues while in therapy. The director had been trained in *The Epley Maneuver.*

What is Epley Maneuver?

The impact threw the crystals out of place in her inner ear – and the had not been able to resettle where they belonged, throwing her off balance.

This treatment is used for a particular type of vertigo, called *benign paroxysmal positional vertigo* (BPPV) infection, which is caused by tiny calcium crystals dislodging in the inner ear and brushing against nerves that control balance. When that happens, the wrong signals are sent to the brain, causing disorientation and dizziness.

VERTIGO

Barb was a "fall risk". She would lose her balance and just fall down. My first concern and question was always *"Did you hit your head?"*

She would lay on the floor, and her PBA would kick into overdrive. She would dissolve into tears, shaking all over and filled with rage at her lack of control when her PBA would kick in. She could not get herself up.

Chapter 28

In the early stages of her recovery, when she would fall and I would have to get a helping hand in order to get her to her feet. It wouldn't work. Her coordination was off. Then she went through a phase where she would become so enraged that she could not be helped.

By the time I would hear her from the other room, and get there, she would be trying all sorts of contortions to get up, most of which were ineffective. She would usually end up on her back like a turtle. She could not right herself – and the frustration and anger overwhelmed her. All that did was remind her that she was helpless, which although a reality – was the last thing Barb wanted to be reminded of. I would talk to her to get her to calm down. I would then remind her of what she had to do in order to help us help her to get up into a chair.

Finally, in February 2012, having been faced with this dilemma countless times, I brought this to the attention of the physical therapist. I explained to them, ***"Your first priority needs to be to teach her how to get off the floor without help! If she falls, and I am not there, she can't get herself up! She gets so frustrated that she can't think what she needs to do, to get herself back into an upright position. HELP!"***

The physical therapist made it a priority to teach her how to get off the floor when she fell. Once she was able to master the steps, she was much better able to cope with any fall, physically and mentally, *achieving a greater sense of independence.* Now, when she occasionally falls, like when she leans into a closet too far and loses her balance, she gathers her wits and asks for a chair. Once she realizes she is not injured, she works to get herself to her feet. It takes some effort, and she huffs and puffs, but she *has mastered the task.*

What had Causes BPPV?

The most common cause of BPPV in people under age 50 is a head injury. The head injury need not be that direct — even whiplash injuries have a substantial incidence of BPPV (Dispenza et al, 2011).

Over a year after her accident it was made clear to us this was partially due to the fact that her head had repeatedly and violently impacted the driver's sides window and steering wheel in her car, causing major injuries to her face and chest, as they took the brunt of the collision. The same impact *threw the crystals out of place in her inner ear – and they had not been able to resettle where they belonged, throwing her balance way off.*

For months after she left rehab, we were unaware that *the cause of her balancing issues* were in our journey through recovery. A number of therapists had hinted at a procedure that only a few therapists were trained to do, **which** *"might" help her*. It was glossed over, and I really didn't understand what they were referring to.

Many therapists have a vague knowledge of **The Epley Maneuver**. Others seem to have more than a vague knowledge of it, however, later it was explained to us that home therapists are not eager to employ it even if they may have been trained in **The Epley Maneuver.** Why? Their reluctance was understandable due to the fact that a significant number of patients throw up on them during or after the procedure. Therapists who visit several patient's homes each day are not anxious to carry extra clothing with them, and it tends to leave *"a bad taste in their mouth"* (pun intended).

The therapist who finally agreed to help Barb by performing **The Epley Maneuver** was head of her department, and had access to a shower and kept extra clothing at work. She knew she would have this request recurring by other therapists employed in her department. She was able to deal cheerfully with it.

Barb had the procedure performed on her three times as part of her therapy on a weekly basis *without nausea* with each procedure. Each time she was instructed to go home and lay very still on her back through the night. *Each time she experienced noticeable improvement.* By the third time it was performed, her balancing issues were significantly better.

Unfortunately, this was not her only balancing issue.

> "We all want to Dare Greatly.
> If you give us a glimpse into
> that possibility we'll hold on
> to it as our vision.
> It can't be taken away."
>
> Brene Brown

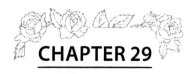

What Did He Say?

February 2012

I was sitting on my bed, the second Sunday in February and I happened to run my hand across my neck on the left side, just above my Clavicle. I stopped! *There was a lump the size of a walnut. That had not been there before.* It was **not** painful or tender, but it definitely was there. *What was it? What could it mean?*

By now, Dr. T was also my primary care provider. I decided just to be safe I wanted to have Dr. T to tell me *it was nothing.*

I had to take Barb for an appointment, so I decided to consult with him. Better safe than sorry, I concluded. As we were finishing up her appointment, he turned to me and said, ***"Okay, what brings you in today?"***

"Well," I remarked, almost in a whimsical way, "I seem to have a small child growing here on my neck. It is probably nothing, but *I want you to be the one who tells me it's nothing."*

His expression changed as he examined the mass on my neck. "Huuuhhh... I am sending you for a CT scan. Let's just be safe. Let's see how that comes back."

His office made the appointment, and I followed through in a few days. Shortly his office called, "Dr. T wants you to go for a biopsy on your neck. We made an appt."

Again, I followed what I was asked to do. I had to go to the hospital and lay very still on the table as the radiologist took five biopsies. I counted them. I told myself she was being careful in ruling out everything. *This biopsy will come back, and we will know, for sure, it is nothing.*

On March 21, 2012, the day after my 65 birthday, I kept the appointment to find out the results of the biopsy. I was still convinced that he was going to give me a clean bill of health. He examined me carefully. The mass had grown from 3.4 cm to 6+ cm. He looked concerned. That is when he laid the news on me.

"Betty, you have Squamous Cell Carcinoma. It is a form of skin cancer, but in your case it is internal. It is classified as a Head and Neck Cancer. Fortunately, it is cancer we know the second most about. This thing seems to be very aggressive. We need to get you over to see the oncologist as soon as possible. I am referring you to Dr. Robert Whorf. You will like Dr. Whorf, and he will tell you what needs to be done next."

I sat there, trying to absorb what he had just told me. I looked at Barb. *Did I hear him correctly? Did he just say I have — **CANCER?***

I had been in denial. I had talked myself into believing he was going to tell me it was nothing.

What happened??? I went numb.

I was sent to see Dr. Bruce Dorman MD, an ENT (ear, nose and throat specialist) for the extensive throat and head biopsies. These had to be done in the hospital under general atheistic. *The objective* was to pinpoint where this cancer had begun. He sent me to the hospital as a day patient. That was the first time that my veins were not readily found. Just before the procedure my IV infiltrated. I ended up having an IV put in my foot, *which I do not recommend.*

Dr. Dorman determined that his findings and the biopsies were *inconclusive.* Wherever cancer had begun, my body had destroyed the initial site. The mass in my neck was from a few random cells that had traveled to the lymph node and attached themselves and began to grow. This did not make it any less deadly!

I had been religiously taking 12 vitamin and food supplements everyday for 5 years. No one admits that was what made the difference. However it is my biased opinion that my immune system was built up so well, my body destroyed the initial cancer site. Dr. Whorf would only say,

"Anything is possible. We just don't know."

> "No one can give us power. If we aren't part of the process of taking it, we won't be strong enough to use it."
>
> Gloria Steinem

CHAPTER 30

Alarming Aggression

❧

"You gain strength, courage, and confidence
by every experience in which you really stop
to look fear in the face...
You must do the thing which
you think you cannot do."
Eleanor Roosevelt
(1884 - 1962)

❧

March 21, 2012

While I was in the diagnostic stage, the cancer was so aggressive that it became visible to onlookers, as it grew from an estimated 3.4 cm (the size of a walnut) to over 6 cm. (I would place my hand on top of the mass, and the entire palm of my hand was needed to cover it.) This *should* have been frightening – however **I had been in denial.**

There were concerned and opinionated people in my life, who voiced that it needed to be surgically removed ASAP. What they clearly understood was that when something like a mass, is threatening your life, you cut it out of your body. I understood this. I had had my share of surgery, and I was not frightened by the prospect of more surgery — if *there was a good reason.*

"Fear is an emotion indispensable for survival."
Hannah Arendt (1906 - 1975)

The location of it raised concerns. It was in a place where it was likely to invade my jaw and my lower throat and tongue, the inside of my mouth.

As the cancerous mass grew, so did my imagination. The chances were that it would spread to my mouth —perhaps my face and brain.

The ramblings of my mind were impassioned, vehement, profuse, and pandemic.

It could invade my Jugular Vein, a major blood vessel in my neck, and I would bleed to death. All in all, this was not a promising prospect. The other possibility was that it would enlarge, blocking my airway, and I would suffocate. Either way I was dead in ways I found atrocious, ominous and inconceivable.

In my years of nursing, I had seen the results of radical head and neck surgery, and the images of the resulting disfigurement. The visual images were daunting and (frankly) horrifying. I had asked myself if *this might not be a fate worse than death.*

The aggressiveness it had already demonstrated meant that this was likely to happen within weeks or months at the most. It was unlikely I would survive to see Christmas 2012 *if it went untreated.*

♌

Philippians 4:6 (ASV)
"In nothing be anxious; but in everything by prayer and supplication with thanksgiving let your requests be made known unto God."

♌

I had to speak Faith into my future.

We can never make it to what God has for us in our lives, until there are "weeds" in our way.

When "weeds" came up in my garden, I knew that Almighty God was testing me to see if I would stay the course and keep The Faith.

I don't think God ever tells us *no.* He gives us options. *Yes,* but not right away, or I have something better in mind. We just have to be patient. Disappointments are just God's way of saying, "I have something better in mind."

Society is filled with a message of instant gratification. We live in "a social media world" where television, radio, and the internet bombard us with messages that translate to "get it now" or "buy it now". **God does not like shortcuts.** He wants us to experience "the process" by demonstrating we believe in Him and trust that when we are prepared and the time is right if it is His Will it will be ours – along with The Kingdom of Heaven.

Be patient.
Live life.
Have faith.
When the time is right
He will reveal himself to you.

Some people would say, "you have to talk the talk and walk the walk."

Chapter 30

𝒬

The Lord's Prayer
King James Version (KJV)

⁹ Our Father, which art in heaven, Hallowed be thy name.

¹⁰ Thy kingdom come, Thy will be done in earth, as it is in heaven.

¹¹ Give us this day our daily bread.

¹² And forgive us our debts, as we forgive our debtors.

¹³ And lead us not into temptation, but deliver us from evil: For thine is the kingdom, and the power, and the glory, forever. Amen.

Matthew 6:9-13

𝒬

Barb's "weeds" had been the greatest challenge I had ever faced, Greater in measure than the death of my 30-year-old husband, David, in 1978. At least that was the conclusion I had foolishly drawn.

What I do know was that God knows who belongs in your life and who doesn't. Trust and let go. Whoever is meant to be there will still be there.

My Faith was again being tested. This is what Faith is about. I had the Faith to believe God would stand with me, and when He is with me, who can be against me?

𝒬

"Coincidence is God's way of remaining anonymous."

Albert Einstein (1879 – 1955)

𝒬

"What shall we then say to these things?
If God is for us, who can be against us?"

Romans 8:31 (KJV)

𝒬

CHAPTER 31

Legal Guardianship Reversed: Applying The Golden Rule

As I pursued knowing more about my diagnosis, I realized that one thing had to be taken care of without delay. My daughter had been confirmed through Dr. James McGovern Ph.D. to be *"cognitively intact."* I had known it, but it was nice to have her tested in July 2011, and again May 2012 and have the tests to confirm what I already knew. (She was to be tested in May 2012, by Dr. McGovern because of a request from Vocational Rehab. and her tests when compared to the first set in July 2011, were scored as higher/improved.)

Barb could now do the tasks my legal guardianship was directed to do for her — manage her finances and make other legal decisions. **She no longer needed a legal guardian**. She only needed a chauffeur.

I called Neil Scott, Esq. and informed him of my diagnosis. He expressed his sincerest sympathy and concern. I explained that I didn't know how this diagnosis was going to play out. The fact was simply that **I could be dead in a matter of months**.

Facing my mortality was a sobering experience.

Legal issues take the time to make their way through the court system, and I didn't know how much time I had. Mr. Scott needed to get a petition filed with the court to *reverse* my legal guardianship, so that in the event of my death, Barb could again, manage her own affairs. There were reasons this could not fall to her siblings.

Mr. Scott took the matter under advisement and informed me of what procedures had to be put into place, to accomplish what we needed. We agreed, and he went to work to achieve this.

I explained to Barb about my intentions, as I had with every choice I had made since she could understand. She was included every step of the way, just as I had done with her from the earliest time she was beginning to understand what had happened to her, after her accident. She felt comfortable with my decision, as it affected her. Always reverberating in the back of my mind was The Golden Rule. *"Do unto others as you would have them do unto you."*

Chapter 31

❧

**Matthew 7:12 (KJV) the Gospel of Matthew in the
New Testament and is part of the Sermon on the Mount.**

**This well-known verse presents what has become
known as The Golden Rule.**

*"Therefore all things whatsoever ye would that men should do to you,
do ye even so to them: for this are the law and the prophets."*

❧

The road to success is always under construction throughout our lives. I clearly knew that my life was now literally on the line and time was ticking.

All my instincts told me to stay the course and trust that God would be there, holding my hand, as I walked through this. I never for one moment lacked the Faith to know that I had to listen to my Instincts. I had to do what I was being directed to do. I knew His path is filled with righteousness, and He can work miracles. I also knew that just like we had needed a miracle to bring Barb back from the brink of death, now I had to call on all my internal strength and my Heavenly Father to keep me from the edge as well.

Bishop J.D Jakes in his 2014 book <u>INSTINCTS: The Power to Unleash Your Inborn Drive</u> states: *"It is a sad thing to live your life without a deep-rooted sense of connection to your purpose. Like a light bulb without a lamp, this kind of disconnect fosters dark and foreboding feelings in the soul.....what matters is that you have been awakened to your purpose and enlightened to the inner fulfillment that it affords."*

Eons ago I remembered discovering that weighing and measuring facts and circumstances can serve me well. I used to tell people who were questioning the decision they should make, *"Ask yourself. Will "it" really matter in 5 years?"* Analyze – and more often than not, the answer is *"not really"*. However, when the answer is a resounding *"YES!"* then you need to understand this decision matters – for the long haul.

❧

**"God does not ask your ability or your inability.
He asked only your availability."**

**Mary Kay Ash
(1918 to 2001)**

❧

I immediately recognized that the choices I had made in Barb's health care _mattered_. Now, I realized that the choices I was making in committing to my healthcare _mattered_! I needed to understand, and without delay. I needed CANCER 101: Treatment and Effect (and Side-effects). The long-term outcome was an unknown, of course.

I dug into the internet, trying to find anything and everything related to **_Squamous Cell Carcinoma_**. I was trusting God. However, I was ignorant of what this was. This was not an area I had worked in nursing, and it was a wake-up call to a whole other level for me.

Squamous Cell Carcinoma is a type of skin cancer.

In my case, it was internal.

I wanted to understand in-depth who this enemy was. To no one's surprise, all I did was get confused when I researched the internet. I tried and tried, to seek out the answers with no success.

❧

It is hard to find the answer, when you don't know the questions.

❧

Finally, confused and frustrated, I told Dr. Whorf what I was doing.

"Stop doing that!" he smiled. "Trust me! Squamous Cell Carcinoma is the one we know the second most about. You are going to be fine. The ENT did biopsies on your Head and Neck. We found nothing that told us where this cancer started. Your body destroyed the original site of where cancer began.

What happened is that a few random cancer cells got into your Lymphatic System, and landed in a lymph node in your neck, and set up housekeeping. They started growing, and that is why you have this mass in your neck. We are going to do 3 cycles of Chemo. These will be scheduled 3 weeks apart."

Then he said something that really caught my attention.

"Half way through the second Chemo, that place is going to disappear."

Disappear?

He said "disappear."

How is that possible?

It is a solid mass — large.

The size of this mass covered the palm of my hand.

This was scary.

Chapter 31

Did I hear him right?

"But," I heard myself protesting. "I watched Mom die when it went to her lymph nodes. When the doctors told us it was in three lymph nodes, we knew it was a death sentence. It was only a matter of time."

"And how long ago was that?" he queried.

"That was 1969, and she died 8 years later in 1977," I answered.

"That was 50 years ago, Betty. We know so much more now, and we have amazing drugs. I promise you, we are going to save your life. Just trust me."

This was profound.

"Just trust me" is a statement people often make in jest.

What I knew was that he was asking me to trust him with the most precious thing I owned — My Life.

Wholehearted Living

Wholehearted living is about engaging in our lives from a place of worthiness. It means cultivating the courage, compassion, and connection to wake up in the morning and think, "No matter what gets done and how much is left undone, *I am enough.* It's going to bed at night thinking, *Yes, I am imperfect and vulnerable and sometimes afraid, but that doesn't change the truth, that I am also brave and woROTHY of love and belonging."*

Brene Brown

FOMO – Killing your mojo –

"The 'fear of missing out' is what happens when scarcity slams into shame. FOMO lures us out of our integrity with whispers about what we could or should be doing. FOMO's favorite weapon is comparison. It kills gratitude and replaces it with 'not enough.' We answer FOMO's call by saying YES when we mean NO. We abandon our path and our boundaries and those precious adventures that hold meaning for us so we can prove that we aren't missing out. But we are. We are missing out on our own lives. Every time we say YES because we're afraid or missing out, we say NO to something. That something may be a big dream or a short nap. We need both. *Courage to stay our course and gratitude for our path will keep us grounded and guide us home.*"

Brene Brown

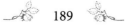

189

ᘒ
AN INTERVIEW WITH GOD

Poem by Hamid Yeganeh

I dreamed I had an interview with God.

"So you would like to interview me?
God asked.

"If you have the time." I said.

God smiled.
"My time is eternity.
What question do you have in mind for me?"

I asked.

"What surprised you most about humankind?"

God answered:

"They get bored with childhood.
They rush to grow up and then long be children again.
That they lose their health to make money
and then lose their money to restore their health.

That by thinking anxiously about the future,
they forget the present,
such that they live in neither the present or the future.

That they live as if they will never die,
and die as though they have never lived."

Chapter 31

God's hand took mine
and we were silent for a while.

And then I asked...
*"As a parent, what are some of life's lessons
You want your children to learn?"*

God replied with a smile

"To learn that it is not good to compare themselves to other.

*To learn that a rich person is not one who has the most,
But the one who needs the least.*

*To learn that it only takes a few seconds
to open profound wounds in persons, we love,
and it takes many years to heal them.*

To learn to forgive by practicing forgiveness.

*To learn that there are persons who love them dearly,
but simply do not know how to express or show their feelings.*

*To learn that two people can look at the same thing
And see it differently.*

*To learn that it is not always enough
that they are forgiven by others,
but that they must forgive themselves.*

And to learn that I am here always."

CHAPTER 32

❧

"Courage is fear that has said its prayers."
Dorothy Bernard
(1890 - 1955)

❧

My Ship had Sprung a Leak

My ship had sprung a leak, and without intervention it was going to sink. What I did not know then, but was to discover as I walked this journey, was that God was already ahead of me.

For a bit, I thrashed around, trying to realize how I needed to act and react — and feel. While I was busy, struggling to find *my own way*, **God threw me a life boat.** I grabbed on, and when I mustered the strength to climb in, my fellow passengers turned out to be the most incredible team of health care specialists I have ever encountered:

Dr. Craig Trigueiro MD (my primary care doctor)

Dr. Robert Whorf MD (oncologist)

Dr. Dwight Fitch MD (radiological oncologist)

Dr. Ivan Rascon MD (gastroenterologist)

Dr. Bruce Dorman MD (ENT)

Dr. Gary Bunch MD (surgeon)

There were countless others doctors, nurses, and technicians, as I worked my way through the maze of medical procedures and circumstances that were required, one day at a time. They were like a well-oiled machine. I would love to tell them all how grateful I am they were there for me. *I would like to thank them all.*

They had a plan for me and my healthcare, **with God at the helm of my ship.** Each has a calling to divine service, and that is their Gift — a Gift they offered to me. Maybe they saw me as "just another patient" but no one made me feel that way.

Chapter 32

There is no way we humans can begin to imagine what God has in store. The world is filled with noise, but God commanded:

ℒ

"Be still, and know that I am God!"
(Psalm 46:10 KJV)

Occasionally, we must shut off "the noise."
and listen –
really listen with our heart –
really listen **to what God is trying to tell us,**
through all that noise.

ℒ

INSTINCTS: The Power to Unleash Your Inborn Drive

Author: *Bishop T.D. Jakes (2014)*
(page 12 ,13,14 -16. 19)

"We are wired to stay alive. Our bodies naturally seek out nourishment (food and water) and protection(such as shelter, clothing and weapons) to survive. You've probably heard of the "fight or flight" response, which is an instinctive reaction to any perceived danger. Many scientists also believe that language is instinctive, or at least the desire to express our responses to both internal and external stimuli. Some researchers believe that we are instinctively spiritual beings as well...

As we grow and mature into mature into men and women, our various instincts also evolve and become more sophisticated and personalized — but so does our reliance on intellect, evidence, and technology. We are assaulted by so much information each day that it's easy to lose touch with the voice inside us, the compelling sense of knowledge, the awareness we have in our gut...

In addition, we're often conditioned to dismiss our instincts as primal and animalistic, subjected and unscientific. We're taught to rely on facts and figures, data and digits, not hunches and gut feelings. Some people may even consider relying on instincts, in the same way, they regard superstitions and mental telepathy: fodder for science fiction and super hero movies.

Sometimes we rely on our instincts without even realizing it... Not one of us is born without instincts. A person is more likely to be born without sight than to be born without instinct... Our instincts speak to us daily, prompting us to pay attention, and to seize the opportunity.

Our Creator designed everything he made to have a purpose. Yet most of us live our lives wondering what our purpose is...

Without understanding the guidance that our innate God-given instincts provide us, we simply adjust to the urgency of circumstances. Deeply spiritual people pray for it to be revealed other people just wander for a lack of it...

When we have the courage to leave the familiar and step into the destiny to which our instincts keep drawing us, we can live the same way...

Instincts in action... the inner compass is guiding us from where we are to where we want to go..."

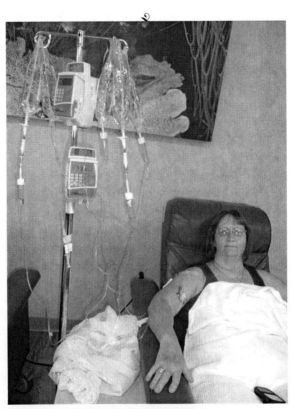

The author in chemotherapy.

CHAPTER 33

Never Whine

April 6, 2012

This chapter in my life like all the others was in God's hands. I began treatment, knowing there was a good chance I would not survive — no matter how much knowledge the doctors possessed.

The second time I showed up in Dr. Whorf's office, I thought it was for more information and additional consultations. I was informed that I would be staying all day. The Chemo would take eight hours and would involve 10 bottles of IV fluids with an assortment of Chemo drugs to be administered throughout the day. There was no TV, but some patients brought their laptops, and kept themselves busy and entertained.

The nurses were magnificent — experienced, poised, knowledgeable, and confident. They were attentive to each individual's needs, and answered every question and addressing every concern, no matter how trivial it might have seemed.

There were 50 recliners in that large room and enough fluids being infused to float a battleship. There was a steady stream of patients going in and out of the restrooms IV poles in tow. There were snacks to munch on, and magazines to read. It was quiet, sometimes to the point that the quiet was deafening.

From time-to-time, someone would strike up a conversation with me or someone in chairs a couple of seats over. It was impossible not to overhear the conversations.

One day "Kay" came for treatment. She took a place next to me, and we began to chat. I estimated her to me in her early seventies. I know it sounds naïve now, but I had not considered that if I got cancer and got "cured" it could happen again! (Yes, I knew they monitor you for 5 years, to make sure there was not a "recurrence", but somehow I never processed that in my mind.) Perhaps an entirely different type of cancer could happen following "the cure."

As a result of this revelation, I have learned to be exceedingly more conscious and aware of my health, now that, *perhaps, I have been given a second chance at life.*

"Kay's" story touched my heart and shook me to the core. She told me that this was her *fifth* diagnosis of cancer since 1997. She had a great attitude. She said that she was still alive and kicking and she was not about to give up. Her attitude was amazing.

I met "Jenny" who told me her cancer was "chronic" and incurable. I saw "Jenny" as mid-seventies. She had been taking chemotherapy for 17 years, and it would be on-going for the remainder of her life.

Watching the **incredible spirit and strength and resiliant attitude** these people possessed and the impact of their outlook was inspirational. I wondered how I would react if I found myself in that situation.

One day "Ivan" came in. He looked to be in his mid-fifties. I had to look twice to make sure my eyes were not deceiving me. He had a fresh surgical dressing in the middle of his face. I remembering being so overcome with emotions, I wanted to cry. He walked past me, and I realized **his nose had been removed.** I thought no matter how bad my diagnosis (Stage 4) seemed, there is always someone facing a worse fate than me. I remember thinking, **"Okay God. We are in this thing together, and I am trusting you, that we will come out of it together in one piece... and I will keep my nose, and other vital parts."**

From that point on the fear lifted, and I submitted to every treatment that Dr. Whorf (and later Dr. Dwight Fitch MD my radiological oncologist) recommended.

**Fear is part of our existence
but is should not dominate our life.
Our fear is for "the unknown".
God will give us the answer,
but we must be still... and listen.
There is no shame in knowing
what God declares in our lives.
You can't be afraid to reinvent yourself.
Keep growing into what God wants for you.
Your calling is your gift.
If you have a goal and vision to share –
and you have been hiding it,
be proud to share it with The World.**

Elizabeth A. Scott (2015)

Chapter 33

There was nothing I could do except hold on to my faith in God, and trust that He would bring people into my life that would help me overcome this enemy, and get on with my life. I remember thinking that I had to submit to God's Will and trust Him to do what was required for me — to live.

> "Let me win, but if I *cannot* win, let me be *brave* in the attempt."
>
> Eunice Kennedy Shriver

> "I don't know how to do this but something inside me does."
>
> From Gratitude and Trust by Paul Williams and Tracy Jackson

> "You can't get to courage without walking through vulnerability. Period."
>
> Dr. Brene Brown

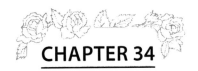

CHAPTER 34

The Gift He Gave to Me

April 2012

**Chemo provided one goal in doing its job — to keep
me alive, while it killed cancer.**

I saw a pattern form; I had had one week to get sick, one week to be sick, and one week to begin feeling better. Then the cycle started again… three times.

My hair began falling out following my second chemo treatment, just about the same time the mass in my neck disappeared. Rather than to look (in my estimation) like some "old hag," we all went out to the patio, and a friend took the clippers and shaved my head. We made light of it. What was the alternative? I was pretty sure my hair would grow back, and the mass in my neck wouldn't. I saw this as a trade-off!

Pantene, the shampoo company, was in partnership with American Cancer Society, to supply beautiful human hair wigs, free of charge. Barb and I made a trip to their office, and I was fitted with a gorgeous auburn shoulder length wig, very close to my natural hair. I was grateful for the generous gift.

The nausea was overwhelming at times. Over time, I dropped 60 pounds, and I felt lousy. I told myself this was the price I had to pay — to live — and that I would come out of this never-ending tunnel triumphant.

I was prescribed drugs for nausea, and even suppositories when I was too sick for pills to stay down. I was in bed most days, and the TV was my constant companion.

My love for sewing and painting gave in to ravaging fatigue. My family stayed near, and they were wonderfully supportive. I was grateful. I did not want to go through this alone. No one should go through chemo/radiation alone.

I was equally grateful that Barb was more than a year into her recovery. She was now pretty much self-care. Although she remained a fall risk, she quickly discovered that she could microwave her meals, and let our pets in and out, because I was not able to. I wondered how we would have managed this "cancer-thing" if I had been diagnosed 1 year earlier. I was grateful we had not had to face that scenario.

I had undergone three cycles of chemotherapy, which took 9 weeks, followed by 33 radiation treatments to my throat. My mouth was full of sores, and swallowing had become a major issue!

I had appointments for labs and saw Dr. Whorf or his ARNP, Loretta, weekly. They were an incredible team of medical specialists, and I could not thank them enough. I saw no reason to burden them with my complaints. All they could do was give me moral support – and I had that at home. I had always heard chemo was dreadful. It is, but that is temporary. When it is over, you begin to recover from chemotherapy.

꙳

It is not so simple with Radiation.

꙳

---

8 CHOICES FOR SUCCESS

(1) Turn your motivation into actions

(2) Learn to take risks

(3) Don't fix the problem.
Find the problem.

(4) Develop your knowledge

(5) Learn to compare

(6) Learn to deal with difficult people

(7) Avoid blaming yourself

(8) Utilize your capacity for
connection…

CHAPTER 35

This Was an Apocalyptic Moment!

Dr. Whorf would later write a report that stated,

"Somewhat anxious appearing; alert, oriented, comfortable. No obvious oral lesions. She has a significant palpable lymph node mass in the left supraclavicular area low cervical chain. No other significant palpable lymphadenopathy in the neck or on the right side… No auxiliary lymphadenopathy. Lungs clear to auscultations. Heart normal S1, S2… the lump has increased in size. She was sent for a CT scan as well as a biopsy at Blake on 3/15/2012… The biopsy showed… complex mass… 3.6 x 3.7 cm, with anterior displacement of the sternocleidomastoid muscle as well as the mass effect upon the jugular vein…"

(1) A 64-year-old female who presents with poorly differentiated squamous cell carcinoma, head and neck evaluation.

(2) … Often in this situation, one cannot find the primary. I think we should have a thorough head and neck evaluation.

I do not think this mass would be resectable, but I would ask the ear, nose, and throat surgeon if he felt that it could be safely removed to try to debulk the disease. I suspect that radiation with radiosensitizing chemotherapy would be the mainstay of treatment to the supraclavicular area. Given the fact that it is poorly differentiated, and there is likely to be a primary elsewhere, we could follow such therapy then with consolidative higher dose chemotherapy in attempts to try and remove residual micrometastatic disease.

(3) She is apprehensive about her renal cyst. I explained to her that I think that is likely to be benign. I would not expect a squamous cell carcinoma to arise from a renal cyst.

(4) …There is no obvious skin involvement by this mass or other skin lesions in the local area that appear to represent squamous cell carcinoma of the skin.

I am going to refer her to both Dr. Bruce Dorman M.D. (ear, nose & throat) and Dr. Dwight Fitch M.D. (Radiological Oncology) for immediate evaluation. The 3 of us work closely together. I think that would make a highly functional multi-disciplinary team. I am going to set her up for a PET scan as well as look for other possible locations. I will see her back on Tuesday, 4/10, and confer

Chapter 35

with Dr. Fitch and Dr. Dorman and go over the PET scan results and come up with a combined treatment plan."

Dr. Robert C. Whorf, MD 4/02/2012

4/06/12 — Park South Imagine Center did both a CT and PET scan. The imagines were fused for the best result.

The resulting observations were as follows: Extensive hypermetabolic, partially necrotic, confluent lymphadenopathy/soft tissue mass left low neck position, within the posterior triangle at the level of the larynx. This measure 43 mm in maximum transverse dimensions and 5.2 mm in maximal superior to inferior dimensions. Marginal and central glucose hypermetabolism to peak SUV 14.0 or immediate imaging. Finding consistent with malignancy. This most likely represents metastatic lymphadenopathy..."

4/13/2012 — Diagnosis: Malign Hypopharynx specified... No obvious oral lesions... Dr. Fitch is checking for the tumor for HPV(*)... PET scan shows confluent lymph node mass in the left neck at about 5.2 cm with an SUV of 14. There is no clear evidence of another metastatic disease, except for possibly some hyper glucose metabolism at the base of the tongue... I explained to her in detail that my predilection, given her young age and her excellent health, is that if this ends up be HPV negative, which implies a worse prognosis, I will favor neoadjuvant chemotherapy followed by chemoradiation given its extreme efficacy in head and neck cancers. This is based on date from Marshal Posner at Mass General Hospital in Boston, Harvard Medical School. If it were HPV positive, this would suggest a better prognosis, and then perhaps chemo radiation would be appropriate... If she does get neoadjuvant TPF, she will need an Infuse-A-Port." Robert Whorf M.D.

4/16/2012 — HPV is a sexually-transmitted disease.

I must interject here that this was the first (and only) time in my life that I was clearly told that having contracted a sexually-transmitted disease had its advantages! It had never occurred to me before this, and somehow I found that amusing that if I had contracted HPV during my life and was unaware of it, I had a better chance of surviving this cancer! In the end the HPV test came back negative, which was not a surprise to me. It also meant the doctors had a much tougher fight on their hands with my treatment.

4/17/2012 — Underwent pan-endoscopy to include the tongue, pharynx, nasopharynx, and esophagus.

4/23/12— Biopsies of tonsils, as well as nasopharynx, were all negative... HVP negative... Given the fact that she is an otherwise very healthy, young, and it being IVA stage with obvious primary, I think it would be reasonable to try neoadjuvant chemotherapy followed by chemo/RT (Radiation Therapy)... certainly the results can be quite astonishing with historical control... I talked with her about more risk with neutropenia and even neutropenic sepsis. Cisplatin can cause auditory problems, cystitis, as well as neuropathy. The fact that this is growing rapidly also raised the possibility of an increasing risk for micrometastatic disease... She is terrified that there could be cancer elsewhere in her body. After discussion, at length she said she would like to proceed... PLAN: PICC line; start TPF with slight dose reduction; prescriptions are given for Compazine, Zofran and Decadron; patient education with the first dose; plan for 3 cycles and then chemo/RT; recommending aggressive hydration to try to help forestall problems.

4/24/2012 –PICC line placement, right upper extremity placed with the tip in superior vena cava, at Blake Medical Center as an outpatient.

5/2/2012 — Follow-up following the 1st cycle of Chemotherapy. Fatigue from Chemo. Very close observation. 2nd cycle of Chemo. Will include a slight increase in dose of both cisplatin and the Taxotere. After 3 cycles of Chemo, we will get restaging scans and see Dr. Fitch.

5/7/2012 –She complained to her primary physician of a sore throat, which is Mucositis grade 1, from chemo. He confirmed that she had Thrush. Given a prescription for nystatin. She had an episode of bone ache. She felt her heart was pumping out of her chest. She felt no improvement in the size of the mass on her left neck. All other aspects are normal. This is a rapidly growing IVA. Overall she has done well.

5/17/2012 – She tolerated her 1st treatment without many ill effects. It was mild. She reported it was horrible... She had no nausea. She is eating and drinking fluids well... She was reminded that mucositis, diarrhea, and nausea are expected. She is prescribed meds...

5/24/2012 – She looks well, but she does look fatigued. Alert, oriented, comfortable. She has now finished her 2nd cycle of Chemo.

NOTE: The lymph node mass in her neck has decreased by 50% in size

Each week there were blood tests. For a period of time, I was given IV's to keep me hydrated during, between, and after cycles of chemo. Because I was developing "chemo veins" once the PICC Line came out, it was difficult for the nurses to find a vein they can sustain an IV effectively.

One day I went into having hydration. Four nurses ended up trying *nine times* to find my vein. They felt terrible for me. I was upset because they were trying so diligently – and I was failing them, because of my "chemo veins". I was a nurse, too!

Diane, one of the nurses, finally succeeded in getting access to a vein. I could feel an audible collective sigh of relief among the staff. From then on, it was Diane who was assigned to me, when I had to come in for hydration. (I have no doubt Diane was thrilled!) I was equally relieved that Diane seemed to possess "the magic formula" for finding a vein they could access.

It was not long before I went back to Blake to get another PICC line installed – giving them ready access to my veins PRN (as needed).

For anyone who might ask, I highly recommend a PICC Line as the best way for accessing your veins when undergoing long-term IV therapy of any type. It is not painful to have installed, and it can remain installed under your arm for extended periods of time (generally) without issues.

CHAPTER 36

My "Point-of-Light"

I was sent to see the radiological oncologist, Dr. Dwight Fitch, MD, and to be fitted for a mask. He was to direct my radiation therapy. I found Dr. Fitch to be a very personable and engaging doctor – one might say he had "great bedside manner." He had earned a degree in engineering in Michigan, prior to deciding to further his education and go on to earn his medical degree and then into the field to become a radiological oncologist.

In the same way as Dr. Whorf had reassured me, Dr. Fitch made me feel that when I was in his presence, I had his undivided attention. He was there to answer my questions and calm my fears. *The importance of a doctor possessing that trait can't be over emphasized.*

The material the masks are fashioned from were initially developed by NASA. It is a white, pliable material. When placed for a time, in hot water, it can be molded to any face. When the mask was molded to my face (since my radiation treatments were on my head/neck) they laid me flat on a table. The technicians told me that they were going to form-fit it to the contours of my head. When it was placed on my face, it had just come out of the scalding hot water. The sensation is shocking – even if you are prepared. It was molded to my specific features. There is nostrils cut. I insisted that my eye openings had to be cut, because I tend to be claustrophobic.

The mask was designed to be locked in place on the table so that my head absolutely couldn't move during the treatments. When I would feel the techs lock my head down to the table, I would close my eyes and start counting down from 1000. Counting kept my mind off the claustrophobia and kept me from feeling too confined. I knew there was no other alternative. No matter how many times, I went through this, I had to keep talking to myself, so I did not freak out during the treatments. I had a total of 33 radiation treatments.

Oh yes! I got my first tattoo — because of medical necessity — a reference point for the radiologist to measure my treatments. It was the size and color of a pencil lead, a point from which the Radiation Treatments were measured and referenced. I now call it my "Point of Light" because that tattoo allowed me to find the light of my new life. This, I reasoned, was one my parents would have approved of.

Chapter 36

June and into July 2012

6/7/2012 — Her blood count is adequate. She is due for her 3rd cycle of chemo. The mass on the left side is now completely resolved

6/14/12 — She is now 1 week after #3 TPF. She feels worn out.

She has waves of nausea, most bothersome at night. She had reflux symptoms and had taken Carafate. The Claritin before Neulasta helped with the bone pain. One positive note, she had had no reoccurrence of abdominal spasms from IBS…She looks run down…

6/21/12 — She is now 2 weeks after #3 TPF. She is actually doing well… tired of the horrible taste… trying PO (by mouth) hydration, and maintaining the taste alteration is bothersome… she had no neuropathy or nausea… Alert and oriented. She looks well, but frustrated… I did encourage she proceed with the scheduled IV hydration today to make sure she had no further occurrence of abdominal spasms from her IBS.

She says she is drinking fluids, although she admitted it is very difficult due to the horrible taste. She was reassured that the taste is strictly from the chemotherapy treatment, and will resolve once she completes therapy. Right now she is concerned about the side effects that she may experience when she ventures on radiation therapy.

6/28/12 – She finished her TPF chemotherapy on 6/11/12… She does have some fatigue… She looks well, alert, oriented and comfortable.

I cannot palpate a lymph node at all… Low magnesium… I will set up a PET scan… D/C PICC line… She is set up to with Dr. Fitch.

7/9/12 – IMPRESSIONS: Dramatic improvement and nearly complete resolution of left inferior cervical lymph node mass compared to the prior exam of April 2012. No PET scan evidence for new metastatic or reoccurring head and neck neoplasm

7/19/14 – …She is recovering nicely from the neoadjuvant chemotherapy. She had a PET scan. She feels reasonably well. She is up and about… active… eating… She looks well, alert, oriented, and comfortable. I cannot palpate a lymph mode at all. Lungs are clear… She had met Dr. Fitch; the mask had been made. She is due to start on radiation sometime next week… I told her that my experience low-dose weekly carboplatin/Taxol is extremely well tolerated and very effective in head and neck cancer. It does come with added mucositis and possible salivary gland damage. We also talked of hypothyroidism given that that may be in the radiation port. I recommended that she speak further with Dr. Fitch about the pros and cons, risks and benefits of radiation based on her anatomy... Following chemoradiation, she will have restaging studies and be placed on observation...Regiment: Taxotere 75 mg., Cisplatin 75mg....

The radiation treatments were 5 days a week. The actual radiation treatment was 4 minutes each session and is entirely painless. The entire process was approx. 20 minutes, plus the 20 minutes each way I would drive. I drug myself out of bed, dressed and drove myself to my first 22 treatments. By the time I returned home, I was exhausted. All I could do was climb back into bed and watch TV until I fell asleep.

> I call it my "Point of Light" because that tattoo allowed me to find the light of my new life. This I reasoned, was one tattoo my parents would have approved of.

"How Did You Loose So Much Weight?"

I'm Glad You Asked!

While enduring chemo and radiation, I dropped 60 pounds. People would come up to me and says,

"Girl, what is your secret to losing so much weight?"

They, of course, wanted to know if I had come up with some magic formula I could pass on to them.

"Chemo and radiation – it works every time!" I would answer.

Then I would add, **"I don't recommend it."**

They would look stunned and bewildered — unsure what to say next.

While I was being treated, the court per our request moved forward. On July 18, 2012, Barb submitted to an interview with Dr. James Slocum MD, who had been ordered by the court to file a report of his examination.

He was the psychiatrist who initially saw Barb when she was a patient at RidgeLake Hospital on Feb. 14, 2011, and was basically unresponsive. He did remember her and was pleasantly surprised to see her in good spirits, walking into his office!

After receiving a report from Dr. T, recommending her rights be restored, he interviewed her and found his experience, "Revealed a personable, alert woman who was oriented to time, place, and person... She interoperated proverbs without difficulty and was able to find similarities between like objects. Her fund of general information was intact, as was her mathematical ability. The judgment did not seem to be impaired by the usual means of problem-solving. She was neither depressed nor anxious. She was not hallucinating and not delusional. She has normal emotional presentation..."

Chapter 36

RECOMMENDED COURSE OF TREATMENT: I believe that all her rights should be restored. Her plans would be to continue to live with her mother, to utilize public transportation, and continue to improve. Consequently, it's my opinion that all her rights should be restored, except for her right to have a driver's license or operate a vehicle.

James L. Slocum M.D.

NOTE:

August 24, 2012, after requested reports were submitted to the court in Sarasota, Florida, recommending my Legal Guardianship was reversed and Barbara was granted restoration of all her Legal Rights again when the court with one exception. She still is not allowed to drive.

8/15/12 — Continue with weekly treatments. Weekly visits. Neupogen to help prevent her missing chemotherapy treatments. Pain medications, supportive care per Dr. Fitch for the radiation. I explained to her that she is going to have taste changes throughout and she may not recover her tastefully. She may also have problems chronically with salivation. She says she is aware, and she is willing to continue.

8/22/12 — She has completed 4th week of radiation... A sore throat is more intense She has received IV hydration; that helped greatly. She had no appetite primarily from taste alterations. In spite of a sore throat, the treatment is tolerable... Continues on Benedryl to help her sleep...Weekly monitoring to assess for treatments related toxicity and adjust supportive measures as needed.

8/29/12 — She has 2 more weeks of radiation. A sore throat is more intense. RT had prescribed fentanyl patch, which is not working. She is unable to tolerate hydrocodone liquid or the magic mouthwash. She has a poor venous accent. She requires 4 unsuccessful venipunctures. She scheduled for a PICC line yesterday but, unfortunately, has to be rescheduled due to insurance issues. The taste alternation is bothersome... *Her platelet count is down to 50,000.* Hold chemotherapy treatment today.

IV hydration today and 2 times this week. Hopefully, this will keep her hydrated and avoid hospitalization. Continue fentanyl patch, concentrating oxycodone 0.5 ml, q4 hrs. to alleviate the pain from the esophagitis. She will meet with Dr. Bunch this afternoon regarding feeding tube placement. She is resistant to the idea. Weekly monitoring to assess for treatment related toxicity and adjust supportive measures... She is looking frail. Weekly monitoring to access for treatment-related toxicity...

Yankee 794 Trauma

8/29/12 — PICC line placement in the upper left arm.

One of the only foods I could tolerate was Yoplait's White Chocolate/ Strawberry Yogurt at the time, and I was eating that consistently. (This was prior to my discovering Boost.)

CHAPTER 37

The Aftermath Was Sobering

September 2012

The radiation burns to my throat, mouth and internally, became significant. My blood work alarmed Dr. Whorf. *My platelet count dipped to 50,000.* (It would normally have been 350,000 – 400,000.) He announced that I was going to be hospitalized for close monitoring, and for blood transfusions – 2 units of platelet and 4 units of whole blood.

At that point, I relented and decided to have a feeding tube installed while I was already a patient at Blake Medical Center. My weight was now down to 138 pounds from 196. (At one point by 2007 my weight ballooned to 225 so 'yes' I have had a weight challenge in my life with my 5'4" height.)

Dr. Gary Bunch MD performed the installation of my feeding tube. I was discharged from the hospital after 4 days and sent home to resume my last 11 radiation treatments.

I contemplated not finishing. I had done all my chemo and 22 radiation treatments. It seemed to me, with all the mental and physical fatigue, *it should have been enough.* I wondered if I just inconspicuously stopped going, maybe I could run "under their radar", and no one would really miss me or notice. By now:

(1) my taste buds were gone
(2) my thyroid was dead
(3) my parotid gland refused to do their job (which was to produce saliva) so I was always fighting severely dry mouth.

I had a fear of driving because I was so fatigued, I was concerned that while driving to and from my radiation treatments I could not react in the split-second I needed to avoid a collision with another car, I was terrified that I would injure or kill someone. A friend stepped up to volunteer to drive me to and from my last eleven treatments, and I completed them in early October.

To add insult to injury, I was forced to look in my bathroom mirror at someone I did not recognize — someone who was bald! It does not sound very appealing, does it? It wasn't, but as I have often remarked "It is what it is, and that's the truth."

I had been prescribed Morphine and Magic Mouthwash to numb the pain of the sores in my mouth and throat. Fentanyl 25 mg. and 50 mg, patches were for pain. I had Morphine Sulfate liquid 100 mg. to be taken every 3 – 4 hours PRN (as needed) but don't remember using any of it. The suppositories for nausea were always readily available in case I could not take anything by mouth.

"Just so you know. I am totally on board for driving you to treatment, cleaning your place, helping you pick out flattering wigs, coming up with bad-ass visualization exercises, and if you twist my arm, I guess I'd also be cool with lying on the couch and watching trashy TV together. I know. It's a sacrifice I'm willing to make."

Emilymcdowell.com

Traumatic Brain Injury Survivors Prayer
God,
I come before You as one whose injury
Cannot be seen by your other children.
While others see me, they know not that
My wounds are invisible.
I come before you as a
Traumatic brain injury survivor.
You alone know the depth of my pain,
Of my despair, of my confusion, of my aloneness,
And of my overwhelming loss of self.
Humbly, I ask of You...
When exhaustion strikes, please
Grant me the strength I need to continue.
When others leave my life, help me to
Remember that You are always there with me.
When unsteadiness causes me to stumble,
Please take my hand and lead me safely forward.
When my memory so often fails me,
Help me to never forget what is really important.
God, so many of your children walk daily with
Challenges that dwarf my own.
By understanding this, I can see my own
Life in a better perspective.
Help me for today to accept my fate in this life
Knowing that if I trust in you,
All will be well.
Amen.

CHAPTER 38

"...I Wish He Didn't Trust Me So Much!"

I kept saying to myself, *"I know God won't give me more than I can handle, but I just wish He didn't trust me so much!"*

The phrase "do not be afraid" is written in the Bible 365 times. That's a daily reminder from God to live everyday fearlessly. Sometimes reminding myself of this helped.

There was some passing speculation that second-hand smoke might have contributed to me developing cancer. I had, in fact, been married to two smokers in past years. I had never smoked nor had I been raised with parents who smoked. I was not in a household where anyone smoked for years. So when I left the hospital, I found it mildly amusing that I received a paper stating, *"Tobacco smoke can be harmful to your health, and second-hand smoke can be detrimental to those around you. Avoid second-hand smoke. If you don't smoke, don't start..."* Now that had not occurred to me!

When I was dismissed from the hospital four days later, I had not had the energy to worry how we were going to buy the formula I would require to stay nourished. Only God knew how long it would be necessary – most likely for months.

While I was in the hospital, the customary trips to SCIL (Suncoast Center for Independent Living) for Barb continued. She had kept them abreast of my reports, and when they came to her with this, it was something more than we could have hoped for.

I actually had not considered what this formula (Jevity and Osmolite) would cost. However, it is about $50 for a case of 24 cans. It is a liquid designed as a supplement with all the vitamins and minerals for a healthy diet when you can't eat. I would have to feed myself 1 eight-ounce can every 4 hours followed by 60 cc of water.

God again intervened in my life.

Barb had been a client of SCIL (Suncoast Center for Independent Living) in Sarasota, Florida, for over a year. It is primarily (but not exclusively) a resource and support system for people with Acquired and Traumatic Brain Injury. The center had just gotten a call that *20 cases* (ten cases of Jevity and ten cases of

Osmolite) had just been donated. The person it was to be donated to was no longer in need of it. The director of SCIL asked Barb if they could donate it to me. She immediately told them 'yes.' That beautiful gift from SCIL allowed me to survive from mid-August, 2012 until the end of January 2013 when I was finally able to have Dr. Bunch remove the feeding tube. Because the feeding formula was donated to me and I had 10 cases remaining, I donated it to The Source Church, who then passed it along to another person who needed it.

> I know God won't give me more than I can handle, but I just wish He didn't trust me so much!

9/26/12 — Alert, oriented, comfortable. She appears quite a bit better. Feeding tube site is markedly improved. Pet scan... no worrisome findings... There is no clear evidence of another metastatic disease... at the base of the tongue... Infection at the G-tube site appears to be under excellent control... Proceeding with last chemotherapy today... DC PICC line... When she has recovered from treatments, in approx. 6 – 8 weeks, repeat CT/PET scans. At this point, she will need ongoing surveillance and ENT evaluations.

10/17/12 — She is recovering from treatments. She finished 16 days ago. She says she is doing well. She is up and about... active. She does have some decreasing hearing because it sound as though she is "hearing things underwater". Weight 159 pounds BP 110/74.... She looks fantastic. No oral lesions... She completed radiation.

10/01/12 — If her hearing does not improve, we will consider ENT evaluation, possibly audiology.

Shortly after this, I saw Dr. Dorman again. My eustachian tubes in my ears had slowly closed due to the swelling created by the radiation burns in my throat, which had extended to my ears. It was so subtle that I had not realized what was happening until I kept having to turn the TV volume up to hear.

I was completely amazed when he informed me there was a simple fix to my problem of pronounced deafness. He quickly placed tubes in my ears. The difference was *instantaneous* and *astonishing*. I asked him when I would need to make an appointment to have the tubes removed. His response was, *"Oh you don't. In about a year, they will fall out on their own."*

12/3/12 — CT/PET scan results with IV contrast administered. There is no evidence of new or enlarged pulmonary mass or nodule.

No CT evidence of metastatic disease or acute cardiopulmonary disease. CT Neck evaluation demonstrated 36 x 37 mm nodal within the left deep jugular position at the level of the larynx... There is:

Chapter 38

(1) No evidence of pathologic enlargement.

(2) No evidence for enhancing nasal or oropharyngeal mass.

(3) No evidence of a skull vase mass or abnormal enhancing.

(4) No focal abnormalities of the salivary glands or para-pharyngeal spaces observed.

(5) No evidence of a dominant thyroid mass or nodule.

(6) Residual left deep jugular soft tissue thickening is stable in comparison to fused PET/CT evaluation of 7/9/12.

(7) No evidence for new or progressive malignant/metastatic focus.

12/7/2012 — Weight 148 – BP 126/86... Clinically she appears well. Problems with her salivation... radiation can have an effect on salivary glands. She is also having some problems with Eustachian tube dysfunction... I am going to set her up to see Dr. Dorman (ENT). Perhaps she could receive a stent if there is some scarring at the Eustachian tubes. She is going to speak to Dr. Fitch further about the salivary gland issue. Repeat scans in 6 months with CBC and CMP at that time.

In early December 2012, Dr. Whorf scheduled me for a CT and PET Scan to see if there was any sign of cancer still in my body.

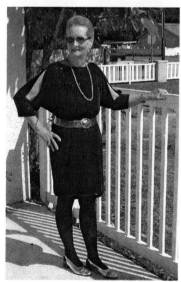

Just after I was told, I was cancer free!

The scans came back NEGATIVE – *I was cancer free!* From that time on, I went every 6 months for CT or PET Scans, just to make sure that no cancer had reoccurred.

It is said that 'no news is good news'. It depends. When it comes to cancer, when you have a scan, indeed, no news is good news. But in a case like this "no news" tells you nothing — and the problem with the dizziness still persisted, not to mention bewildering, as it coninued to plague me. The specialists don't tell you all this. The reason is that no two people are going to have the same symptoms. Why alarm you when it may not even happen? Why worry them unduly, when nothing can be done to stop the side-effects? It is just a lot of wasted energy that accomplishes nothing.

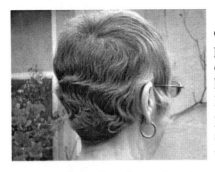

This is a photo of my hair when it grew back. I had never had curly hair in my life but was told that when your hair first regrows after Chemo/Radiation, it will be curly. Also, I was not allowed to color my hair for more than a year.

In the meantime Barb could not exercise, and she had mindlessly been packing on the pounds. I had become concerned about her weight and other health issues that might be looming. Her 5'2" frame was now supporting 235 pounds. I brought my concerns to her attention. She had been aware she had a weight issue early in her adult life, and had tried various "diets" with limited short-term success. I had a treadmill and she repeatedly asked to begin exercise using it. I was afraid she would lose her balance and fall. So I flatly refused to allow her to use it. Not long after that she got an exercise bike and began to ride. She began to measure and weigh all her food, cutting out all but 1200 calories a day. Between the exercise and calorie regimen the weight began to disappear.

By the time this book was ready for publication, Barb's weight (along with her adding an emphasis to decreasing fats and proteins) over two years dropped to 153. It became commonplace for her to ride two hours (18-24 miles) which also strengthened her legs and back. Her general outlook on life improve as she saw her goal wight of 135 become close and closer… a total weight loss of 100 pounds!

God gave us the strength and we give God the glory!

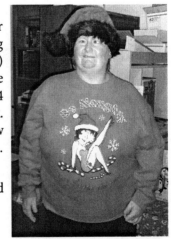

*Barb – Christmas 2012
Just at the beginning of her
weight loss at 233 pounds.*

Chapter 38

𝒬

God placed you in my path
when I began my unexpected personal odyssey.

YOU WERE HERE

To the incredible team of doctors
who mapped out a strategy to save my life.

YOU WERE HERE

the journeymen who stayed the course,
and remained constant
propping me up when
I was anxious, fearful,
and when I was too frail or weak to continue.

YOU WERE HERE

when I needed questions answered, and
to bring me through "the storm" and back to health.

Dr. Craig Triguerio MD
Family Medicine

Dr. Robert Whorf MD
Hematology & Oncology

Dr. Bruce Dorman MD
Ear, Nose, and Throat

Dr. Dwight Fitch MD
Oncology Specialist (cancer), Radiation Oncology

Dr. Gary Bunch MD
General Surgery

𝒬

Because of you,
I am alive.

THANK YOU

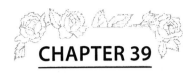

CHAPTER 39

Grand Mal Seizure

January 2013

January 20, 2013, twenty-five months after her accident, for no apparent reason, Barb had her first (and only) Grand Mal Seizure. It happened one evening as she was eating dinner.

Although I am well aware of the protocol teaches you to place the person having the seizure on the floor, I opted, under the circumstances, not to follow that. We had tile floors, and she was seated at the table. I was afraid to attempt to move her to the floor, while she was having a full-blown seizure. I was more concerned that she did *not* hit her head! We held her in the chair as I called 9-1-1.

The dispatcher who initially answered my call and alerted the ambulance, kept telling me to put her on the floor. I tried to explain to him that we were holding her where she was to keep her from hitting her head because of her TBI. He had a hard time understanding why I didn't seem to be following his directions.

Fortunately, the 9-1-1 responders were at our home within 5 minutes, and four medically-trained responders (God bless them!) were then able to lift her, and place her on the gurney to transport her to Blake Medical Center. She was halfway to the hospital before she woke up and realized what had happened to her.

The ER doctor ordered an MRI of her brain but came up with nothing new. He reported observing a black area in her brain the size of a walnut. That was the central location for a lot of the damage that happened during her accident. Nothing specifically pointed to the cause for a Grand Mal Seizure, other than (as he so eloquently put it), ***"She has TBI. I am surprised it didn't happen before now."***

The following day we scheduled an appointment to see Dr. Frank Loh M.D., her neurologist. He immediately placed her on Tegretol, which she will be required to remain on for the rest of her life.

Going through her test results the doctors had been impressed. Dr. T and Dr. McGovern *independently* had been discussing what types of employment Barb could realistically aspire to with her disabilities, at some point in the future. After all, she was only 39, and we all wanted to encourage her.

Chapter 39

The two doctors voiced their confidence in her. These two like-minded doctors, who she respected and revered, had independently suggested that in time and given the right training, each was confident she would be capable of working in the field of medical administration in a health care facility. Her background and experience, they reasoned, would be an asset in developing her overall outlook in this type of position.

Barb was encouraged by what she saw as their confidence in her abilities. *She made up her mind to go back to college!* We discussed doing online campus, but Barb felt strongly she needed to be face to face in a classroom with her professors to ask questions. I had always encouraged her. How was this any different from any other place she had ventured in her life?

At first, reluctantly, I cheered her on. The chatter at SCIL was that it was too soon, and she was "jumping the gun" on her recovery.

On the other hand, I decided who was I to insist it was all too early? How could we know if she did not try? Either way it was going to be a yardstick for determining just what she could and couldn't do. *She had decided it was time to step into her new forever reality.*

In September 2012, she began the process by making a trip to the local college to apply for a Pell Grant. When that came back approved, we made a trip to speak to a guidance counselor to determine what classes she already had credit for, and how to map out a strategy for her success. Twelve hours of classes were scheduled per week. We purchased books and a small suitcase with wheels so she could tow it behind her Go-Go Scooter.

She applied for transportation through Manatee County, and she was approved. This allowed Barb to be picked up each day that she had a class. She would be returned home each day after classes. I would not be going with her. (I admit I was tempted!!)

In January 2013, I held my breath and prayed that she could overcome what I sensed would be significant unforeseen obstacles that would pop up along her journey. *Wasn't that a description of what we had been doing since her accident?*

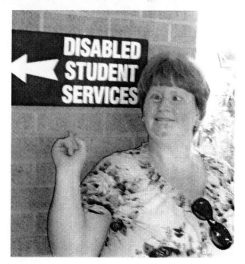

The transportation system could deliver her to and from the campus, however, while she was on campus, she was on her own. This could only be defined as "trial by fire." I realized afterwards that we should have done a practice run to iron out issues that she later encountered. Like so many trials and tribulations in life, you live and learn.

Monday was her first day. Immediately there were issues that I was not present to help solve. Her book bag, which her GoGo Scooter was towing, would hit a crack in the sidewalk and would flip over. She was still in the early stages of walking and unsteady on her feet, with only one working arm and hand. Her vision and perception issues remained. It was nearly impossible for her to manage this situation – *and no one would stop and assist her!* She would be late getting to her next class, and with her PBA in full-blown mode, it immediately became overwhelming for her.

By Wednesday, my tenacious and determined daughter's "enlightened spirit" had flickered, and was in danger of being extinguished! It was one of those "coming to Jesus" moments. She told me,

"Momma, it's too hard to manage. I think I need to withdraw and try again when I am stronger!"

After we had discussed it, and I could see how overwhelmed she was, I agreed. In order to preserve her Pell Grant, classes had to be withdrawn and books had to be returned – and it all had to be done by Friday.

Barb concluded that the stress of going back to school too early in her recovery might have been the catalyst for that seizure. She now takes a daily maintenance dose of Tegretol, and she will do so for the rest of her life.

> My tenacious and determined daughter's enlightened spirit had flickered, and was in danger of being extinguished!

February 2013

I continuously marvel that Barb had found her own way back to walking without a cane three years into her recovery. I saw her go from bed to a wheelchair, to a walker, to a cane. Each step along the way was a triumph for her and thrilling for me to watch.

Finally, there came a point where she was no longer using her cane to navigate our home. Instead, she used a method called, "furniture cruising." The cane sat still by the door as if waiting for her when she would leave the house.

One day, she braved the world without her cane. I had been aware that, by now, she was strong enough not actually to depend on it for support. When she got brave enough one day to leave the house without it, I asked her if she had forgotten something. She grinned at me and stated, *"Nope. I think I am fine. The only reason I take that cane out in public is because people don't see me, Mama. They just pay no attention to me being physically challenged. I figure if they are going to knock me down, they are going with me! I see the cane as an alert to people. When they see me, they are alerted to walk around me, instead of running into me."*

Now back to my story. For me, it turned out that one year after being diagnosed with Stage 4 Squamous Cell Carcinoma I was given some incredible news.

3/11/13 — CT scan of the neck with and without a contract. Nothing to report. It was clean. No cancer.

At this point, I began to breathe a sigh of relief feeling that the worst was behind me and was confident it would be smooth sailing ahead.

I was on the road to full and complete recovery!

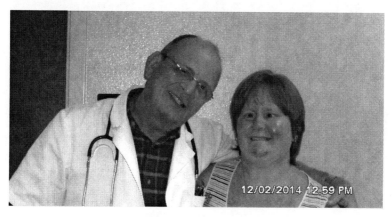

Dr. T and Barb – December 2014

> "It's as simple as this: you are here to
> honor something called
> *THE MIRACLE OF LIFE."*
> Paulo Coelho

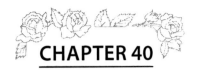

CHAPTER 40

Déjà Vu

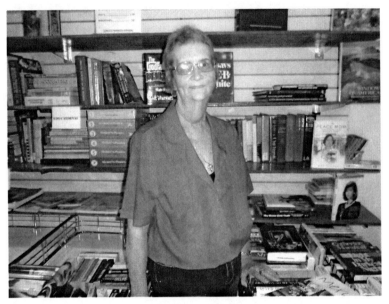

April 2014

Barb and I were volunteering at The Source Church City Reach Thrift Shop organizing their books while I was in recovery from chemo/radiation. My second illness, May 2013, was a complete unwelcome jolt.

May 26, 2013

I was again hit, this time with a necrotic bowel. I have almost no memory of the next month of my life. I apparently became violently ill at home. I was taken to Blake Medical Center ER and admitted. It was more than a day before they concluded I was dying — there in front of their eyes. No one knew why.

I had a history of IBS (Irritable Bowel Syndrome) and hernia surgeries going back to 1978. The problem was chronic. Periodically I would have "an episode" and infrequently it would become acute, and I would land back in the hospital after I became extremely ill. I had six Hernia surgeries through the past 15+ years, and my "problem" had now gotten to the place, where if

Chapter 40

my bowel strangulated and died, so would I! A necrotic (strangulated) bowel undiagnosed and untreated **will lead to death!**

My surgeon, Dr. Gary Bunch MD, was finally called to the hospital. When he took a look at me, read my chart, and got the report, he immediately realized I was dying. My BP had dropped dangerously low to 40/0.

Dr. Bunch told my family, ***"She's trying to die, and I don't know why. She needs to go to surgery right now. I don't know if I can save her."***

Dr. Bunch is a wonderful guy with a great bedside manner and sense of humor, but when he looked at me, there was nothing to joke about.

He knew it was a race against time to find and correct my problem. He did not know if I would live through the procedure, however without it, *there was zero chance I would survive.*

It took him 2 ½ hours to remove my gallbladder which was long overdue to come out, as well as to cut through many adhesions (scar tissue from previous surgeries) just to get to where he could hunt for my problem. He said that after three hours struggling, he finally stopped and called in his surgical associate to help him!

During five hours of emergency surgery, he resuscitated me three times, while he searched methodically for what was killing me. He pulled my colon out of my abdomen and examined it inch-by-agonizing-inch. Finally, in the very back of my small bowel, he located a three-foot section that was black and dead.

He masterfully crafted a resection of my small bowel and completed my surgery – with me still clinging to Life. Even though I don't remember any of it, ***I know God was with Dr. Bunch and me that day***!

"Lady you had me worried! It generally takes me an hour to fix a hernia!" he told me later.

To add insult to injury, pushing IV fluids on me in surgery, to keep me hydrated and alive, also threw me into septic shock — which had to be dealt with in ICU.

What Is Sepsis?

- Sepsis or septic shock is systemic inflammatory response syndrome (SIRS) secondary to a documented infection. This response is a state of acute circulatory failure characterized by persistent arterial hypotension despite adequate fluid resuscitation or by tissue hypoperfusion (manifested by a lactate concentration >4 mg/dL) unexplained by other causes.

After miraculously surviving the first 48 hours at Blake, I am told I spent three weeks in and out of ICU.

I have only flashes and glimpses of my stay there. My family kept vigil. Barb later joked, *"Mom you should have seen me, with only one functioning side, trying to get in and out of all that isolation garb!"*

I would be conscious for 2-3 minutes, but never long enough to really grasp what had happened until after I got to rehab toward the end of June. I was told that I pulled out a catheter to my heart! Because of me pulling this stunt, (and apparently other outrageous behavior that I don't recall.) I do remember being aware that I was restrained and wearing mittens as part of my stay in ICU.

Another time, I remember two wrestler-type guys who were working around my bed doing something, when one of them exclaimed, *"You got me good that time!"*

I had the horrifying and distinct feeling I had bitten him! This type of behavior was arbitrary – totally out of character for me!

Some time later, after I returned home, I asked my family about those two wrestler-types. Did they exist or was I delusional? I was informed that they were most assuredly real and that either one of them could have carried me across the hospital without breaking a sweat!

Another vivid memory I had was a man in a black suit and a clerical collar that came about the same time each day. He was soft-spoken with piercing blue eyes. He was caucasian, handsome, well-groomed, average build and 5' 10" tall, with short sandy brown hair. He was perhaps approaching his 50's – certainly younger than me. He had a reassuring smile that gave me the impression he could see right through me, and "the stuff I was made of." His voice was reassuring. When he was with me, I sensed that no matter whether I lived or died, I was going to be at peace.

Each day, he would come to my bedside in ICU and sit and talk to me. I got the distinct impression we had very rational conversations and each day before he left my side, we would pray. There was something about his presence I can't define.

I never saw him after I was transferred out of Blake. To this day, I didn't know his name and if he was on the team of clergy at Blake — or if he was my guardian angel. I do know that if I ever saw him again, I would instantly recognize him.

For anyone who might want to ask, no I did not ever feel I had traveled into "The Light." Most of that month of my life is blank.

CHAPTER 41

Out of Rehabilitation

❧

*"You have to accept whatever comes and
the only important thing is that you meet it
with the best you have to give."*

**Eleanor Roosevelt
(1884-1962)**

❧

June - July 2013

When I arrived at Bradenton Healthcare, a rehabilitation center, I felt like Rip Van Winkle, who is said to have slept for 100 years. Gradually I became aware of my surroundings.

Unknowingly, I was assessed by a team of therapists that evaluated me for speech, occupational and physical therapy. They wrote reports estimating that I was going to be there for three months, relearning all the essential skills. I had been down this road 18 months earlier with Barb! If she could make it back, so could I!

When an otherwise healthy person like myself goes into "a state of suspended animation" where they lay in bed 24/7, after about a week, the human body begins to produce an enzyme that breaks down your muscles. By the time, I reached rehab. I was totally dependent on others.

I could do nothing for myself – nothing as essential as controlling my bowels and bladder, dressing and undressing, taking a shower. *They were all gone!* To add insult to injury when I set up at a 45-degree angle, I got dizzy! It was dreadful — and I was unprepared to deal with it.

I woke to discover that my major swallowing issues from the radiation treatments that I had completed in October 2012 were still there. In fact, they had been *assaulted* by the tracheotomy I had at the hospital for a time while in ICU.

I found that actions that were previously effortless were now impossible, like lifting myself off the toilet. My legs were not strong enough to support my weight. When I explained to the therapist my dilemma, they got me an elevated seat so I could lift myself from the toilet without assistance, but that was half way thru my stay.

I felt it was absurd and humiliating to have to ask for assistance for a shower, and yet that is what I had to do. The CNA's didn't mind, because they expect "old and frail people" to need help – and I was surrounded by them!

I refused to be "old and frail" and yet somehow I had "gone to sleep" back in May, a physically fit and completely independent person, and woke up to find I fit right in. My mind found this fact repugnant. My dogged determination kicked in.

Fortunately, I had some redeeming qualities left, tenacity and perseverance and let's not forget *instincts*. Luckily those inborn traits were still kicking and screaming! Unlike my health and the use of my muscles, these had not failed me.

> They wrote reports estimating I was going to be there three months relearning all the essential skills.

They remained firm. I knew of only one option. I had to fight my way back to complete independence and health.

Dr. Bunch had told my family I might die. Since, I didn't follow his prediction, now, I didn't have time for this nonsense. Daylight was burning. My determination kicked into overdrive.

I had been totally independent before this happened, and I would be totally independent again, a lot sooner than they all estimated!

"Three months…" they predicted.

"Bah humbug!" I declared.

I sat in a wheelchair in the hall, and I looked around at all those aging souls, who seemed forever lost to time and family, in this skilled nursing facility. I had been one of the nurses who had, for years, compassionately cared for and "looked after" the elderly — those who were now too old and infirm to do so for themselves. Many of them had been accomplished and proud and now they were simply being "warehoused" until they died. Their lives were now suspended — except that their hearts still beat. Many were shattered by 'abandonment' from their "loved ones".

I spent a lot of time thinking while surrounded by them. It was hard not to when I was totally surrounded 24/7. Now I had inadvertently become one of them. How did that happen? I wanted to cry - not for myself, but for the

Chapter 41

unnamed millions who seemed to have been forgotten, and had no hope of recovering and returning to an independent life again.

Didn't they have anyone who cared? I came to wonder, in a simplistic way, if those who were diagnosed with late-stage Dementia or Alzheimer's were, perhaps, the lucky ones. They were no longer aware of their plight. They left the stress and worry to those left behind – if they were fortunate to have anyone left behind who cared. They weren't concerned any longer about how the bills would get paid, or if their children were doing well. All of that was gone. They unintentionally lived in a delusional world that they had created in their minds. They wandered aimlessly, asking the same question they had asked five minutes ago because their mind could not retain the answer that they had just given.

I recognized this first hand because I witnessed my Grandad Acie, and later my father tragically diagnosed with Dementia, after years of having countless small and seemingly insignificant TIA's (Transient Ischemic Attacks or mini-strokes.)

Dad was admitted to a nursing home in 1999, due to balancing issues initially, after the TIA's corrupted the balancing mechanism in his brain. As time marched on, he became less and less coherent. His phone conversations with me were vague and disjointed. Sometimes, when I would call him, I realized that he was talking in riddles, and did not know who I was.

At first it was infrequent, but over time it became more and more evident that he was losing his memory, and some would say "his mind." As he slipped further and further into "never-never land", I wondered if he would know me when I saw him again. It had been a while.

Finally in June of 2004, I made a trip from Florida back to Missouri.

I had mixed feelings about seeing him. I loved him as much as I had ever loved anyone. Yet, I dreaded seeing him – not knowing if he would know who I was.

I had a reverence for this man, and yet the past 27 years, since Mom's death, we had drifted apart for his self-imposed reasons, I never fully understood.

I dreaded visiting him for a lot of reasons that are very personal. (I cover in my 2nd book **A Search for Judith Ann**.)

On the one hand, I adored and revered this lion heart of a man who had raised me with steadfast loyalty, perspicacity (intelligence), rational comprehension, perseverance, honor, and compassion. These were the same qualities his patients admired in him as a compassionate and down-to-earth physician they knew.

Yankee 794 Trauma

There was nothing you could describe as "wishy-washy" about him. He had been an incredibly compassionate father, steadfast in his beliefs, as my character was being formed in the 1950's.

As a child, his six-foot, 180-pound frame towered over me, representing protection and wisdom. I adored him like no other in my life since.

At five years old, my dad could fix anything, heal any hurt, and make unpleasant things go away! He represented the morally-upright virtues that I was raised to embrace.

I knew that with God and Dad on my side, all was right with the world.

On the reverse side, my unwavering father had an uncanny ability to ostracize those who were in obvious disagreement with his beliefs. He clearly saw it as "a selection process."

Fiercely aware of what he perceived as "right" and "wrong" in God's Eyes, he taught me to respect those like-minded people who represented authority, honor, and charity. He often repeated a saying Grandma Vena, his mother, had taught him as a child.

"A bird with a broken pinion never flies so high."

I came to understand his interpretation of its meaning, and what it represented to him, as I reached (what he would have referred to as) "the age of accountability." Unfortunately, forgiveness was not a virtue high on my father's priority list.

He used this saying, **"A bird with a broken pinion never flies so high."** to reinforce his beliefs.

Ah yes! Dr. Vena Herbert Moore, my grandmother, was a remarkably strong and independent lady possessed of fortitude and perseverance, accompanied by a great faith in God.

She had been my father's savior and fortress (*from his father*) going back to childhood. Her funeral was the first I remember attending. She died when I was five in 1953.

To this day, I can still visualize that petite, vigorous, stable, self-reliant lady's looming presence. She had proudly forged her own successful path in life. Certainly, she would have been a hard act to follow!

Long before it was fashionable to educate women, she and her four sisters (Lula, Erie, Martha and Alice Herbert) were a remarkable family of doctors. Their parents have been educators and had stressed the importance and value of education for women in the 1890's. She could be a seething spitfire, and left an indelible influence on our family. (More about her and this family in my second book **_The Search for Judith Ann._**) *She was my hero.*

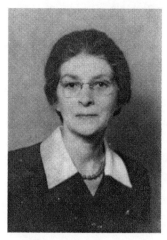

Dr. Vena Herbert Moore,
my grandmother

Grandma Vena loved riding trains, and since Grandpa Acie was a telegrapher on the railroad for many years, she rode free. It was a well-known fact that when she and Grandpa Acie would have a disagreement, she would hop a train and visit one of her four sisters, sometimes for extended periods of time. They were married for over 40 years, yet I have only two memories of seeing them together.

When I was a toddler, she would come by train and would stay two weeks with my parents and me. When she would go back to my grandparents home in Little Rock, Arkansas, she would take me with her on the train for a visit. A few days later my parents would make the trip to retrieve me.

Dad once told me, *"Betty. if there is ever a time you doubt the existence of God, just look around and see all the amazing things the man didn't create. Ask yourself how it all happened. All I had to do with delivering a baby and listen to its cry. Something had to flip a switch and turn it on. This is one of God's real miracles."*

But I digress… back to my trip to Missouri. I spent three days, staying with a friend, knowing I had to "face the music." That is the only way I can describe my feelings about visiting my father. I was compelled to visit Dad before I returned to Florida.

I dreaded going. Somehow seeing him in the flesh, knowing the fragile comings and goings of his mind was tricky for me. What I was experiencing with his mental state was best described as escaping down a rabbit hole where no one could follow.

I wanted, more than anything, to remember him as a vibrant, curious, proud and gifted man – a doctor now retired. He had a sense-of-humor that some described as dry, but my description went beyond that to *dusty.* From my earliest memories, I watched with envy as he honed this skill.

He loved working with his hands, restoring his two old cars. His first, a 1929 Model-A Coupe, he appropriately named "Henrietta". He expressed that it seemed only right since Henry Ford was her creator.

Some of the most memorable times we had together were when I was a teenager, and he would be looking for a part for an antique car that he was restoring. He invited me to accompany him to swap meets. I stood in awe of his ability to wheel-n-deal for what he knew he wanted.

He loved judging old car shows, which had been an enjoyable pastime in his retirement. He loved his woodworking shop where he created with his mind and hands when too much of the world was closing in. He loved driving his "fine automobiles" and going on trips, and enjoying the world God made.

He used to tell me in a prophetic way, *"You spend half your life acquiring all the stuff you think you can't live without, and the second half of your life getting rid of all the stuff you really never needed."*

All that was now gone (lingering only in my memories I cherished) – along with his mind, much of the time. I ached for what both of us had lost. He was now a shell of the man he had once been, as age had taken its toll – extracting its price for having lived such a long and abundant life.

He was 88 now, increasingly frail and mentally lost. There were still occasional episodes of the former man. I prayed I would glimpse him one more time with this visit. I strongly sensed it would be the last time I would see him alive.

I drove up to the building and parked my car. He had no clue I was coming. What difference now? If he was in full-blown Dementia, he would not know me. That was going to break my heart all over again. If he did know me, it would be a pleasant surprise, my visiting now.

I turned off the ignition and sat quietly for a moment, saying a prayer that no matter how I found him, I would be able to have a memorable visit. Taking a deep breath, I exited my car and slowly and deliberately made my way into the building and then to his room.

There he stood. He had yet to see me. Would I see that smile of recognition – or the look that told me, he was trying to disguise his confusion, searching his already-mostly-gone mind, attempting to find recognition for the lady standing in his doorway?

The unavoidable was now slapping me in the face. I stepped into his room.

"Dad?"

He turned to the direction of the voice, and *he lit up!*

"Betty! Well, well, what's brings you by?"

It was as though we had only just seen each other. *He knew me!* The feeling of euphoria was overwhelming.

I moved up to him, and we hugged — a long, affectionate and loving embrace. I would cherish that memory for the rest of my life. *He actually knows me!*

We sat in his room for a while chit-chatting about everything and nothing — all the stuff fathers and daughters talk about. At one point he said, *"Come with me. I want to show you something."*

Wheelchair-bound now, due to his balancing issues, he took the lead and we moved down the hall and past the nurse's station.

He led me to the other end of the lobby which was brightly lit from panorama windows that overlooked the facility's grounds. There he requested me to sit with him on a bench next to the wall.

"This is where I spend my time now...watching the birds."

As I turned around he pointed out a large glass atrium. It encompassed the entire wall behind me, floor-to-ceiling, and ten feet wide. It was massive and about three feet deep. Within were an array of brilliantly colored finches and doves, flitting about the enclosure, which had been decorated with a forest scene. He explained, *"I sit here for hours watching the birds. In Spring, they build nests and sit on eggs. When the babies hatch, I watch them as they learn to fly."*

He kept staring at the atrium and watching the many tiny birds flitting around the space. They were all quite busy with their activities, and completely oblivious to my father's intense gaze. His eyes were fixed as they followed every flutter and move.

I kept watching him and I silently cried, *"I am here with you! Can't you stop staring at those birds and just look at me. Dad, it's me. I am here with you."* I said nothing.

My mind flashed back as I remembered a time sixty years earlier when his eyes might have been fixed on his one baby bird, as she flitted around the house, or backyard, intently watching her every move.

My father, who loved TV so much, was now reduced to watching birds flittering around an enclosure because his mind could no longer follow the story line. It made me want to cry.

Those were a great few minutes as we shared memories, and we talked about everyone and no one.

Then he was gone...

I witnessed his change in his expression, his conversation, his tone, and his manner, as I gradually becoming aware of our conversation slipping away.

I pushed this shell of the man I had loved so much, back to his room, realizing that I had quickly morphed into a kind visitor whom he really did not know.

I said a loving goodbye – knowing it was most likely the last goodbye I would say to him. I sat in the parking lot, and I cried and cried for the loss

> Just when things look impossible,
> you asked for God's help,
> and thru your faith in our Heavenly Father,
> you will find that anything is possible.
> God is your vindicator,
> and God will bring the right people into your life,
> when they are required!
> What is supernatural to men,
> is simple to God.

I was now grieving. I think I cried on and off most of the drive back to Florida. I knew reality had hit me square in the face – and there was no escaping it now. To this day, when I tell the story, I still cry.

My illnesses, and that of my daughter, Barb, looked overwhelming to many people. However, we put this into God's Hands, and we trusted Him to heal us.

> *We currently stand tall today*
> *as testimony to the fact*
> *that faith works.*
>
> *Faith activates God's Power.*
>
> *I know, beyond a shadow of a doubt, that there are no limits. He controls the entire Universe. He created. It is what God calls Great Faith. All the power was in God's Hands. He spoke Worlds into existence. When you have The Faith to ask, and believe, and you realize you are not alone,*
>
> *He will show up to do Miracles.*
> *You have to take the limits off God.*
> *Your faith will help you to prosper*
> *My daughter and I are proof positive,*
> *that God can do anything you have faith to ask of Him*
>
> *He can move mountains.*

Chapter 41

As my days in rehabilitation progressed, I did one thing that kept my eye on the prize. I prayed that God would bring me back to health.

On the occasional days when my spirits were down, I would look around, and I could always find someone that was far worse off than I was. That gave me a realistic perspective on my ordeal, and where I needed to be heading — home to my life.

> "One only gets to the top rung of the ladder
> by steadily climbing up one rung at a time,
> and suddenly all sorts of powers, all sorts of abilities
> which you never thought belonged to you –
> suddenly become within your own possibility and you think,
> 'Well, I have to go too.' "
>
> Margaret Thatcher (1925-2013)

At one point, I began sitting in my wheelchair and became aware of silent conversations going on in my head with God. It went something like this:

God:
"Betty, I want you to write the book.
You know what I am talking about."

Betty:
"But God,
I have no talent to write the book
you want me to write.
You deserve magnificent. You deserve perfection.
You deserve words that will move mountains.
You'll find someone better equipped
to do the book justice, besides me."

God:
"Betty, I have already given you the way,
and you need to use what I have equipped you with."

Betty:
"But God,
I am nobody. I don't believe I can do what you
asked. I do not have self-esteem, or faith in myself, to
accomplish what you are asking. I am sure you can find
someone, that is better equipped, talented and qualified."

God:
"You have an inspirational story in your head that you have
lived. It needs to be shared. It can be an inspiration to many,
when you witness to them. You sit down at the computer,
and the words will come to you, trust me.
Have some faith in Me."

Betty:
"But God!
What if I spend a year of my life, researching and
documenting. What if I pour my heart and my soul, into this
book, you want me to write, and then I have no money to get it
published? No one will ever see it. How is that supposed to help anyone?"

God:
"You do as I ask, and have faith that in time –
the way will be made clear."

Betty:
"Okay God.
You're the boss. Show me the way."

**The moral of this story:
No one should argue with God.
You're fighting a losing battle.
He is always the winner!**

☙

Romans 10:17 (KJV)

17 "So then faith cometh by hearing, and hearing by the word of God."

☙

At the end of 6 weeks, I had made so much progress my therapists called
me "a miracle." I really didn't understand what all the fuss was about. After all, I
felt that if I could do this, anyone could do this. Maybe they just underestimated
me? All my life people have been doing that, so it was not all that surprising.

God gave me the strength and I gave God the glory!

Nothing happens randomly.

Chapter 41

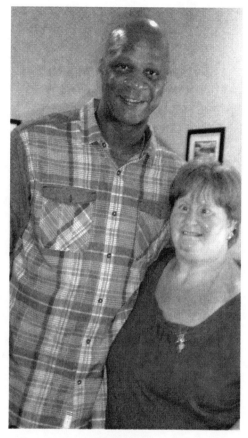

June 2014
Barb with Darryl Strawberry

"The key is recognizing that you
are more beautiful than you dare to
imagine and that you have to be
afraid of nothing in sharing
yourself with the world."

Timothy Shriver

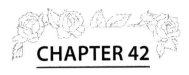

CHAPTER 42

Four goals for a meaningful life:
seek out a need of the world work, forget self, trust God.

Jennie Fowler Willing
(B: 1834 – D: 1916)

Words, Deeds, and Promises

"Things That Are Taught and Things That Are Caught."

June 2014 – May 2015

While still in recovery from the "double whammy", I'd began to consider my future and the fact that both Barb and I were going to live.

Barb had come through more than four years of recovery and was still progressing, and it seemed to me she represented a testament to God's Grace and healing power.

I had begun working on writing this book. The two of us were attending church regularly, and living in a three bedroom apartment in midtown.

With the exception of me acting as her chauffeur to doctor's appointments, shopping, and SCIL, Barb was almost entirely independent, except for an occasional fall.

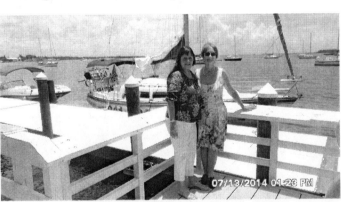

My fabulous friend, Jacqueline Cook with me June 2014. We drove out to Anna Maria Island, Florida

I decided that I would turn this over to God, and see if He had anyone in my future who would be *"the right one"* with whom I might share my life.

Chapter 42

He obviously had a plan for me, and if I needed to find a meaningful future with a partner, He would be leading the way.

It's called Blind Faith.

I was having one of my frequent chats with God when I challenged Him.

"As you know God, my luck with Love does not seem to be very efficient or accurate. Perhaps my priorities are misplaced. I am giving this over to you.

If there is a partner with whom you think I should share my life, I am through trying to do this by myself. You need to bring him to me. Amen."

I had given a great deal of thought to what I wanted and needed in a partner. More importantly, what I did *not* want, was also on my list. I spent some time crafting a number of personal advertisement which I put on the internet, along with a current photo.

It read:

Critical Spirit Need Not Apply — 65 (Bradenton)

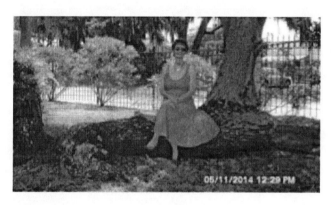

Read my profile… it was thoughtfully written.

If you feel we are a match, then contact me with your favorite food in the header.

Facts about me:

I am single and sincere. You must also be.

I'm a cancer survivor and consider each day I wake up, a Gift from God.

FREE of gambling, drugs and smoking. You must be as well.

Rarely consume alcohol; only on special occasions and then in moderation.

I was widowed at 29 and raised three children.

They are now responsible and productive adults.

I have dedicated the majority of my life to a career in healthcare.

I am a practicing Christian, who deserves a partner who is also a practicing Christian, and is willing to attend every Sunday services with me.

One who lives by The Golden Rule and desires a partner who understands that.

He must understand the need for "random acts of kindness" when appropriate.

I seek a one-woman-man who believes that means a monogamous relationship.

I am an avid news watcher, both morning, and evening, and so I am able to carry on an intelligent conversation.

I thrive when confronted with a stimulating conversation on many topics.

I am an animal and parrot lover (ran a parrot rescue for 6 years) who is a country girl at heart.

I believe that secrecy, in a relationship, will foretell its downfall.

My heart is waiting for that 60+ romantic, considerate, financially responsible, trustworthy, reliable, dedicated partner, who seeks a lady who is his equal.

__His goal__: to make that lady feel so loved and cherished that when they walk into a room with 1000 other people, there is not one woman in that room who feels more valued behind closed doors

__Definition of Fun__: Farmers markets, bar-b-ques, estate sales, garage sales, sailing, day trips, photography, animals, volunteering, cruises and watching TV with my favorite person!

__Music preferences__: Country (old and new), Oldies, Big Band Era… No Rap!

I enjoy expressing my Art (pastels, chalk, charcoal, acrylic painting) when I feel creative & need to relax. I also have taken classes in stained glass construction and knew how to lay tile and hardwood floors.

__He must__: seek a LTR (long-term relationship) with a genuine marriage partner. (Not commitment-phobic.)

Willing to help around the house. An honorable and creative cook is a big plus! Seafood and bar-b-ques are my favorites.

He should understand the need for nurturing the passion for the things she loves, such as creative ART. In turn, I will respond in kind.

A man willing to play (or learn) Canasta is another big plus.

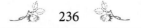

Chapter 42

He needs to understand that a willing and joyful heart is the key to living day-by-day.

I belong to a non-denominational Christian church whose primary focus is not on the "legalese" of religion but rather on community service and the individual. I do volunteer for them when there is a need – which is much of the time.

My photo was taken Mother's Day 2014, and so is current.

PLEASE do not answer this ad if you are a SCAMMER. I know the signs.

PLEASE only answer this ad if you feel we might be a MATCH for an LTR.

The result of my advertisement?

I must have gotten, literally, about 100 responses to the ad over the next few weeks. I laughed because the red dress seemed to take on a life of its own. It developed its own fan club, which I found more than a bit amusing!

Some men wrote me and rudely told me (in no uncertain terms) that I was too old and set in my ways and I should just give up and get over it. I was a way to bossy and no man worth his salt would answer such an advertisement.

Among the ones who responded including one from a 4-Star Army General, who "claimed" to be divorced with one son. He was retiring after a 38-year career, and was willing to relocate if he found "the right companion."

This peaked my curiosity. I took the detailed two-page letter and the photo he sent, and I Googled him. I discovered the *true* 4-Star Army general was *very much* married with 4 daughters. That was a not-so-subtle giveaway. At one point, it occurred to me that The Pentagon, where he worked, might find this "impostor" interesting to investigate.

I read and reread the letters which came in my e-mail from all over the US, as well as Americans claiming they were living/working in several other countries.

Occasionally, I even got one who sounded as if his first language might have been English! To say the least, it was a mixed bag. Fortunately, I had the time to deal with this.

I embarked on this venture knowing, that although I was likely to get many responses, frauds abounded, and impostors were clever. I made it my business to find the words and phrases that were a tip off – and I watched diligently for those. I investigated.

I also felt that I had to "put myself out there" in order for God to be joined with His choice of partners. I had never been one to hang out in bars or clubs. I do not drink alcohol nor smoke and did not want this man to do so either.

I preferred a widower who could grasp the commitment of staying for the long haul and missed having a companion.

How was he supposed to find me? It all boils down to one word: *FAITH* I was sure if it were meant to happen, God could make it so.

It was a well-guarded secret that there were a few ground rules that were not in my advertisement:

1. The man had to be a Christian and attend church regularly with me, as well as in the way he lived his life.

2. I was not having sex or co-cohabiting with any man until and unless we were married.

3. He needed to *volunteer* the fact that, "Your daughter will always have a place to live," and they would have to learn to love and respect one another.

I felt that if I could find *this* man – maybe, just maybe, we could look at a future together. I felt the chances were remote – but worth waiting for *if he existed*.

"Oh and by-the-way God, if he happens to be an IT guy, it won't hurt!"

One day after running several ads. on Craiglist, I opened my e-mail, and there was a letter from a man who lived in Cape Cod, Massachusetts. Keep in mind, I was in Bradenton, Florida.

To The Lady Posting on Craiglist:

Thank you for your latest posting. Not to scare you, but I have been following your posts....

They continue to intrigue me for various reasons.

First of all, we seem to both be seeking the same thing... companionship and love (LTR).

To introduce myself, my name is Thomas, and I presently am staying at my home on Cape Cod in Massachusetts. I am in the process of transitioning back to Florida. In fact, I have recently returned here to Massachusetts after purchasing a "fixer-upper" mobile home in Bradenton, FL.

I am 66 years old but have my next birthday early in August.

I am widowed. My late wife passed away five years ago after a long, but courageous battle with cancer. We lived in Bradenton, Florida for five years, and I got accustomed to the area. That's why I am returning.

My favorite food is Chicken Salad. I grew up on steaks and potato, but for my health I need to continue to improve my diet.

I am a Christian man. Let me put it this way, my faith and belief is strong, but currently my practice is weak. I would be happy to escort you to church. My late wife encouraged me to become Catholic, by the example of her strong faith.

Canasta – I have not played in many years, but would look forward to relearning the game.

I would certainly promote and encourage your passion for art.

Sorry, but I'm not much of a cook. We can work on that.

I promise to hold no secrets from you.

Well, I have told you a little about me. If any of this intrigues you let me know.

Sincerely, Thomas

I read and reread his response to my personal ad, and I found myself fascinated. He had included a good deal of significant information. Certainly there was enough for me to chew on and digest. There was something "different" about him. He was widowed in Jan. 2009, and was now retired from Massachusetts Mutual Insurance Company, where he was *an IT subcontractor.*

He was a Vietnam veteran, just turning 67 in August, and was tired of being alone. I was 66. Statically, the odds of either of us finding a compatible companion were not in our favor, but *that's for people who don't know what happens when you team up with God!*

Tom's wife of 16 years had died of cancer in January 2009. He, too, had been diagnosed with cancer — and had survived.

At this point in his life, he had been finalizing a decision to sell his home on Cape Cod, where he had spent a lot of his life, and move to the town where I lived. What were the odds of that?

We both had grown children and grandchildren, and we valued the worth of family and friends… so I responded, and he wrote again. That is how my relationship with Thomas John Leab began.

Early in our e-mail conversations, I discovered that he had been living in Bradenton from 2001 – 2006 with his late wife, Mary Ellen. He had fallen in love with the area and the semi-tropical climate.

Yankee 794 Trauma

When Mary Ellen became ill, she was initially misdiagnosed. She insisted on returning home to her family in Connecticut, to see her doctors there. Pursuing a further diagnosis, it was discovered she to have advancing colon cancer.

Mary Ellen died in January 2009, at the age of 49, after a valiant fight with stage 4 colon cancer, leaving Tom alone.

To keep himself busy and active, Tom had joined Lion's Club in Cape Cod. He was an active member, working to promote and serve their cause. For the past four years, he had kept busy fixing friend's computers and joining other charitable endeavors.

It was readily apparent that he had a caring and compassionate heart, and he fully understood the implications and complications of long-term relationship — on both the part of my daughter and myself, as well as the special considerations required.

At first our correspondence was all by e-mail but it was not long until we were on the phone talking and laughing, and getting to know each other. Conversations were remarkably easy. *Perhaps* we could be friends when he moved back to my area. Still, I was skeptical.

I had been "the fixer" of all things that went wrong, and I was forever frustrated and wanted that role to change with no idea how that would happen. I look back and realize that I had taken my parent's motto of, "The only value you have in this life, is the value in serving others," and twisted it to suit my own interpretation without being aware of how I had inadvertently chosen to apply it.

"There are things that are taught, and things that are caught."

I guess this one fell under the later. I had, for years, offered nearly unconditional pardon and acquittal to friends and family, and chosen to overlook many troublesome and annoying characteristics of those who kept creating problems and drama in my life. I made excuses for my "frenemies" – (people whom I saw as friends, but who, in fact, were counter-productive) to my becoming who I needed to be in order to reach my full potential in God's world. I needed to separate myself from that bad habit and to get on with where my life was now heading. Really, it was a simple process once I realized where I was going.

My unspoken expectations only serve to disappoint. I had come to realize that if I had no expectations, I couldn't be disappointed with the behavior of others. I had learned through many years of disappointment and broken promises, not to get excited about "events to come." I came to realize and understand that my "near-death" experience was a powerful turning point in my life.

I remember Oprah Winfrey advising once, *"never lend money."* She had gone on to explain that if a person came to you and asked to borrow money, never do that because it sets up an expectation that the money will be paid back. If you have the money to loan, and you feel that the person is sincere, give the money to them as a gift. *Never anticipate they will return the money.* If they sincerely can and want to pay you back, they will. But if you expect the money to be returned, and they don't return it; *you will likely lose that friendship.*

The same is true of favors and advice. So I began to give advice only when asked, and I did favors when I saw benefit as **a random act of kindness.**

Once you discover the true spirit and gift of giving, you will find joy in serving others for the act in itself.

Charity for the sake of giving is its own reward.

The primary thing to remember in charity is that *all we have belongs to God, and all we give is a response to His love for us (1 John 4:19).*

When we see our resources not only as God's provision for us but as tools He desires us to use to care for others; we begin to understand the vastness of His love and sovereignty. As spiritual children of Abraham, "We, too, are blessed to be a blessing" (Genesis 12:1-3).

We are invited into relationship with God and with His people. When we care for those He loves we care for Him.

> *"Give, and it will be given to you.*
> *A good measure, pressed down, shaken together and*
> *running over, will be poured into your lap.*
> *For with the measure you use, it will be measured to you."*
>
> *(Luke 6:38)*

I was emotionally exhausted by the role I had unconsciously misunderstood and backed into many years earlier.

I had stepped up many times in situations where others seemed to lack that ability or desire. One person's neediness was starting to look unremarkable and indistinguishable from another – and I found myself moving to create distance from this trap, as I recovered from cancer.

People's under-developed sense of loyalty, perseverance and *downright ignorance of what they don't know that they don't know,* was undisputed.

It had begun to irritate me, like an itch that I could not scratch.

I had found a kind of serenity — a new maturity. I didn't feel better or stronger than anyone else however it seemed no longer important whether everyone loved me or not. My need to be needed took on a new and more prominent role — in an entirely different way, and *I stopped being a people-pleaser!*

One person told me in an accusing tone, *"You have changed in the past six months!"*

My reply was, *"Yes, I am different. Things feel different now that I finally got my priorities straight."*

She was not happy that I was not offended by her observation and gave me a rather annoyed look. Her reaction did not phase me and when I stopped to reflect. *I realized that I had changed*.

Many Christians use the "tithe" (ten percent of income) as a reference point for their giving. This is fine as long as it's understood God has the right to request more of us besides financial giving.

Your tithe can also be in the form of giving of time and personal physical resources such as energy. God designed us to possess so many more resources than our wealth in spendable cash. He intended us to *spend time and energy to help those* who are less fortunate than ourselves.

Maybe it could be as simple as running into a friend or family member and sensing they are having a bad day. Using your time (God gave you) to lend a sympathetic and compassionate ear when you really felt you could not spare the time is a form of tithing. Who know? Perhaps their day was turning into a lemon, and your giving of your time turned it into lemonade!

Can you imagine how different our world (God's world) would look if everyone would climb on board this concept enthusiastically, and a truly giving heart, spending God's resources giving back to his or her local community?

Barb has 60 days out of her life where she has no memory. I experienced waking up to find I had no memory of three weeks out of my life. In each case what happened to us was astonishingly unexpected and sudden, and there was a point in time where each of us could (and should) have died – according to the calculations of man's world.

When you come back from "a near-death experience", you realize *time and energy are precious*, and not to be wasted.

Having been faced with sudden death, as well as significantly diminished energy and time and having to fight my our back, Barb and I realized the value of these which fall into the category of "God's currency." I now understood that I had "misspent" much of the currency God had given me throughout my life.

I became less tolerant of those who see themselves as 'victims,' as I distanced myself and my previous surroundings from drama every time I saw it coming. I began to close ranks to include fewer and fewer people as close friends – and acquaintances became primarily members of my church family and organizations where I chose to volunteer.

I found I paid very close attention to the people that entered my life now. I have become acutely aware of a small and but significant and vibrant few of them who were there because they have a message to bring to me – or they have a purpose in impacting my life. The rest come and go.

Time, energy, talent and endurance (health) are authentic gifts from God. They allow a person to move about our world seeking a way to distribute God's gift to others.

How you choose to spend God's time, and energy is how you will measure your ability to spend the resources you possess through Almighty God. Choosing to seek out ways to spend God's currency (time and energy) he has given you, is no different that the change you carry around in your pocket. It is spendable currency and must be given thoughtfully. *This too is a form of tithing.*

Barb and I volunteered at our church first in organizing a new thrift shop and then organizing the church kitchen. We also work with Welcome, Auditorium, and Nourish (food giveaway) Ministry Teams. Where we saw a need, we tried to fill it.

We discovered joy.

I had been raised by Christian parents in "the church" and was saved when I was sixteen. My children had been raised in the church. However, as the kids left home, and I experienced a type of "Empty Nest Syndrome", I became a bit indifferent and had spent years trying to find my own way.

When Barb survived what should have been a fatal auto accident, and then I survived what should have been a death sentence from stage four cancer, plus another close call with The Grim Reaper, I felt that God was trying to give me a message. I thought I had better "listen up" and heed the call, whatever that was. Apparently God had something in mind I had yet to fulfill before my life was done.

ℒ

"More important now, was for me to love them.

Sincerely feeling that way
turns your whole life around;
living becomes the act of giving.
When I do a performance now,
I still need and like the adulation of an audience,
of course, but my real satisfaction comes from what I
have given of myself,
from the joyful act of singing itself."

Beverly Sills
(B: 1929 D: 2007)

ℒ

When Barb felt comfortable staying alone for a few hours, I joined a creative writing group, as I began writing this book. Occasionally she would attend with me. I also stepped up my acrylic painting, which brought a new-found joy and relaxation to my life.

I refused to step into situations and be the peacemaker, just for the comfort of others. The natural progression of this resulted in bringing order and tranquil prayer into my world. I deliberately elected to distance myself from allowing disruption and chaos near my and Barb's world.

There were people in my life who felt that I had turned against them. Most of them were addicted to the adrenaline rush of turmoil and histrionics. For many years, I accepted drama as an unavoidable part of my life – not realizing that certain people around me were intentionally creating and feeding on it.

I chose to open my eyes and see who was disrupting our lives, and I evaporated from their lives as we turned toward new people, new goals, and new adventures, searching out what God's Will was for our lives. In fact, all I had really done was quietly turned away from what I no longer wanted –— turmoil and disruption —- and those who were the center of it. My change in my perception quieted my surroundings. It was a conscious and authentic decision I made, as I built on my inner strength. I now viewed my place in the world differently.

Barb and I were alive, and it was not to be wasted on nonsense!

I found making mindful, and deliberate choices allowed God to remedy past behaviors, bringing people into my life that enriched both of us.

Chapter 42

God's true character came to me in a message one Sunday when Pastors Ralph and Joanne Hoehne explained:

Omni-potent

The ability and power to do anything.

Everything is in harmony with God's perfection. His power flows through us — His believers — who exercise free will. However, when God gives us free will, there can be consequences in our imperfect world. Satan does not create anything. Satan can only imitate.

God is big enough to handle all our problems.

Omnis-stent

He knows all.

There's no hiding from God in shame or anguish. If you come to Him and ask, He will forgive you. He can fully navigate you. God does not always tell us the overview — but God knows what your future holds.

Omni-present

He is everywhere at all times

God is always watching and is willing, ready and able to meet you – when you go to Him. God loves us intimately. There is no running from God. You do not have to go through rituals to reach God. Quietly go and ask. He is always there to hear and answer your prayer

Omni-benelivant

John 3:16-18 (KJV)

[16] For God so loved the world that He gave His only begotten Son, that whosoever believeth in him should not perish, but have everlasting life.

[17] For God sent not His Son into the world to condemn the world; but that the world through Him might be saved.

[18] He that believeth on Him is not condemned: but He that believeth not is condemned already, because he hath not believed in the name of the only begotten Son of God."

**If He did not love what He had created,
He would have hit the "reset" button long ago.**

If we are not living in His Love, it is our fault. God came to give you life and life abundantly. In the same way parents set rules for a child's protection, we are God's Children, and he sets rules for our protection not for our misery.

God is amazing, promising to give us life in eternity. God's Grace is available anytime you ask Him for forgiveness. He is slow to anger and has mercy and compassion — because He knows our every flaw and imperfection we possess. If we confess our sins, He will forgive — **no matter what the sin is.**

If there is a void in your life, He can heal your broken heart and forgive your sins. He is big enough to handle all our problems. In order to allow forgiveness —*remember something had to die.*

One night I voiced this to Tom. His response was one that came from a man with courage, self-worth and conviction — a man of few words.

ৼ

WORDS

Words are the most powerful weapon we possess.

Words can kill a spirit or make it soar.

Words can magnify good or evil.

Words can give knowledge and provide insight.

Words can undercut a well-meaning act to the core —
taking all positive meaning away.

Words can give insight into the very heart
of who a person truly is.

All you have to do is cultivate
the ability to stop and listen —-
to be a compassionate communicator.

When words are chosen with thought
and with healing, giving spirit –

They can signify a path for change in your life
and that of those you influence.

Author: Unknown

ৼ

I sensed a quiet, steadfast leadership, as well as guidance in this modest man, who knew how to guide his compassionate heart. He was centered with confidence in his own identity, *"You are going to find out I am the real deal,"* he told me. My response was, *"I certainly hope so."*

With that, I said good night over the phone.

Chapter 42

There was an unexplained and unmistakable peace that came over me with his few well-chosen words that I found reassuring and comforting. It was almost like an invisible safety net had been dropped over me to cover and protect me. The idea that God might have brought this man to me was more than I could have ever hoped for!

One evening, early in our conversations Tom asked, *"What are you doing with yourself since you aren't working?"*

Almost without giving it a second thought, I said,

"I am writing a book."

"You are writing a book?" he repeated in a surprised tone.

"Yep, I am," I acknowledged.

"What's the book about?" he quizzed.

I began to explain to him what my memoir was about. His next statement stunned me.

"What if I publish your book for you?" he asked.

I sat in silence remembering back to the conversation I had with God sitting in rehab all those months ago when He told me,

"You write the book, and I will make a way for it to be published."

"Well, let me send some of it to you by email. You read it and see what you think," I replied.

As the days progressed, e-mails were flying back and forth. We compared notes on fundamental values, and he asked to read more and more of my writing.

I watched Tom with his quiet steadfastness and resilient spirit. He had a spontaneity that mirrored mine. I would throw out some dry sarcasm — a gift I had developed at the feet of my father, and he turned into it without hesitation, responding with some unexpected bit of humor or wisdom that made me smile.

Occasionally, he would erupt with an unmistakable pearl of wisdom that made me stop and think, *"Who is this guy—really? Seriously... seriously God?"*

We found we agreed on most everything fundamentally significant for a meaningful relationship. We found the same things to be nonsense, and we laughed a lot which, we all know is good for the soul.

He told me one Sunday afternoon in July, *"Now if I could just sell my house, I would be on my way to Florida – and my new life. I guess I should call the realtor and get a sign placed in my front yard."*

My response was, *"Tom, all you have to do is turn it over to God. Pray about this."*

Tom took my suggestion to heart. He hung up the phone and said a prayer. No one in his neighborhood knew he was considering selling his home.

Two hours later a young man knocked on Tom's door. He was inquiring whether Tom's house was for sale. His parents lived next door, and he was newly married. He wanted it for a summer home.

It took no more than a couple of weeks for them to come to an agreement! Tom was apparently selling his house "as is." Tom's money was in his hands, and he was overjoyed! He never even had to go through a realtor. *He simply opened that door with Faith and a prayer – and God answered.*

He called his attorney friend who specialized in real estate law and asked him to draw up the papers. It was a done deal.

Tom wrote me and asked, *"I've made the trip to and from Florida and I hate driving alone. If I send you a plane ticket, will you fly up here, and drive back with me?"*

I had never even *met* this man. I had to think long and hard about such a move. I do admit deep down; I am the perpetual optimist.

I would have to make arrangements, so there would be friends checking in on Barb. I had been a protective Mother Hen, keeping my chick under my wing. I had never gone away and left her since her accident, three and a half years ago. This would be a real trial by fire for both of us, yet I knew she was now independent enough that she and I could do this — with the help of concerned neighbors and friends. There was also her sister living only a few blocks away checking in.

Tom offered to fly me from Bradenton-Sarasota International Airport through Atlanta, and on to Providence-Hartford, Connecticut. where he would meet me. He then suggested, *"Half way through the drive back to Florida, we should 'take a break.'"*

I looked at the map and suggested that we do The Smithsonian in D.C. He countered with, *"How about Nashville?"*

I was puzzled and stopped to ponder and ask, *"Since when is Nashville half way between Cape Cod and Bradenton?"*

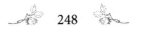

Chapter 42

"I don't care! I want to go to The Grand Ole Opry!" came back the answer. Being a big fan of country music also, I was sold immediately!

Spontaneity is a big factor in my life — and it would need to be one of the traits I would seek in a new partner, whomever I envisioned as that partner. I agreed to fly up and drive back with him.

Tom ordered a new car, and we agreed it should be blue metallic. He took delivery just four days before my arrival.

My daughter Andrea, delivered me to the airport in time to make the 6:00 AM flight. I am happy to report my flight was uneventful.

Tom and I spent the next four days packing up his house and loading his car. He also took me whale-watching, sailing out of Cape Cod, which was an incredible adventure. I think I suspected then that he may have fallen in love with me, but we never discussed it. We just became friends.

We decided to drive to Hershey, Pa. and take the tour, as well as go to the antique car museum. We walked through The Hershey Company's gift shop, and the smell of chocolate was intoxicating. I had never before been surrounded in all directions by chocolate! I could cross THAT off my bucket list. This was better than any perfume shop I had ever visited! I guess you could describe me as *"a kid in a candy store."* I was smitten.

Once we arrived in Nashville, we visited The Parthenon, and took in The Grand Ole Opry on Friday night with reserved seats.

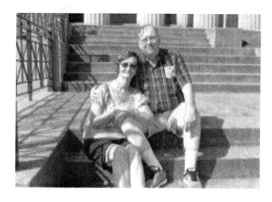

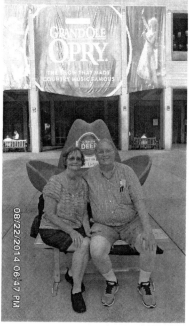

When we got to Atlanta, Ga. we toured the world-famous Aquarium, before returning to Bradenton.

All of this was shared with photos for friends on our Facebook pages. While driving for hours, we talked, laughed and began to get to know each other on a far more emotionally intimate level.

By the time we reached Bradenton, we felt like old familiar friends who had just reconnected after years of separation.

I was raised Baptist, and Tom's parents did not attend church. He had converted to Buddhism when he married his first wife who was a native of Thailand after serving in Vietnam. When they divorced in 1990, and then he met Mary Ellen, he converted to The Catholic faith when he married her in 1994.

I had mentioned to him earlier, that he could go to his computer while he was still living in Cape Cod, and follow the same Sunday morning service I was attending. He began to watch our services from Cape Cod. *http://www.tapintothesource.com* with my Pastors Ralph and Joanne Hoehne each Sunday.

When we arrived back in Bradenton, he began to attend with me each Sunday and started to make friends with this church and community. It was not long before he was volunteering to help when the church needed volunteers and then was ask to step up to be co-head of Nourish, our church's food giveaway. He couldn't get over the vibrant and thriving youth ministry that we had developed as a vital part of our church ministry, along with community outreach.

❧

We hate "religion" but we love The Lord.

❧

THE SOURCE CHURCH

Bradenton, Florida is a non-denominational Christian church

http:///www.tapintothesouce.com

The following is copied/pasted from The Source website:

Chapter 42

We believe
that the Bible is God's Word.
It is accurate, authoritative and applicable to our everyday lives.

We believe
in one eternal God, who is the Creator of all things.
He exists in three Persons:
God the Father,
God the Son and
God the Holy Spirit.
He is totally loving and completely holy.
We believe that sin has separated each of us from
God and His purpose for our lives.

We believe
that the Lord Jesus Christ as both God
and man is the only One, who can reconcile us to God.
He lived a sinless and exemplary life, died on the cross in our place,
and rose again to prove His victory and empower us for life.

We believe
the church functions through representation
of all the spiritual gifts given by the Holy Spirit.

We believe
in divine healing through the prayer of faith,
laying on of hands, and anointing with oil for all believers today.
We believe in the baptism of the Holy Spirit.

We believe
that faith and obedience are the doors to all of God's blessings.
God desires to bless us in each and every area of our lives with abundance.

Yankee 794 Trauma

We believe
in water baptism and in the regular taking of Communion as an act of remembering what the Lord Jesus did for us on the cross.

We want you to realize the truth of Jeremiah 29:11

"I know the plans I have for you."
said the Lord.
"Plans to prosper you, and not to harm you.
To give you hope and a future."

❧

Tom had been sitting alone in Massachusetts talking to God about finding a companion, at the same time that I had. The more time we spent together, the more we realized there was no doubt God had brought us together.

I constantly remained vigilant of his attitude and treatment of me as a person — as well as female. At every opportunity, he treated me with dignity and respect — and I returned the gesture.

Tom began attending my creative writing meetings with me, and I started attend his Lion's Club meetings with him.

When our discussions began to inch toward talk of a more permanent arrangement as a couple, I told him that I thought a man choosing an engagement/wedding ring for a woman was ridiculous. After all, she has to love it and wear it — not him. I also told him I wanted a "proper wedding" with friends and family gathered in our church. He agreed.

Tom voiced concerns that my three children be agreeable to our marriage. My son had been deployed to Iraq in October 2014. Tom spoke to him on instant messenger on Facebook. He wanted them to get acquainted, before asking for my hand.

With both my parents having passed away, he felt he should ask for my son's permission for my hand. I thought that was outstanding that Tom was concerned about my family's acceptance, and an enormous step in the right direction. He understood the value of being part of my family. He wanted my children's blessing, and he got it!

One of the discussions we had been our fundamental belief about the distribution of wealth.

"Money is never to be squandered or spent ostentatiously. Some of the greatest people in history have lived lives of the greatest simplicity. Remember, it's you inside that counts. Money doesn't give you any license to relax. It gives you an opportunity to use all your abilities, free of financial worries, to go forward, and to use your superior advantages and talent to help others."

Rose Fitzgerald Kennedy (B: 1890–D: 1995)

Oct. 30, 2014 – Tom asked me to marry him. I accepted.

I joked that I did not want him to get down on one knee, due to age and health issues because I was afraid he would never be able to get up! We made the same joke about him carrying me across the threshold after we were married. We agreed that those traditions are for the young (with good backs and knees), and I would forgive him for breaking tradition. After all he was 67, and I was 66.

We went together to choose my ring. It is a magnificent top-quality one karat Marquis diamond with a halo of diamonds around it. It was breathtaking, and I wear it with pride!

He had asked me to accompany him to New Orleans, La. for a few days to attend a family gathering on March 26-27, 2015. He didn't have to ask twice. New Orleans is one of my favorite cities in the whole world!

When I asked him how long he thought we should be engaged before we marry, his answer was immediate.

"I think we should be married before we go to New Orleans."

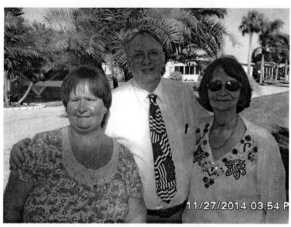

By then we would have known each other nine months. We figured if nine months was long enough for God to grow a whole baby, it should be long enough for two senior citizens to start a meaningful and lasting relationship. Besides, I used to tell inquiring minds, *"If we wait too long, we will both be dead!"*

2014 — *Our first Thanksgiving together.*

I sometimes would add, *"Tom and I have talked about almost everything. We just haven't decided how many children we want yet!" That would usually bring a chuckle.*

We set the wedding date for Sunday, February 15, 2015, at 1:00 PM at our church, The Source. Tom agreed to pay for everything – and he kept his word. I asked Barb to be my Maid-of-Honor, and she agreed.

Now the challenge was getting my tomboy daughter in a dress! That turned out to be the biggest challenge of all! We finally accomplished that after 10 stores in three weeks! For Barb, shopping is like watching paint dry. After all *we came as a "package deal" — Barb and me.*

Even though we had both jokingly expressed a fear of her falling on her face trying to navigate the four steps at the front of the sanctuary, that fear faded when Jeff, Barb's best friend, agreed to escort her up the aisle as Tom's best man. I knew I could trust Jeff *never* to let Barb fall.

In January, we sent out invitations to friends and family. Our church bulletin carried an open invitation for the church congregation to join in our special day. "No gifts expected."

Pastor Ralph remarked that he felt a lot of the congregation would attend because, he reasoned, *"You know women are suckers for a wedding, and a great piece of cake!"*

Our colors for our wedding were our favorites: Blue — with white and aqua accents.

Our co-pastors, Ralph and Joanne Hoehne, agreed to perform the ceremony. Tom and I wrote our entire wedding ceremony including our vows. Rather than the traditional wedding music – we chose YouTube music videos that had words which were meaningful to us as a couple.

With my son, Mark, overseas and unable to attend to give me away, it was suggested we have him SKYPE in for the ceremony. The problem was we had no I-Pad, and we were not sure where to get one.

The day of the meeting to finalize wedding plans with the pastors, we walked away unsure of how to accomplish this. I prayed that somehow this could be accomplished. It meant a lot to have my son with us that day. Having all three of my (adult) children present was the ultimate goal! The answer came in a very unexpected way.

God again stepped in and answered our need.

Being a TBI survivor, Barb had been put on a list of which we were totally

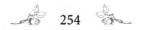

254

unaware. There was a group in Colorado that refurbishes and gifts I-Pad's to TBI patients. To this day, we have no clue how they got her name.

Immediately following the meeting at the church, when Barb opened her e-mail there was correspondence from an organization saying, *"You are next on our list to receive an I-Pad. We need confirmation that you still want the I-Pad and a current address."*

Barb was astonished. She returned her response with a resounding "Yes!" and our current mailing address. The next day she got a conformation e-mail with a tracking number for the package that had been shipped to her.

She wrote back to ask, *"How long have I been on your waiting list?"* and discovered it had been nearly three years. She has no clue how she ended up on a waiting list from a group in Colorado that works with people that have TBI when we live in Florida.

The timing could not have been more perfect. The I-Pad, a 2012 4th generation with a leather carrying case, arrived looking like new.

God showed up again – just as we were praying for some way that my son, Mark, who was half way around the world, could be at my wedding, to give me away.

As was to be expected, glitches showed up, and *so did God*.

Two weeks before our wedding, just when it appeared every detail of our wedding was finalized, the photographer totaled her car and had to cancel!

Barb and I put out a request on Facebook for recommendations for a replacement. The next day we found one that was available on our day, Joni Dusek! www.jonidusekphotography.com

She was a professional photographer with 20 years of experience, from Sarasota. Her husband was an author with a ministry taking them worldwide. Our story touched Joni's heart. What a gift that turned out to be – *God working in mysterious ways* – again!

February 9, 2015 — Tom and I applied for and received our marriage license today.

Everything seemed to be pretty much on schedule. Honeymoon reservations and plans completed for Marathon Key, Florida.

One day I told Tom on the phone,

"I am feeling a little funny."

"What do you mean?" he inquired.

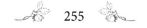

"You know... wedding is getting close."

"Butterflies?" he asked.

"Yes, I guess," I responded.

His comeback was, *"Oh I have the exterminator here. I will ask him what we do."*

Since this was not my first marriage, I chose a sapphire blue floor-length dress that was embellished with crystals at the waist.

My choice of flowers were dark red roses, (in memory of my mother).

Tom and I were married.

DATE: February 15, 2015 @ 1 PM
LOCATION: THE SOURCE CHURCH,
5412 East SR 64, Bradenton, Florida 34208

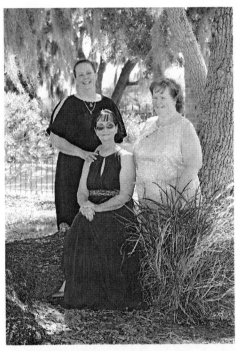

Andrea and Barb behind me.

Having my beautiful daughters with me on my wedding day to Tom meant so much!

Chapter 42

The ceremony included U-Tube Music Videos:
"Everything Happens For A Reason"
"When You Say Nothing At All" — Allison Kraus
"My Valentine" — Martine McBride & Jim Brinkman
"The Prayer" — Celine Dion & Josh Groban
"You'll Be In My Heart" — Phil Collins

The reception followed in an adjoining room, and everyone had amazing wedding cake and Ginger Ale. One of the wonderful ladies at our church, Kim

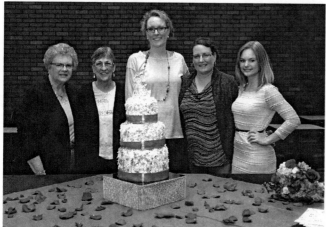

George, agreed to make us a three tiered coconut cake, my favorite, as the centerpiece of the reception.

A crystal bride and groom stood at the top of our cake. Ginger

Linda, Cam, Kim, Kalley, Rachel

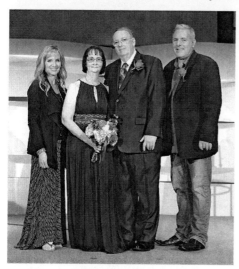

Pastors Ralph and Joanne Hoehne after our wedding.

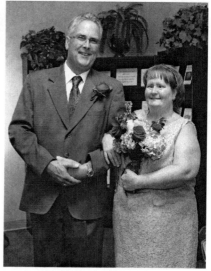

Jeff Valpel and Barb after our wedding.

Ale, I later presented each of them an acrylic painting I created, as a token of my appreciation.

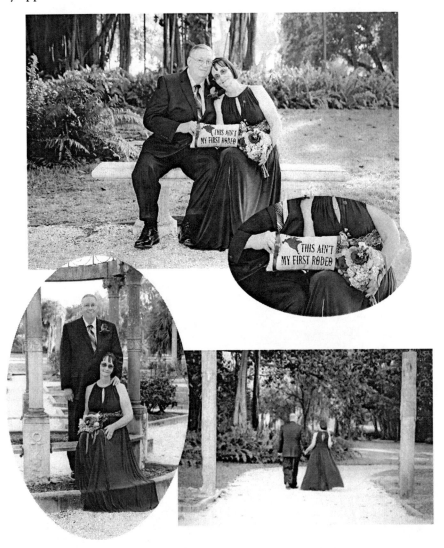

Following that, twenty-four close friends and family members joined us at a local restaurant for dinner.

Then we departed for formal portraits at The John & Mabel Ringling Estate in Sarasota, where the 100-year-old Banyan Trees and Rose Garden make for a perfect backdrop for wedding photos. The weather turned out amazingly perfect.

Chapter 42

Tom and I decided to spend the night in town because we were both exhausted from the full day of activities.

The following morning we left for a week-long honeymoon in The Florida Keys. Tom had never driven to The Keys, and I feel everyone should have that experience at least once. The drive is scenic and spectacular. Leave it to us to have picked the coldest days since records have been kept: 42 degrees and the wind blowing at 25 MPH. We did have a room with an ocean view.

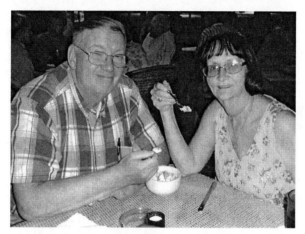

Tom and me on our honeymoon in The Keys.
As is traditional we were consuming Key Lime Pie.

Not long after we got back from our honeymoon, Tom sponsored me to be a member of Lion's Club International/Bradenton Chapter. This was just after he became Membership Chairman.

On March 25, 2015, we left for New Orleans and stayed at the Sheraton/ Metairie. Tom's family was waiting to welcome us when we arrived, and they treated me as "the newest bride" in The Beckwith Family.

Our time was memorable. Tom had never been to New Orleans, and it is one of my favorite cities. I had the privilege of going with him on the two-hour trip south to Venice, LA to experience a boat tour of The Beckwith Family Trust holdings in The Gulf of Mexico.

Introducing him to the incredible hospitality of the people who have lived in that area for generations was a highlight of our trip.

Early Sunday morning we headed for The French Quarter and sampled New Orleans's famous Beignets at the word famous Café D. Monde in The French Quarter. We stopped to enjoy the variety of street performers, and

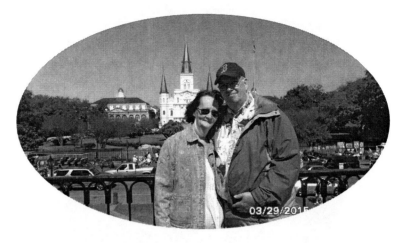

03/29/201_

the astonishing array of art that was on display for sale. We joined the family in the afternoon for a late brunch at 300-year-old world famous Court of the Two Sisters for a scrumptious buffet – a combination of real world food Creole and Cajun selections with historic surroundings. We enjoyed The Steamboat Natchez when we experienced The Jazz Cruise that evening on The Mississippi River that night, before returning to Florida.

My next great challenge, which I took on with excitement was finding a place we could call home. Tom sent Barb and me out to look, and we located a place we thought was perfect — with three bedrooms, plus a private office (so I could have a tranquil place to write) and a saltwater pool. At the end of May 2015, we moved to our home place.

> "Surround yourself only with people
> who are going to lift you higher."
> Oprah Winfrey

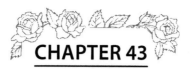

Triumph Comes Out of Tragedy

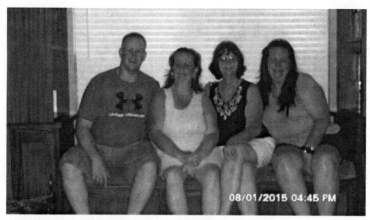

Mark, Barb, Betty, Andrea – My family together in August 2015.

When it came time for me to find someone to edit this book, God brought two amazing believers into my life – both via Craigslist.

For those readers who have never written a book, it is never a good idea to edit your own work. Sometimes sentence structure is off, and you need other people to find that. You need fresh and microscoping eyes to find and correct errors — lots of errors — errors you are not able to see because you are too emotionally invested in your project. This requires line and content editors

I also found GRAMMARLY.com, which is an internet program that finds little things you have overlooked — and helps you fix them. It's a process. Anyone who is involved in "the process" will tell you that a book is 20% writing and 80% editing, plus other details that have nothing and everything to do with writing the book.

I had gone to Craigslist to place an advertisement for an editor. The first person I met was Barbara, who I interviewed on by phone. She immediately caught what I was doing. Remember I said, *"Some things are taught, and some things are caught?"* I rest my case.

I felt compelled to ask one question in my interview, *"Are you a Christian?"*

I sincerely believed that if an editor was not a believer they would not be able to do justice to editing my book. In other words, an atheist or agnostic would not "get" the message of my book. Again, "Some things are taught, and some things are caught."

I could send a chapter to Barbara, and shortly she would e-mail it back to me — rewritten. A word or phrase here or there can make an immense difference in the way a sentence rolls off your tongue.

I would read what she had returned and the small but significant changes were dramatic and made my book flow better. She never changed the meaning of any sentence or thought. She just made it read in a more polished way. I loved it. She made me look smarter! She took my book and made it new and improved! I have to tell you when we can accomplish that, it is a miracle! People who write books use this all the time — and never admit it, or they just assume everyone knows about the process. I didn't, and now I do!

The second person I found was also through Craigslist. I had a dilemma about the text and structure of the book.

In placing all the chapters I realized that I had read and reread the text so much I saw double — duplicates were springing up, and I was unable to find and delete them — without help. That is when I met Joseph Schroeder, who answered my call for help.

I met Joseph at Dunkin' Donuts, and we had an instant connection. He has written his own book, _**My Little Miracle Story**_. He had been a pastor for more than 30 years and understood the power and pull of creating a book you have been called to write. He was well aware of the process that it took to write and publish a book.

We began working on chapters in my book adding suggestions and bringing corrections to my attention. As we got to know one another, it came to light that the tree that Barb hit was in the front yard of the church that he now serves! There was a true revelation! What were the chances? God works in mysterious ways.

He was able to understand when I told him I had locked onto the journey of getting this book completed. Yet, it seemed that each time I thought I was finally going to finish it, there were obstacles that arose in my path. I would become discouraged, however after taking a break, I possessed the desire and dream that is God's journey. You have seasons of learning in your path. God can take the bad and turn it into good, if you will open your heart to him — and believe.

> I knew this book was not just going to be just a good thing. It was going to be a God-thing.

Chapter 43

Sink into your destiny, I remained locked onto His promise and didn't get distracted. His Will is going to become a reality if you **plug in and get turned on.**

James 1:3-4 (NKJV)

*[3] knowing that the testing of your faith produces patience.
[4] But let patience have its perfect work, that you may be perfect and complete, lacking nothing.*

I knew in time; God would help me to overcome those barriers and forge ahead. I knew if it was truly God's will it would come to pass. The journey is part of the process and a waiting game. God allows you to go through it for your own protection.

Hebrews 12:2 (NLT)

[2] We do this by keeping our eyes on Jesus, the champion who initiates and perfects our faith.[a] Because of the joy[b] awaiting Him, He endured the cross, disregarding its shame. Now He is seated in the place of honor beside God's throne.

If your heart is truly lead by God, you must stay the course and finish what you start. The simple fact is that in life, stuff comes at you and you have to push through it.

John 16:33 (KJV)

[33] These things I have spoken unto you, that in me ye might have peace. In the world ye shall have tribulation: but be of good cheer; I have overcome the world.

Thanks to Barbara Flewelling and Joseph Anthony Schroeder for their help and support in editing my book. I was blessed to have God bring you into my life just when I needed you most!

"I know for sure that love saved me, and that it is here to save all of us."

Dr. Maya Angelou

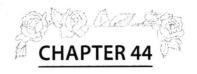

CHAPTER 44

Kindred Spirits:
Our Four Year Journey

If you found my first book a compelling read, my second book is a prequel and answers the burning question "Why did I stay?" in a different way. It is the story of my search, as an adoptee, for my birth family, and the results of that search. It is about my journey, as I meet Life's challenges.

It is filled with the hope you will find inspirational, heartwarming, down-right-funny, and relatable to anyone who's life it touches.

The Search for Judith Ann (2016)

Writing the second book allowed her to connect the dots; leading her on a journey of self-discovery, and the answers to her many questions about self-awareness regarding why she stayed with her daughter, Barb, when she was grievously injured in a near-fatal auto accident, that she did not realize prior to penning the second book *The Search for Judith Ann* (2016)

People who know Elizabeth and Barbara Scott's incredible story have asked her questions about how she and her daughter Barb got through those four plus years (2011-2015). To answer those questions requires knowing fully who they are. She had to go back to "before" so you, Dear Reader, could understand the "after."

Yankee 794 Trauma (2016) revealed details of the mystery of how Elizabeth and Barb Scott's journey of discovery unfolded. It is a story of undying love, dedication, passion and commitment – and above all Faith in God.

Her story reveals how, in the face of the greatest challenges of their lives, She asked the right questions and made choices that mattered; how she evolved and educated herself to a medical knowledge and vital resources.

It is a story of the people that touched both the lives of a daughter, Barb, and herself, the author/caregiver/mom, as well as events that brought her to be the person who she is today.

Elizabeth made hard choices that she was forced to make ... leading to the outcome that is told in their memoir *Yankee 794 Trauma* (2016).

The Search for Judith Ann (2016) her second memoir is a prequel to

Chapter 44

Yankee 794 Trauma. It chronicles the heartfelt and amazing odyssey of the author, Elizabeth A. Scott, in her prior years.

Born at Booth Home for Unwed Mothers in St. Louis, Missouri in March of 1948, Elizabeth's journey reveals the story of how she ended up in "legal limbo" for a time following her birth. At some point, she was relinquished for adoption against her young mother's will.

Assigned to an orphanage, Children's Home Society of Missouri, the task was undertaken of matching her with the right set of adoptive parents. Soon after arriving she developed a case of Whooping Cough, which was often fatal for infants. This is altered her path to adoption. An "alternative" couple was asked to take her because of her immediate need for medical care.

Her placement, at 10-weeks-old, to a young doctor and his wife, William and Katherine Moore, and her unconventional upbringing, are told with unquenchable curiosity, humor, passion, conviction, and most all, with loving and endearing first-person memories.

Elizabeth's journey revealed her two mothers. Betty Lou, her young birthmother, and Katherine, who yearned for a child that she could nurture, however, was denied, due to her inability to conceive.

Both Mothers loved her unconditionally. Certainly her birth grandmother, Josephine, by all accounts, was mentally unstable throughout her life — and in fact, may have been a homicidal maniac — directly resulting in her untimely death in 1949 at age 39.

God intervened to conjoin baby Elizabeth to a wonderful and God-fearing couple whose childless journey allowed her to be accepted and cherished. Through their hearts and minds, she experienced an ambrosia of life — filled with a constant fragrant atmosphere of active and ambitious expectations and experiences. Grafted into a tree whose genealogy was unrelated, her new parents impacted her life in ways she still finds immeasurable.

The major players in this odyssey in addition to Elizabeth were:

Dr. William Herbert Moore D.O., her adoptive father, who was accomplished and dedicated to being a small town middle-American doctor. He also cultivated a social smokescreen that he created for his own protection and survival. This hid a complex and conflicted childhood with a dark and smoldering secret — never before revealed.

Rose Katherine "Katie" Moore, her adoptive mother, herself an only child. She possessed amazing qualities of unfailing loyalty, selflessness, unconditional love, and enduring commitment which sustained the family through good times and times of adversity.

Dr. Charles J. Moore, her dad's only and younger sibling who was an optometrist by profession. Elizabeth and he developed a mutual admiration and adored each other. Through his eyes and presence, she found a loving, conflicted, and kindred spirit unequaled. He too felt like "a square peg in a round hole." Ultimately, he became a shame on the family name, in his brother's eyes, and had his own demons to fight through his life.

Her parent's motto:

> ***"The only value you have in this life,***
> ***is the value you have in serving others."***

In 1959, leaving her heart in the small mid-American town of Argyle, Mo., and her family relocated to California, Missouri, where her values and outlook on life were forged. She went on to a lifetime calling in Nursing and community service. She married, had three children and became a widow in eleven years.

It was a slower, kinder, and quieter 1950's post-war America, one that had faded from public view, consciousness, and memory,her story begins.

Her earthy and gripping memoir tells of the life and subsequent, inevitable death in 1977, of her adopted mother, with which she shared an acceptance, appreciation, recognition, and unconditional love. That was followed several months later by the untimely and shocking death of her 30-year-old husband, David, just as she was due to give birth to their third child and only son.

Having experienced profound loss and grief, followed by the joy at the birth of her son, she found herself compelled to seek her roots. The journey lead to more questions than answers, spurring her to explore hidden and unexpected places, times, and people.

This book is an experience that will propel you, the reader, into uncharted territory as she seeks to unveil her circumstances of her birth, and where her genealogy would evidently lead her.

Her quest is an eye-opening search for her biological family tree — an ancient tree with untold gnarled and twisted branches. In the end, her search, which took three years, resulted in more strange twists and turns than a mountain road. The results could not have been predicted or imagined. It would shake her to the very core of who she thought she was, and help her to realize a new truth. It led her to a renewed faith in God, as she discovered that the truth is, indeed, stranger than fiction.

℘

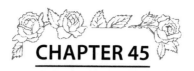

CHAPTER 45

Lost & Found:
What Brain Injury Survivors
Want You to Know

Barbara J. Webster, Lash & Associates

I need a lot more rest than I used to. I'm not being lazy. I get physical fatigue as well as a "brain fatigue." It is very difficult and tiring for my brain to think, process, and organize. Fatigue makes it even harder to think.

My stamina fluctuates, even though I may look good or "all better" on the outside. Cognition is a fragile function for a brain injury survivor. Some days are better than others. Pushing too hard usually leads to setbacks, sometimes to illness.

Brain injury rehabilitation takes a very long time; it is usually measured in years. It continues long after formal rehabilitation has ended. Please resist expecting me to be who I was, even though I look better.

I am not being difficult if I resist social situations. Crowds, confusion, and loud sounds quickly overload my brain, it doesn't filter sounds as well as it used to. Limiting my exposure is a coping strategy, not a behavioral problem.

If there is more than one person talking, I may seem uninterested in the conversation. That is because I have trouble following all the different "lines" of discussion. It is exhausting to keep trying to piece it all together. I'm not dumb or rude; my brain is getting overloaded!

If we are talking and I tell you that I need to stop, I need to stop NOW! And it is not because I'm avoiding the subject, it's just that I need time to process our discussion and "take a break" from all the thinking. Later I will be able to rejoin the conversation and really be present for the subject and for you.

Try to notice the circumstances if a behavior problem arises. "Behavior problems" are often an indication of my inability to cope with a specific situation and not a mental health issue. I may be frustrated, in pain, overtired or there may be too much confusion or noise for my brain to filter.

Patience is the best gift you can give me. It allows me to work deliberately and at my own pace, allowing me to rebuild pathways in my brain. Rushing and multi-tasking inhibit cognition.

Please listen to me with patience. Try not to interrupt. Allow me to find my words and follow my thoughts. It will help me rebuild my language skills.

Please have patience with my memory. Know that not remembering does not mean that I don't care.

Please don't be condescending or talk to me like I am a child. I'm not stupid, my brain is injured and it doesn't work as well as it used to. Try to think of me as if my brain were in a cast.

If I seem "rigid," needing to do tasks the same way all the time; it is because I am retraining my brain. It's like learning main roads before you can learn the shortcuts. Repeating tasks in the same sequence is a rehabilitation strategy.

If I seem "stuck," my brain may be stuck in the processing of information. Coaching me, suggesting other options or asking what you can do to help may help me figure it out. Taking over and doing it for me will not be constructive and it will make me feel inadequate. (It may also be an indication that I need to take a break.)

You may not be able to help me do something if helping requires me to frequently interrupt what I am doing to give you directives. I work best on my own, one step at a time and at my own pace.

If I repeat actions, like checking to see if the doors are locked or the stove is turned off, **it may seem like I have OCD** — obsessive-compulsive disorder — **but I may not.** It may be that I am having trouble registering what I am doing in my brain. Repetitions enhance memory. (It can also be a cue that I need to stop and rest.)

If I seem sensitive, it could be emotional lability as a result of the injury or it may be a reflection of the extraordinary effort it takes to do things now. Tasks that used to feel "automatic" and take minimal effort, now take much longer, require the implementation of numerous strategies and are huge accomplishments for me.

We need cheerleaders now, as we start over, just like children do when they are growing up. Please help me and encourage all efforts. Please don't be negative or critical. I am doing the best I can.

Don't confuse Hope for Denial. We are learning more and more about the amazing brain and there are remarkable stories about healing in the news every day. No one can know for certain what our potential is. We need Hope to be able to employ the many, many coping mechanisms, accommodations and

Chapter 45

strategies needed to navigate our new lives. Everything single thing in our lives is extraordinarily difficult for us now. It would be easy to give up without Hope.

Created with the assistance of the "Amazing" Brain Injury Survivor Support Group of Framingham, MA.

Excerpted from **Lost & Found: A Survivor's Guide for Reconstructing Life After a Brain Injury** by Barbara J. Webster. © 2011 by Lash & Associates Publishing/Training Inc. Used with permission.

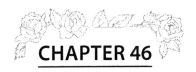

9 Things NOT to Say to Someone with a Brain Injury

Marie Rowland, PhD, EmpowermentAlly

Brain injury is confusing to people who don't have one. It's natural to want to say something, to voice an opinion or offer advice, even when we don't understand.

And when you care for a loved one with a brain injury, it's easy to get burnt out and say things out of frustration.

Here are a few things you might find yourself saying that are probably not helpful:

1. You seem fine to me.

The invisible signs of a brain injury — memory and concentration problems, fatigue, insomnia, chronic pain, depression, or anxiety — these are sometimes more difficult to live with than visible disabilities. Research shows that having just a scar on the head can help a person with a brain injury feel validated and better understood. Your loved one may look normal, but shrugging off the invisible signs of brain injury is belittling. Consider this: a memory problem can be much more disabling than a limp.

2. Maybe you're just not trying hard enough (you're lazy).

Lazy is not the same as apathy (lack of interest, motivation, or emotion). Apathy is a disorder and common after a brain injury. Apathy can often get in the way of rehabilitation and recovery, so it's important to recognize and treat it. Certain prescription drugs have been shown to reduce apathy. Setting very specific goals might also help.

Do beware of problems that mimic apathy. Depression, fatigue, and chronic pain are common after a brain injury, and can look like (or be combined with) apathy. Side effects of some prescription drugs can also look like apathy. Try to discover the root of the problem, so that you can help advocate for proper treatment.

3. You're such a grump!

Irritability is one of the most common signs of a brain injury. Irritability could be the direct result of the brain injury, or a side effect of depression, anxiety, chronic pain, sleep disorders, or fatigue. Think of it as a biological grumpiness — it's not as if your loved one can get some air and come back in a better mood. It can come and go without reason.

It's hard to live with someone who is grumpy, moody, or angry all the time. Certain prescription drugs, supplements, changes in diet, or therapy that focuses on adjustment and coping skills can all help to reduce irritability.

4. How many times do I have to tell you?

It's frustrating to repeat yourself over and over, but almost everyone who has a brain injury will experience some memory problems. Instead of pointing out a deficit, try finding a solution. Make the task easier. Create a routine. Install a memo board in the kitchen. Also, remember that language isn't always verbal. "I've already told you this" comes through loud and clear just by facial expression.

5. Do you have any idea how much I do for you?

Your loved one probably knows how much you do, and feels incredibly guilty about it. It's also possible that your loved one has no clue, and may never understand. This can be due to problems with awareness, memory, or apathy — all of which can be a direct result of a brain injury. You do need to unload your burden on someone, just let that someone be a good friend or a counselor.

6. Your problem is all the medications you take.

Prescription drugs can cause all kinds of side effects such as sluggishness, insomnia, memory problems, mania, sexual dysfunction, or weight gain — just to name a few. Someone with a brain injury is especially sensitive to these effects. But, if you blame everything on the effects of drugs, two things could happen. One, you might be encouraging your loved one to stop taking an important drug prematurely. Two, you might be overlooking a genuine sign of brain injury.

It's a good idea to regularly review prescription drugs with a doctor. Don't be afraid to ask about alternatives that might reduce side effects. At some point in recovery, it might very well be the right time to taper off a drug. But, you won't know this without regular follow-up.

7. Let me do that for you.

Independence and control are two of the most important things lost after a brain injury. Yes, it may be easier to do things for your loved one. Yes, it may be less frustrating. But, encouraging your loved one to do things on their own will help promote self-esteem, confidence, and quality of living. It can also help the brain recover faster.

Do make sure that the task isn't one that might put your loved one at genuine risk — such as driving too soon or managing medication when there are significant memory problems.

8. Try to think positively.

That's easier said than done for many people, and even harder for someone with a brain injury. Repetitive negative thinking is called rumination, and it can be common after a brain injury. Rumination is usually related to depression or anxiety, and so treating those problems may help break the negative thinking cycle.

Furthermore, if you tell someone to stop thinking about a certain negative thought, that thought will just be pushed further towards the front of the mind (literally, to the prefrontal cortex). Instead, find a task that is especially enjoyable for your loved one. It will help to distract from negative thinking, and release chemicals that promote more positive thoughts.

9. You're lucky to be alive.

This sounds like positive thinking, looking on the bright side of things. But be careful. A person with a brain injury is six times more likely to have suicidal thoughts than someone without a brain injury. Some may not feel very lucky to be alive. Instead of calling it "luck," talk about how strong, persistent, or heroic the person is for getting through their ordeal. Tell them that they're awesome.

Written by Marie Rowland, PhD, EmpowermentAlly. Used with permission.
http://www.brainhealthconsulting.com/.

> "We cannot change the past, but we
> can change our attitude toward it.
> Uproot guilt and plant forgiveness.
> Tear out arrogance and seed humility.
> Exchange love for hate, therby,
> making the present comfortable
> and the future promising."
>
> Maya Angelou

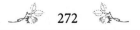

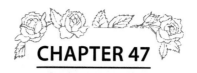

CHAPTER 47

Famous People Who Suffered With Traumatic Brain Injury

What do George Clooney, Della Reese, Gary Busey, Barbara Mandrell, Bob Woodward, and Fantastic Frank Johnson have in common? George Clooney, Della Reese, Gary Busey, Barbara Mandrell, Bob Woodward, and Fantastic Frank Johnson have all had some form of a brain injury.

George Clooney, was filming a torture scene for the movie "Syriana" in 2005, when the chair he was strapped to was accidentally kicked over. When he fell backwards, his head was hit so hard that brain fluid leaked out of his nose. He suffered short-term memory loss from the accident.

Della Reese, had a hemorrhagic stroke in the middle of singing Pieces of Dreams on Johnny Carson's Tonight Show in 1979. An aneurysm burst in her brain, bringing her to her knees and then unconscious on stage.

Gary Busey, had a serious head injury in 1988 during a motorcycle accident. He was not wearing a helmet. A friend saved his life by pressing on a hole in his head until help arrived. After a critical operation that night, couldn't talk, walk, or swallow.

Barbara Mandrell, suffered a head injury during a 1984 car accident in which her two children were told at the scene that she was dead. The 19 year old driver of the other car died. She wrote of her survival in her autobiography *Get to the Heart: My Story.*

Bob Woodward, suffered severe head injuries in 2006 from a roadside bomb, despite wearing a helmet. He was traveling with the Iraqi Army unit as a reporter.

Fantastic Frank Johnson suffered a traumatic brain injury when he was trapped in a fire.

My point is that any one… that is ANY ONE can become a member of the largest group of minorities in the United States at any time, which is people with disabilities. It does not have to be a brain injury,

I just chose these celebrities because I can identify with every one of them!

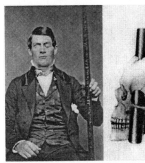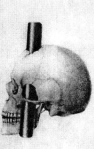

Brain case study: **Phineas Gage**

Phineas Gage (1823–1860) is probably the most famous person to have survived severe damage to the brain. He is also the first patient from whom we learned something about the relation between personality and the function of the front part of the brain.

He was the victim of a terrible accident in 1848. His injuries helped scientists understand more about the brain and human behaviour. Holly Story gets to grips with the grisly tale and its place in the history of neuroscience.

Phineas Gage, whose story is also known as the 'American Crowbar Case', was an unwitting and involuntary contributor to the history of neuroscience. In 1848, when he was just 25 years old, Gage sustained a terrible injury to his brain. His miraculous survival, and the effects of the injury upon his character, made Gage a curiosity to the public and an important case study for scientists hoping to understand more about the brain.

In 1848 Gage was working as a foreman on the construction of the Rutland and Burlington Railroad in Vermont, USA. Workers often used dynamite to blast away rock and clear a path for the railway. On 13 September, Gage was using a tamping iron (a long hollow cylinder of iron weighing more than 6 kilos) to compact explosive powder into the rock ready for a blast. The iron rod hit the rock, creating a spark that ignited the explosives. The rod was propelled through Gage's skull, entering through his left cheekbone and exiting through the top of his head. It was later found some 30 yards away from Gage, "smeared with blood and brain."

Despite his horrific injury, within minutes Gage was sitting up in a cart, conscious and recounting what had happened. He was taken back to his lodgings, where he was attended by Dr. John Harlow. The doctor cleaned and dressed his wound, replacing fragments of the skull around the exit wound and making sure there were no fragments lodged in the brain by feeling inside Gage's head with his finger. Despite Harlow's efforts, the wound became infected and Gage fell into a semi-comatose state. His family did not expect him to survive: they even prepared his coffin. But Gage revived and later that year was well enough to return to his parents' home in New Hampshire.

In 1850 Henry J Bigelow, Professor of Surgery at Harvard University, reported Gage to be "quite recovered in faculties of body and mind".

Chapter 47

It seems that physically, Gage made a good recovery, but his injury may have had a permanent impact on his mental condition. Although accounts from the time are sometimes conflicting and often unreliable, numerous sources report that Gage's character altered dramatically after his accident. In 1868 Harlow wrote a report on the 'mental manifestations' of Gage's injuries. He described Gage as "fitful, irreverent, indulging at times in the grossest profanity... capricious and vacillating" and being "radically changed, so decidedly that his friends and acquaintances said he was 'no longer Gage.'"

The damage to Gage's frontal cortex caused by the iron rod seems to have resulted in a loss of social inhibitions. The role of the frontal cortex in social cognition and decision making is now well-recognized; in the 19th century, however, neurologists were only just beginning to realize these connections. Gage's injuries provided some of the first evidence that the frontal cortex was involved in personality and behavior.

One of the pioneering researchers in this field at the time was David Ferrier, a Scottish neurologist who performed extensive experimental research into cerebral function. In a lecture to the Royal College of Physicians in 1878, Ferrier observed that in his experiments on primates, damage to the frontal cortices seemed to have no effect on the physical abilities of the animal but brought about "a very decided alteration in the animal's character and behavior." He used the experience of Phineas Gage as a case study to support his claims.

The details of Gage's life after his accident are unclear. It is known that he worked as a coach driver for several years in New Hampshire and then in Chile and that in 1859 his health deteriorated and he returned to New Hampshire to live with his mother. He died in San Francisco in 1860 after suffering seizures that resulted from his injury. His brain was not examined after his death, but in 1867 his body was exhumed and his skull was sent to Dr. Harlow to be studied. It now resides, along with the tamping iron, at Warren Anatomical Museum at the Harvard University School of Medicine.

Since then, scientists have made various attempts to use the skull to reconstruct Gage's injury and establish which areas of his brain were damaged. Most recently, a team led by Jack Van Horn of UCLA's Laboratory of Neuroimaging (part of the Human Connectome Project) created a new digital model of the rod's path. It suggested that the damage to Gage's brain was more extensive and severe than had previously been estimated: up to 4 per cent of the cerebral cortex and about 11 per cent of the total white matter in the frontal lobe were destroyed.

The model also indicates that the accident damaged the connections between the frontal cortex to the limbic system, which are involved in the regulation of emotions. This would seem to support some of the contemporary reports of Gage's behavior.

In the 19th century, Gage's survival seemed miraculous. Fascination with his plight encouraged scientific research into the brain, and the continuing research into Gage's condition is proof that this same curiosity is still alive today

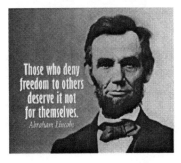

Abraham Lincoln will be remembered for a lot of other things too. He was the President that guided our nation through a civil war and also helped end it. He was one of four presidents in US history to ever be assassinated, the other three were James A Garfield, William McKinley and of course John F. Kennedy. There are a lot of other facts about Lincoln that we will leave to the biographers. But there is one little known fact about the famous President that we wanted to share.

Did you know that Abraham Lincoln suffered a traumatic brain injury as a boy?

According to a variety of reports he was approximately 10 years old when he was kicked in the back of the head by what was either a mule or a horse. Some bystanders alleged that he lay in a coma unconscious for some 24 hours. Some thought he had died and come back to life. According to doctors who have looked at the case, they blame the TBI for causing defects on the 16th President's Lincoln's vision and depression later in life, which was known at that time as melancholia. It also likely caused Lincoln to have what is known as a "lazy eye."

Fortunately Lincoln recovered with all of his cognitive abilities intact. But there's no doubt that he did not have the resources or the knowledge then that we have today. We've seen the research and witnessed firsthand the debilitating effects of a traumatic brain injury. We've observed families and their search for help for a loved who has suffered a TBI.

A Brain Injury can happen to anyone… At Anytime.

Did you know… These people have all suffered Brain Injuries?

Chapter 47

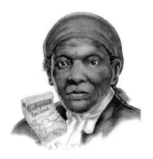

Harriet Tubman
Abolitionist and Organizer
of the Underground Railroad
(c. 1822-March 10, 1913)

Harriet Tubman was an African-American abolitionist, humanitarian, and Union spy during the U.S. Civil War. After escaping from captivity, she made thirteen missions to rescue over seventy slaves using the network of antislavery activists and safe houses known as the Underground Railroad.

Head injury

One day, when she was an adolescent, Tubman was sent to a dry-goods store for some supplies. There, she encountered a slave owned by a different family, who had left the fields without permission. His overseer, furious, demanded that Tubman help restrain the young man. She refused, and as the slave ran away, the overseer threw a two-pound weight from the store's counter. It missed and struck Tubman instead, which she said "broke my skull." She later explained her belief that her hair – which "had never been combed and... stood out like a bushel basket" – might have saved her life. Bleeding and unconscious, Tubman was returned to her owner's house and laid on the seat of a loom, where she remained without medical care for two days. She was immediately sent back into the fields, "with blood and sweat rolling down my face until I couldn't see." Her boss said she was "not worth a sixpence" and returned her to Brodess, who tried unsuccessfully to sell her.

She began having seizures and would seemingly fall unconscious, although she claimed to be aware of her surroundings even though she appeared to be asleep. These episodes were alarming to her family who were unable to wake her when she fell asleep suddenly and without warning. This condition remained with Tubman for the rest of her life; Larson suggests she may have suffered from temporal lobe epilepsy as a result of the injury. The severe injury left her suffering from headaches, seizures and sleeping spells that plagued her for the rest of her life.

This severe head wound occurred at a time in her life when Tubman was becoming deeply religious. As an illiterate child, she had been told Bible stories by her mother. The particular variety of her early Christian belief remains unclear, but Tubman acquired a passionate faith in God. She rejected white interpretations of scripture urging slaves to be obedient, finding guidance in the Old Testament tales of deliverance. After her brain trauma, Tubman began experiencing visions and potent dreams, which she considered signs from the divine. This religious perspective instructed her throughout her life.

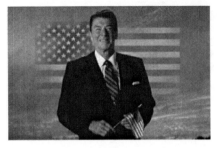

Ronald Wilson Reagan (February 6, 1911 – June 5, 2004) was the 40th President of the United States (1981–1989) and the 33rd Governor of California (1967–1975).

Reagan left office in 1989; in 1994 the former president disclosed that he had been diagnosed with Alzheimer's disease earlier in the year. He died ten years later at the age of ninety-three, and ranks highly among former U.S. presidents in terms of approval rating.

Complicating the picture, Reagan suffered an episode of head trauma in July 1989, five years prior to his diagnosis. After being thrown from a horse in Mexico, a subdural hematoma was found and surgically treated later in the year. Nancy Reagan asserts that her husband's 1989 fall hastened the onset of Alzheimer's disease, citing what doctors told her, although head trauma has not been conclusively proven to accelerate Alzheimer's. Reagan's one-time physician, Dr. Daniel Ruge, has said, however, it is possible, but not certain, that the horse accident affected the course of Reagan's memory.

Vice-President Joseph "Joe" Robinette Biden, Jr.

In February 1988, after suffering from neck pains, Biden was hospitalized and underwent lifesaving surgery to correct two brain aneurysms, one of which began leaking. The hospitalization and recovery kept him from the Senate for seven months. The aneurysm taught him that "it's a hell of a lot easier being on the operating table than in the waiting room."

LEAD: Senator Joseph Biden was released from a hospital today after surgery to correct an aneurysm near his brain. The 45-year-old Delaware Democrat underwent surgery May 3 at Walter Reed Medical Center for his second aneurysm since February. Mr. Biden, chairman of the Senate Judiciary Committee, dropped out of the Democratic Presidential race before the first aneurysm was discovered.

Senator Joseph Biden was released from a hospital today after surgery to correct an aneurysm near his brain. The 45-year-old Delaware Democrat underwent surgery May 3 at Walter Reed Medical Center for his second aneurysm since February. Mr. Biden, chairman of the Senate Judiciary

Committee, dropped out of the Democratic Presidential race before the first aneurysm was discovered.

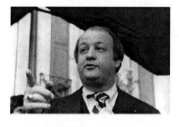

James Brady (8/29/40 – 8/4/14) of Centralia Illinois White House Press Secretary to President Reagan, suffer brain damage during an assassination attempt on President Reagan. Look for book *Thumbs Up The Life* and ***Courageous Comeback of White House Press Secretary Jim Brady.*** The 1991 made for TV movie *Without Warning: The James Brady Story*. For 25 years, the image of President Ronald Reagan and Jim Brady being shot in Washington has remained etched in the public mind. Jim was shot and grievously injured, but, with his wife Sarah by his side, he courageously survived. Not long after Jim was gunned down, Sarah was outraged all over again when her then six-year-old son Scott found what he thought was a toy gun in a relative's pickup truck. In fact, it was not a toy. It was a fully-loaded handgun.

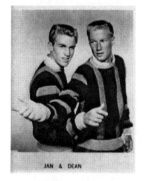

JAN & DEAN

Golden boy **Jan Berry**, 62, overcame a strange twist of fate. On 12 April 1966, Jan Berry received severe head injuries in a motor vehicle accident.

Jan and Dean were a very successful singing duo that had the 1960s surf-music hits Deadman's Curve and Little Old Lady from Pasadena .

If Brian Wilson was the king of the California dream regime, Jan & Dean were the crown princes — and the jesters. Composer/producer/lead singer Jan Berry and partner Dean Torrence manufactured enticing, comically exaggerated myths of the West Coast surf-and-hot-rod lifestyle of the early '60s.

Surf City, Drag City, Ride the Wild Surf, Sidewalk Surfin' and Dead Man's Curve form the soundtrack for the era with the Beach Boys' indelible hits, while The Little Old Lady (From Pasadena) wittily mocked the macho hot-rod culture. Berry's car wreck and its aftermath: 1966-1968 Jan Berry's near-fatal auto accident in Berry pulled out to pass a slow-moving vehicle and slammed full-speed into a truck that was unexpectedly parked at the curb. The Paramedics that arrived on the scene thought Berry was dead. Checking his vital signs, they found he was alive, and rushed him to the UCLA Hospital. There they found Jan's brain had been severely damaged and even numerous major brain surgeries could not completely repair the damage. Not expected to live, Berry was in a coma for months and awoke unable walk, speak and was paralyzed on the right side.

But beneath the blithe surface of the hits there was much more to Berry, who died Friday at 62 in Los Angeles after years of health problems stemming from a 1966 auto accident. His wife, Gertrude, said he suffered an apparent seizure at his Brentwood home; the cause of death was not disclosed.

Growing up in Los Angeles' wealthy Bel Air neighborhood, he was an overachiever who at 17 scored a top 10 hit, Jennie Lee (before the Beach Boys were formed), and had 11 hits before 1963's Surf City crested the surf-music wave.

On 12 April 1966, Berry received severe head injuries in a motor vehicle accident, ironically just a short distance from Dead Man's Curve in Los Angeles, California, two years after the song had become a hit. Jan was on his way to a business meeting when he crashed his Corvette into a parked truck on Whittier Drive in Beverly Hills.

Berry traveled a long and difficult road toward recovery from brain damage and partial paralysis. He had minimal use of his right arm, and had to learn to write with his left hand. Doctors said he would never walk again, but with a persistent refusal to give up, Jan made it through. Torrence stood by his partner, maintaining their presence in the music industry, and keeping open the possibility that they would perform together again.

Berry returned to the studio in April 1967, one year to the month after his accident. Working with collaborators, he began writing and producing music again

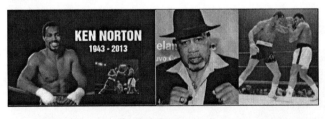

Ken Norton Boxer although he fought Muhammad Ali in the 1970s, received permanent physical disabilities from an automobile accident among them being a Brain Injury. In 1986, Norton was in a car crash that left him with a fractured skull, jaw, and broken leg and no recollection of what had happened. Through it all, he remained a positive thinker and would not accept any prognosis but his own. His doctor told him that he would not walk or talk again after the accident, but Norton refused to accept any prediction that did not include what he visualized. Norton said "At first they thought I might die, and if I didn't die, I wouldn't be coherent. Now I'm talkin' and walkin' and I can even chew gum at the same time." The power of positive thinking led Norton by the hand through his rehabilitation, with determination and drive, Norton regained the ability to walk, talk, laugh, and even to chew gum.

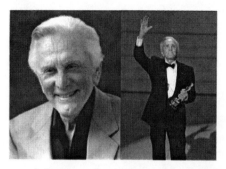

Hollywood legend **Kirk Douglas**, who grew to appreciate more of life after suffering a stroke.

Kirk Douglas finds silver lining after stroke. Most people dread the thought of major life changes being thrust upon them. And fewer still would credit an unexpected health challenge as a bit of good fortune. But actor Kirk Douglas reports that the stroke he suffered in 1996 changed him in ways that enriched his life, and ultimately became the subject of his recent book, *My Stroke of Luck*.

"You know, stroke is a very interesting thing, although at times I wish I didn't have it," says Douglas. "It makes you appreciate things. For instance, the 'simple' miracle of speech — we have no cognizance of the many intricate movements it takes to communicate verbally until it is taken away from us."

Douglas didn't consider his fate to be improved during his initial struggles with recovery. Among other problems, he had to contend with the reality that, initially, he could not talk.

"What is an actor who can't speak — do you wait for silent movies to come back?" jokes Douglas. But the Hollywood great found that even this difficult challenge was a small part in an overall struggle to reclaim his life.

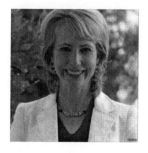

01/08/2011 - The Huffington Post/AP

Rep. Gabrielle Giffords of Arizona was shot in the head Saturday when an assailant opened fire outside a grocery store during a meeting with constituents, killing six people and wounding 13 others. The assassination attempt left Giffords in critical condition — *the bullet went straight through her brain.*

UPDATE: May 22, 2011 — "It's not surprising that today Gabby was doing what she always does, listening to the hopes and concerns of her neighbors," Obama said. "That is the essence of what our democracy is about. That is why this is more than a tragedy for those involved. It is a tragedy for Arizona and a tragedy for our entire country."

UPDATE: January 6, 2016 — On January 8, 2011, a gunman entered a constituents' meeting being held by U.S. congresswoman Gabrielle Giffords outside of Tucson, Ariz. The 22-year-old gunman, Jared Lee Loughner, killed 6 people during the attack including federal judge John Roll and 9-year-old Christina-Taylor Green. 13 people were injured during the rampage including congresswoman Giffords who was shot in the head at point-blank range.

The popular congresswoman was only the third woman from Arizona ever elected to Congress. Although Giffords survived the assassination attempt, she was left her with a severe brain injury. The congresswoman spent months in rehabilitation relearning how to walk and talk. In May of 2011, Giffords traveled to the Kennedy Space Center to support her husband astronaut Mark Kelly in the launching of the final flight of space shuttle Endeavour.

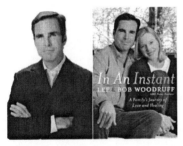

Bob Woodruff — News Journalist

On Jan. 29, 2006, a roadside bomb detonated next to the vehicle carrying ABC News anchor Bob Woodruff in Iraq. The shock wave from the explosion propelled jagged shrapnel and rock, traveling at a deadly velocity, toward his head. In less time than it takes to read this sentence, his brain was forever changed. Woodruff awoke more than a month later, only to begin a long road to recovery. His journey is one that is shared by an estimated 80,000 to 90,000 Americans each year who suffer traumatic brain injury, or TBI. While at least some degree of recovery is possible for many of these patients, the progress back to the people they once were is gradual and uncertain. And many do not make it back.

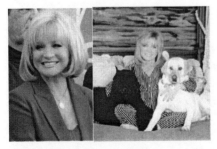

Barbara Mandrell was born December 25, 1948 in Houston, Texas. Mandrell showed musical promise from a very early age.

American country singer Barbara Mandrell scored No. 1 hits with "Sleeping Single in a Double Bed" and "Years."

Barbara Mandrell caught the attention of country stars Chet Atkins and Joe Maphis when she was 11 years old, and toured with Patsy Cline when she was 13. She became the only female country musician to win the CMA 'Entertainer of the Year' award, twice.

Near-Death Experience — Mandrell's faith would be tested by a brush with death. She was involved in a serious head-on car collision while driving on the freeway and barely survived, suffering multiple fractures, lacerations, and memory loss. Her two children were riding in the car with her; she had an intuition just before the crash to remind them to buckle their seat belts, which saved their lives.

The accident changed the course of Barbara Mandrell's life. Mandrell's recovery from her injuries was a difficult one; she was often moody and volatile, suffering temper outbursts as a result of the post-traumatic stress. In 1986, she gave birth to son Nathaniel. That year she stopped recording completely, performing only in live shows, which she continued with some success until she officially retired from country music in 1997. Ever since, Mandrell has focused solely on family, spending most of her time on her ranch with her husband, children, garden, and pets. In 2009, Mandrell won induction into the Country Music Hall of Fame.

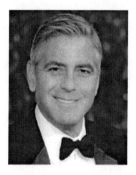

Head Injury Drove Clooney To Think of Suicide

Saturday 22 October 2005 21.11 EDT

Last modified on Saturday 9 January 2016 01.01 EST

George Clooney has revealed how he contemplated suicide to escape horrific pain he was experiencing **after suffering a brain injury** in an accident while shooting a scene for a forthcoming film. The 44-year-old star of 'Ocean's Eleven' and 'From Dusk Till Dawn' said he battled against excruciating headaches and serious memory loss after falling and banging his head while filming Syriana, a thriller set in the Middle East which is due out in January. The actor was tied to a chair for a scene in the $50m Warner Brothers film, based on former CIA agent Robert Baer's book *See No Evil*.

"There was this scene where I was taped to a chair and getting beaten up. The chair was kicked over and I hit my head," said Clooney. "I tore my dura, which is the wrap around my spine that holds in the spinal fluid. But it's not my back; it's my brain. I basically bruised my brain. It's bouncing around my head because it's not supported by the spinal fluid," the former ER star added.

He suffered constant pain and splitting headaches as doctors initially could not identify the problem. He could not take painkillers in case he became addicted to them; several members of his family had suffered that fate. Instead, he had to prepare mentally through therapy that taught him to forget his own pain.

"Before the surgery it was the most unbearable pain I've ever been through, literally where you'd go, 'well, you'll have to kill yourself at some point, you can't live like this'," explained Clooney. He blamed himself because he had piled on 38 pounds in a month to play the main role of Baer.

After the accident, Clooney began trying to encourage his memory to return by doing repetitive counting exercises, and even had to write his lines on scraps of paper for his next project, as director-actor in 'Good Night, and Good Luck.'

Despite doctors' initial puzzlement, a neurologist eventually identified the problem and Clooney underwent a series of operations that banished his headaches.

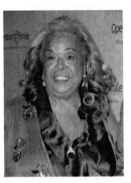

Della Reese shines at 'Stars for Stroke'

Della Reese (born Delloreese Patricia Early; July 6, 1931), is an American nightclub, jazz, gospel and pop singer, film and television actress, one-time talk-show hostess and ordained minister, whose career had spanned six decades. She had also appeared as a guest on several talk shows and as a panelist on numerous game shows.

Reese's long career began as a singer, scoring a hit with her 1959 single "Don't You Know?" In the late 1960s, she had hosted her own talk show, Della, which ran for 197 episodes. She also starred in films beginning in 1975, and included playing opposite Redd Foxx in Harlem Nights (1989), Martin Lawrence in A Thin Line Between Love and Hate (1996) and Elliott Gould in Expecting Mary (2010). She achieved continuing success in the television fantasy drama 'Touched by an Angel' (1994 – 2003), in which Reese played the leading role of Tess. In more recent times, she became an ordained New Thought minister in the Understanding Principles for Better Living Church in Los Angeles, California.

Della Reese only partially remembers the day in 1979 when she was singing Pieces of Dreams on Johnny Carson's Tonight Show. But what she does recall includes a terrifying, life-changing moment.

Chapter 47

"I was in the middle of the song when my body began to twitch uncontrollably," Reese recalls. "Before I knew it, I fell to my knees in front of everyone and was suddenly unconscious." What no one knew at the time was that Reese was suffering a massive hemorrhagic stroke as an aneurysm burst in her brain.

She was moved to three different hospitals before doctors correctly diagnosed her condition. "At first, doctors were looking in everywhere but the right place. I suppose because I'm an actress and entertainer, they initially presumed I was suffering from some sort of alcohol or drug problem. That was more than insulting, it was a potentially fatal misperception."

Two weeks later, when Reese was treated surgically, doctors discovered two additional life-threatening aneurysms about to rupture. She credits prompt surgical intervention on these hidden aneurysms with saving her life.

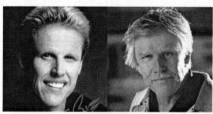

Gary Busey Ministers To Brain Injury Community

No one knows better than Gary Busey that life's road takes unexpected turns.

"I had a nearly fatal motorcycle accident on Dec. 4, 1988," says the actor and musician. "And almost no one expected me to recover."

But Busey was able to come back from the brink, and today he says he's compelled to spread his message of caution. "I want people to understand that life is very important. And that if you're riding a motorcycle, skateboard, or bicycle without a helmet, you're challenging the face of death."

Riding without a helmet is a gamble everyone is bound to lose, sooner or later, he says. "When the odds finally catch up with you, fate will steal your life and the hearts of everyone who loves you."

Busey had just picked up his bike at a repair shop when he slid on a patch of gravel at 40 mph, flipped over the handlebars, and hit his unprotected head on a curb. "I landed at the feet of a police officer and was rushed to an emergency room with a hole in my head the size of a half dollar," he says.

Doctors subsequently told Busey that had he arrived even three minutes later, he would not have survived. As it was, Busey fell into a coma for over four weeks, while family and friends stood by his side.

"I remember being aware of only two things during that ordeal," says Busey.

"The first was that I entered and returned from a spiritual realm, and that experience has been the foundation of my faith ever since. The second, and equally important experience was feeling the healing love and support of the people who surrounded me."

Busey regained consciousness on Jan. 6, 1989, and although heavily medicated, his will to live and recover surfaced almost immediately. And to the astonishment of the medical staff, Busey left the hospital under his own power only five weeks later.

After a period of recuperation and rehabilitation, Busey returned to his film career and has since worked continuously as an advocate for traumatic injury treatment and prevention.

The silent epidemic

An estimated 5.3 million people in the USA currently live with disabilities from traumatic brain injuries (TBI). The Centers for Disease Control and Prevention (CDC) reports that 80,000 Americans are disabled each year, and that over 50,000 others die as a result of TBI.

Vehicle crashes are the leading cause, accounting for 50% of all TBIs. Violence, falls, and sports injuries are the next most common sources of brain injury. The CDC reports that men's risk of suffering TBI is twice that of women, and that overall risk is highest in adolescents and the elderly.

TBI can affect a person in many ways.

- Cognitively, as memory loss, trouble concentrating, communication difficulties, and impaired judgment.
- Physically, with seizures, vision problems, speech impairments, spasticity, fatigue, and pain.
- Emotionally, including anxiety, depression, and mood swings. Patients may also exhibit agitation, impulsive behavior, and difficulty initiating activities.

Dr. George Zitnay, director of the John Jane Brain Injury Center in Charlottesville, Va., states that many people with brain injuries have difficulties with problem solving, making critical decisions, and with complex reasoning.

"What people need to understand is that patients can have trouble with something as simple as dressing themselves," says Zitnay. "It can come down to what goes on first, the shoes or the socks?"

Long-term rehabilitation is often required — a fact that many find hard to accept. Rehabilitation can be as basic as recovering range of motion in an injured limb or regaining bladder control, to more complex goals of occupational therapy and independent living.

"TBI patients are the most untreated and most unemployed group I'm aware of," says Zitnay. "That doesn't mean we should give up or ignore them. An increased commitment to funding and extended treatment is morally necessary and within our means as a country."

Zitnay says that the rehabilitation process for TBI patients should be individualized for each person's unique needs. "Just as no two people are identical, no two brain injuries are exactly alike," he says.

"There is still much that is unknown about brain injury and rehabilitation," says Zitnay. "And while there is no cure for brain injury, the goal of rehabilitation is to help people regain the most independent level of functioning possible."

"Prevention is by far the most efficient way we can deal with this problem in the near future," says Busey, who has visited many hospitals to talk with other brain injury patients. "So many of these injuries are completely preventable. Helmets and seatbelts are easy and convenient methods of protecting yourself."

Busey's commitment to help others resulted in his instrumental role in the creation of the federal Traumatic Brain Injury Act. The legislation, which provides for treatment and tracking of this underserved problem, is the first of its kind to address this issue on a national level.

"The greatest gift we can all receive is by giving," says Busey. "I've learned to pray for the best, prepare for the worst, and to expect the unexpected. My advice to everyone is, don't live in the past, accept what is, take the reigns, and move into the future."

"No matter what happens, no one can take away our ability to live with openness, honesty, and love."

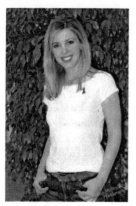

Leean Hendrix — Former Miss Arizona 1998

In 2002, Leean Hendrix was on top of the world. The 26-year old former Miss Arizona was confident, ready to take on any challenge. That all changed when a stroke robbed her of movement on one side of her body, stripped away her self-confidence and erased her memory. "It was like the muscles behind my eyes had broken," Hendrix explained. "It's not even a dizziness. It's almost like I didn't have any control over my eyes."

Leean knew she was having a stroke as she viewed the entire right side of her body drooping and lifeless.

Leean spent six hours at a Phoenix' hospital floating in and out of consciousness as medical teams tried to diagnose her problem. She tried to convince doctors and nurses that she had experienced a stroke. Instead she was asked repeatedly what type of drugs she had taken. Leean tried to explain that she was Miss Arizona and had never used drugs or alcohol. Days passed and she was transferred to a neurological institute where an expert identified her stroke and began treatment. Had she gotten tPA (medication) in the first three hours she probably would have walked out of the hospital a day or two later. Instead, she went home after a week, an invalid confined to a wheelchair, unable to feed or bathe herself or use the bathroom unattended, communicating only in baby talk.

It took a year from Leean to regain the use of her right side. She had to re-learn to walk and even how to brush her own hair. Leean continues to suffer headaches and both long and short-term memory loss. She was a singer and loved to be on stage and yet her goals of past are far different from her goals today. While she has had struggles since her stroke, she isn't bitter or resentful. Instead she uses her story to educate and inspire and is a positive force helping other stroke survivors by sharing information. Her story has been featured on Larry King Live, NBC's Today Show, Ladies Home Journal, LA Times, among others.

May 11 and June 22, 2008

She was a queen—and had the crown to prove it. Leean Hendrix was a former Miss Arizona, 26 years young with a world of possibilities ahead. Then, it happened: "I was folding laundry and I remember just becoming extremely dizzy. My vision became extremely blurry," she recalls. Hendrix looked in the mirror—and knew. When she first arrived at the hospital, doctors didn't believe she was having a stroke because of her age. But in truth, 30 percent of all stroke victims are women under 65. Jim Baranski with the National Stroke Association says women have all the same risk factors men do for stroke—hypertension, obesity, diabetes, and smoking – with an added risk factor from birth control. There are two types of stroke: ischemic, caused by a blood clot in the brain, and hemmoragic, caused when a blood vessel in the brain breaks. Hendrix had none of the risk factors—her stroke was caused by a blood clot that formed in her heart and moved to her brain. Turns out she had a clot due to a hole in her heart she was born with and knew nothing about. There are some amazing new treatments for stroke, including a type of catheter device that literally works like a corkscrew to break up clots. The best treatment for stroke is to know the signs and symptoms. Weakness or numbness on one side of the body, difficulty speaking, problems with vision, a sudden headache, or sudden dizziness. For 5 years, Leann had to take what she calls a hiatus from her life and learn how to be an adult again. She had to start over from scratch—everything from eating to brushing her own hair, her teeth, and taking a bath. Hendrix has climbed back and is now living a life in many ways even more fulfilling than before

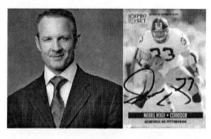

Merril Hoge

The Pittsburgh Steelers selected Hoge in the tenth round of 1987 NFL Draft with the 261st pick overall. He became a key member of the offense and led the team in rushing and receiving in four of his seven years. He is one of only two Steelers to rush for more than 100 yards in back-to-back playoff games (the other was Franco Harris). Hoge was named the Steelers' Man of the Year in 1989 and 1990, and was named to the All-Madden team in 1989.

After seven seasons with the Steelers, Hoge signed with the Chicago Bears as a free agent in 1994, but played in just five games with only six carries and 13 receptions. **He retired after suffering a series of concussions.** He gained 3139 rushing yards and 2133 receiving yards, along with 34 touchdowns, playing fullback for the Steelers two-back offense. *Merril Hoge Ex-Steeler gets serious about head injuries.*

Monday, July 30, 2001

By Dan Gigler, Post-Gazette Staff Writer

The lights go out. Everything is swimming. Names of family, the president or the year don't register. Then there's the vomiting, a loss of coordination and consciousness. That's what can happen when the brain plays bumper cars with the skull.

In 1994, after suffering two consecutive concussions — and the third of his career — former Steelers running back Merril Hoge was faced with a predicament. Keep playing football and risk debilitating memory lapses, **brain damage** or even sudden death, or **quit in the midst of successful NFL career.**

Hoge chose the latter. Now an analyst for ESPN, Hoge, who still makes his home in Pittsburgh, was part of a panel discussion yesterday at the Pittsburgh Hilton and Towers Downtown on **prevention of sports-related concussions.**

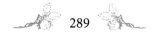

Hoge said the cataclysmic moment that made him decide to retire came when he could not remember where he lived.

"I couldn't find my way home. I was two blocks from my house and it was like I was in the Mojave Desert. I was lost in my own neighborhood," Hoge said.

He also said he had gaps in his memory and had to relearn how to read. Hoge was something of a pioneer when he retired because of head injuries. Before then, athletes didn't consider those injuries to be a reason to quit playing.

"I remember **Dave Wannstadt** said to me, 'No one will think less of you as a player — they know how tough you are,'" Hoge said. "And I thought, why would anyone think less of me? But the mentality in the early '90s was that head injuries didn't end careers."

Attitudes have changed. In the past two years, future hall-of-fame quarterbacks **Troy Aikman** and **Steve Young** also retired due to the number of head injuries they had sustained during their careers, while much has been made of Eric Lindros' decision to continue his hockey career after having sustained more than a half-dozen concussions.

Hoge said that he would never discourage anyone, even his own son, from playing football, but he wants to spread the word that, *"concussions are serious injuries. Not sissy injuries."*

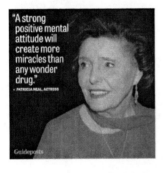

"A strong positive mental attitude will create more miracles than any wonder drug."
- PATRICIA NEAL, ACTRESS

Guideposts

Patricia Neal (1/20/26 – 8/8/10) – award-winning actress of stage and screen.

On February 17, 1965, when she was three months pregnant, she suffered a series of strokes which left her partially paralyzed. Undaunted, Miss Neal began a successful struggle through years of rehabilitation. Her fifth child, Lucy was born healthy. On August 4, 1965, she gave birth to a healthy daughter, Lucy.

Neal was offered the role of "Mrs. Robinson" in The Graduate (1967), but turned it down, feeling it had come too soon after her strokes. She returned to the big screen in "The Subject Was Roses" (1968), for which she was nominated for an Academy Award.

Chapter 47

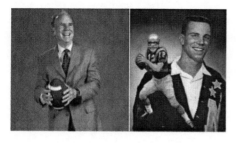

Roger Staubach, also known as Roger the Dodger, Captain Comeback, and Captain America

Staubach ended his Cowboys career with four Super Bowl appearances, including wins in Super Bowls VI and XII. In Super Bowl VI, Staubach was named the game's Most Valuable Player. Following the 1979 season, **Staubach retired, fearing the after-effects of recurring concussions.**

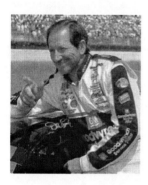

Dale Earnhardt (4/29/51 – 2/18/2001)

Skull Injury Killed Earnhardt, Autopsy Confirms

Ralph Dale Earnhardt known professionally as Dale Earnhardt, was an American race car driver and team owner, best known for his involvement in stock car racing for NASCAR. He began his career in 1975 in the World 600 as part of the Winston Cup Series. NASCAR Xfinity Series career — 136 races run over 13 years.

Considered one of the best NASCAR drivers, Earnhardt won a total of 76 Winston Cup races over the course of his career, including one Daytona 500 victory in 1998. He also earned seven NASCAR Winston Cup championships, tying for the most all-time with Richard Petty. His aggressive driving style earned him the nickname "The Intimidator."

On February 18, 2001, during the Daytona 500 at Daytona International Speedway, Earnhardt was involved in a final lap crash and died of a basilar skull fracture at age 49. He has been inducted into numerous halls of fame, including the inaugural class of the NASCAR Hall of Fame in 2010.

Dale Earnhardt – The Aftermath

He Also Broke Eight Ribs, His Breastbone And An Ankle And Had Blood In His Ears And Chest.

February 20, 2001|By Amy C. Rippel and Beth Kassab of The Sentinel Staff

DAYTONA BEACH — **Dale Earnhardt died from a severe fracture to the base of his skull** that caused bruising and bleeding to the soft tissue in his brain.

Yankee 794 Trauma

When his race car smashed into a concrete wall at an estimated 180 mph Sunday at Daytona International Speedway, it broke eight ribs, his left ankle and his breastbone. There were several scrapes on his body. He had blood in his ears and chest and partially collapsed lungs.

A preliminary autopsy report released Monday evening finds that Earnhardt, 49, died of **blunt-force trauma to the head and neck**, but the report won't be finalized for several weeks, after blood tests are completed.

Earnhardt was pronounced dead at Halifax Medical Center at 5:16 p.m. Sunday after his car slammed into a concrete wall in the final turn of the Daytona 500. Volusia County spokesman Dave Byron said at a news conference Monday morning that the autopsy showed Earnhardt was killed as soon as he hit the racetrack wall.

"My understanding is that the death was instant," Byron said. "He died at the scene."

The autopsy report shows that the **deadly skull fracture circled the base of Earnhardt's skull, extending from the bottom of the skull to the sides. There was a significant amount of internal bleeding at the base of his brain. He had blood in his ears and mild brain swelling from the skull fracture.**

Basal skull fractures have killed four race drivers — Earnhardt, Adam Petty, Kenny Irwin and Tony Roper — in the past year and at least 12 of the 15 drivers killed in auto racing since 1991. They are caused by **violent head movement in which large blood vessels at the skull's base tear, creating immediate and severe blood loss.**

Essentially, it is violent whiplash. With the body held immobile by over-the-shoulder seat belts, only the head can move. Once blood vessels tear, the driver can die in seconds.

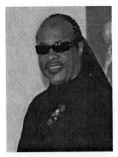

Stevie Wonder — 1973 Car Accident

It was 6th August 1973 and the prodigious 23 year old singer, songwriter, musician and producer was heading north on Interstate 85 on a hot dry Monday afternoon after a performance the night before in Greenville, South Carolina. As they approached the town of Salisbury at around 1:40 p.m., just ahead of them was 23 year old Charlie Shepherd in his 1948 Dodge flatbed farm truck.

A sleeping Wonder was wearing headphones, and Harris, distracted by something, failed to notice the flatbed truck ahead of them.

Chapter 47

There have since been conflicting accounts of the series of events that led to the injury of Stevie. One of the more popular reports that still pervade books and the internet was that a log came flying off the truck, crashed through the windshield of Wonder's car and hit him on the head, sending him into a coma. He said the bed of the truck crashed through the windshield and hit him in the forehead with "great force." As a result of the collision, Stevie was unconscious, however his cousin, John suffered cuts to his thigh and had glass lodged in his fingertips from the shattered windshield. Soon members of the band, traveling in the two cars behind, arrived at the scene and stopped in a panic. One of his brothers rushed to the car, which had come to rest in the median, and noticed immediately that Stevie was unresponsive and bleeding from his forehead and scalp. Stevie was transferred to one of the other cars. Asking directions to the nearest hospital - Rowan Memorial Hospital, they headed off with the unresponsive singer.

Three days into his hospital stay Stevie was able to talk enough to answer simple questions and was making slow, steady progress." The next day he was being fed liquids by mouth, instead of intravenously, though he remained in intensive care. Stevie stayed at N.C. Baptist Hospital for two weeks, including a week in intensive care. As a result of the injury Stevie temporarily lost his sense of smell and was left with a scar on the right side of his forehead

With a new sense of mortality, Stevie left Baptist Hospital Aug. 20, 1973, to convalesce at the University of California at Los Angeles Medical Center. His mother, three brothers, a registered nurse and Abner accompanied him.

"What happened to me was a very, very critical thing, and I was really supposed to die," he said. When plastic surgery was suggested to remove the mark left by the crash, he said, "I will leave it as one of the scars of life I went through."

As recent as November 2008, Stevie returned to Carolina for a concert at the RBC Center in Raleigh. Stevie opened the night with a short speech, giving thanks to God as well as the doctors in Winston-Salem who saved his life after the 1973 crash.

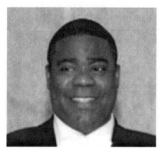

Tracy Morgan Still Struggling to Recover, Battling 'Traumatic Brain Injury'

Comedian Tracy Morgan had to put his life and career on hold in early June 2014, after he was involved in a fatal six-car crash in New Jersey.

The accident left him with a broken femur, leg, nose, ribs, and, perhaps most notably, a traumatic brain injury (TBI).

Morgan tabled the FX series he was developing to focus on improving his health, and has only been seen in public a handful of times since the accident.

There are no reports of Morgan's exact injury. However, both a moderate and severe traumatic brain injury require time for healing and recovery, says Robert Cohen, Psy.D, a neuropsychologist at Orlando Health and director of neuropsychology at Compass Research.

"After a severe traumatic brain injury, the brain has the ability, over time, to heal on its own," Cohen tells Yahoo Health. "The blood, swelling, toxic chemicals and hormones take a long time to pull back. After a severe injury, by and large, depending on the parts of the brain involved, it can take two to two-and-a-half years to get to a place where you'll peak."

However, that timeframe differs dramatically from person to person, which is why docs hesitate to give a prognosis early on during treatment. Usually, though, after roughly two to three years a person with a more severe injury will see a plateau, says Cohen.

The body and brain are miraculous, and will heal some of the TBI on their own, but various therapies will make all the difference — and will last as long as it takes. "It's so important to be reasonable with a person's progress," says Cohen. "We never want to put a limit on someone's rehab potential, but the expectation can't be that they will go back to the same level they were before the accident."

"When you have a traumatic brain injury it takes a very long time to find out how you're going to do and how much you're going to recover," Morelli said. "You just don't know. So that's where he is. He's still fighting and trying to live his life at the same time and trying to get better, and he's just not better. We're hoping and praying to get him back to where he was. But the jury's out."

The list goes on and on…

Domestic Violence and Traumatic Brian Injury

National Statistics

Women who face domestic violence (DV)
have more TBI and CTE than NFL football players.

This is a public health epidemic.

Between 600,000 and 6 million women 4% of all violent crime

3 women and 1 man are murdered each day (1247 women and 440 men)

Intimate partners MURDERS: 30% of women and 5% of men

50% of men and women who assault their partners also abuse their children.

Women who are abused often suffer injury to head, neck, and face.

Repeated injuries to the head decrease the likelihood of
healing and my cause DEATH.

Studies suggest: 3.3 – 10 million witness domestic violence.

1. Every 9 seconds in the US, a woman is assaulted or beaten.

2. Nearly 20 people per minute are physically abused by an intimate.

During one year, this equates to more than 10 million women and men.

3. 1 in 3 women and 1 in 4 men have been victims of [some form of] physical violence by an intimate partner within their lifetime.

4. 1 in 5 women and 1 in 7 men have been victims of severe physical violence by an intimate partner in their lifetime.

5. 1 in 7 women and 1 in 18 men have been stalked by an intimate partner during their lifetime to the point in which they felt very fearful or believed that they or someone close to them would be harmed or killed.

6. There are more than 20,000 phone calls placed to domestic violence hotlines nationwide in a given day.

7. The presence of a gun in a domestic violence situation increases the risk of homicide by 500%.

8. Intimate partner violence accounts for 15% of all violent crime.

9. Women between the ages of 18-24 are most commonly abused by an intimate partner.

10. 19% of domestic violence involves a weapon.

11. Domestic victimization is correlated a higher rate of depression and suicidal behavior.

12. Only 34% of people who are injured by intimate partners receive medical care for their injuries.

13. 2% of the population or 5.3 million Americans are living with disability caused by Domestic Violence

14. All cultural, religious, socioeconomic and ethnic backgrounds are effected.

15. 33% of police time is spent responding to disturbance calls.

16. 57% of cities site domestic violence as top cause for homelessness

17. 86% of victims of abuse are by boyfriend or girlfriend are women

18. 74% of Americans personally know someone who is or had been abused.

19. 75% of Americans fail to connect domestic abuse with economic abuse.

20. 6 out of 10 Americans agree that lack of money and steady income cause domestic violence.

THE INTERSECTION OF BRAIN INJURY & DOMESTIC VIOLENCE

The head and face are among the most common targets of intimate partner assaults, and victims of domestic violence often suffer head, neck and facial injuries.

Common forms of physical assault that can cause brain injury include:

1. Forcefully hitting partner on the head with an object

2. Smashing her head againist a wall

3. Pushing her downstairs

4. Shooting or stabbing her in the head

5. Shaking her which moves her brain in a whip-lash motion

6. Obstructing her airway, causing loss of oxygen to the brain

7. Strangling her (choking)

8. Trying to drown her

9. Forcing her to use drugs or eat foods to which she is allergic

Chapter 48

BATTERERS SELDOM ASSAULT THEIR PARTNES ONLY ONCE, SOME VICTIMS SUFFER REPEATED HEAD INJURIES.

92% hit in the head by partners

83% both hit in the head and severly shaken

8% had been hit in the head more than 20 times.

RAPE

1 in 5 women and 1 in 71 men in the United States has been raped in their lifetime. Almost half of female (46.7%) and male (44.9%) victims of rape in the United States were raped by an acquaintance. Of these, 45.4% of female rape victims and 29% of male rape victims were raped by an intimate partner.

STALKING

19.3 million women and 5.1 million men in the United States have been stalked in their lifetime. 60.8% of female stalking victims and 43.5% men reported being stalked by a current or former intimate partner.11

HOMICIDE

A study of intimate partner homicides found that 20% of victims were not the intimate partners themselves, but family members, friends, neighbors, persons who intervened, law enforcement responders, or bystanders.

72% of all murder-suicides involve an intimate partner;
94% of the victims of these murder suicides are female.8

CHILDREN AND DOMESTIC VIOLENCE

1 in 15 children are exposed to intimate partner violence each year
90% of these children are eyewitnesses to this violence.

ECONOMIC IMPACT

Victims of intimate partner violence lose a total of 8.0 million days of paid work each year. The cost of intimate partner violence exceeds $8.3 billion per year. Between 21-60% of victims of intimate partner violence lose their jobs due to reasons stemming from the abuse. Between 2003 and 2008, 142 women were murdered in their workplace by their abuser 78% of women killed in the workplace during this timeframe.

PHYSICAL/MENTAL IMPACT

Women abused by their intimate partners are more vulnerable to contracting HIV or other STI's due to forced intercourse or prolonged exposure to stress. Studies suggest that there is a relationship between intimate partner violence and depression and suicidal behavior. Physical, mental, and sexual and reproductive health effects have been linked with intimate partner violence including adolescent pregnancy, unintended pregnancy in general, miscarriage, stillbirth, intrauterine hemorrhage, nutritional deficiency, abdominal pain and other gastrointestinal problems, neurological disorders, chronic pain, disability, anxiety and post-traumatic stress disorder (PTSD), as ell as non-communicable diseases such as hypertension, cancer and cardiovascular diseases. Victims of domestic violence are also at higher risk for developing addictions to alcohol, tobacco, or drugs.

SYMPTONS of TRAUMATIC BRAIN INJURY FROM DOMESTIC VIOLENCE

Headaches

Double Vision

Imbalance

Decreased motor ability

Problems with memory, planning and learning

Agitation

Irritability

Depression

Memory Problems

Difficulty concentrating

Poor judgement

Feeling overwhelmed

Need HELP? Call 1-800-799-SAFE (7233) for the Domestic Violence Hotline

> "It's easy to convince ourselves that if we stay busy enough, the truth of our lives won't catch up with us."
>
> Brene Brown

CHAPTER 49

CTE = Chronic Traumatic Encephalopathy

Chronic traumatic encephalopathy (CTR) is a degenerative disease that stems from sustained multiple concussions and results in symptoms like depression and agitation.

From Wikipedia, the free encyclopedia

Chronic traumatic encephalopathy (CTE), a form of tauopathy, is a progressive degenerative disease found in **people who have suffered repetitive brain trauma,** including sub-concussive hits to the head *that do not cause immediate symptoms.* The disease was previously called dementia pugilistica (DP), i.e. "punch-drunk," as it was initially found in those with a history of boxing. CTE has been *most commonly found in professional athletes* participating in American football, association football, ice hockey, professional wrestling, stunt performing, bull riding, rodeo, BMX Biking, and other contact sports who have experienced repetitive brain trauma.

Individuals with CTE may show *symptoms of dementia, such as memory loss, aggression, confusion and depression,* which may appear years or many decades after the trauma. In the case of blast injury, *a single exposure to a blast and the subsequent violent movement of the head in the blast wind can cause the condition.*

In September 2015, researchers with the Department of Veterans Affairs and Boston University announced that they had identified CTE in 96 percent of NFL players that they had examined and in 79 percent of all football players.

What are the classifications of chronic traumatic encephalopathy (CTE)?

The clinical symptons associatedwith CTE vary in severity depending on which clinical state the individual is in (McKee, A.C. et. Al. 2009).

Initial symptons include the following:

Disorientation, confusion, dizziness, headaches, lack of insight, poor judgement, overt dememtia, slowed muscular movements, staggering gait, impeded speech, tremors, vertigo, deafness.

CTE: The facts about chronic traumatic encephalopathy

CTE has been confirmed in many high profile athletes.

By: Alex Ballingall News, Published on Tue May 12 2015

What is CTE?

The verbose way to say it is Chronic Traumatic Encephalopathy. It is defined by experts at Boston University, home of the CTE Centre research facility, as a "progressive degenerative disease" that is **found in people who've suffered repeated head trauma.** Researchers say it can stem from major, debilitating concussions as well as repeated hits to the head that don't result in noticeable symptoms.

The condition is known to affect contact sports athletes, primarily boxers and football players, though it has been linked to professional wrestling, soccer, cheerleading, gymnastic, and horseback riding as well. **People who hit their head repeatedly** during epileptic seizures and victims of domestic abuse can also develop CTE, according to a review of confirmed CTE cases published by the Journal of Neuropathology & Experimental Neurology in 2009.

What does CTE do?

People with CTE often start exhibiting signs of the disease in their 40s, years after they suffered the bulk of their concussions or head trauma. The first symptoms involve memory loss, confusion, and impaired judgment. Over time, people with CTE can also start behaving aggressively and exhibit signs of depression and dementia.

In about 42 per cent of cases from the 2009 review, those with the disease developed trouble with motor skills. These include staggering or shuffling their feet, slurred speech and trembling. These symptoms progress gradually over several years; some boxers examined after death were determined to have lived with CTE for more than 40 years.

When was it discovered?

Researchers point to a 1928 study by New Jersey pathologist Harrison Martland as the first time CTE was described medically. At the time, however, the disease was linked exclusively to boxers, and was called "punch drunk" or "dementia pugulistica." It wasn't until the late sixties the term CTE became the accepted name of the disease.

Why does it happen?

It's still not clear. **Boston University** experts point out that head trauma and CTE symptoms, obviously, don't always mean that one will develop the disease, and that genetics may play a role.

What is known is that CTE can be confirmed only in a post-mortem examination of the brain. The crucial sign is buildup of a protein called "tau," which appears in special tests as dark brown splotches on brain tissue. This protein is meant to stabilize tiny structures in the brain called microtubules, but when someone has CTE too much of it gets released in the brain, causing "neurofibrillary tangles" that damage portions of the organ and contribute to its deterioration. A similar process occurs in the brains of people with Alzheimer's.

What athletes have had CTE?

The disease isn't limited to professionals; it has been found in people who didn't play sports since college or high school, according to the CTE Centre. That said, CTE has been confirmed in several high profile athletes, most recently former NHL defenseman Steve Montador. Former WWE wrestler Chris Benoit, who killed his wife and son before hanging himself in 2007, was shown to have tau tangles in his brain. So did NHLer Bob Probert, who died of a heart attack five years ago and Dave Duerson, a member of the 1985 Super Bowl champion Chicago Bears.

Boston University and the **Krembil Neuroscience Centre in Toronto** are accepting brain donations from deceased athletes to advance CTE research.

Sources: Alzheimer's Association, Boston University, Journal of Neuropathology & Experimental Neurology, **Sports Legacy Institute**

Suicide in Professional Athletes: is it related to the sport?

July 26, 2012

J. John Mann M.D.

Columbia University and New York State Psychiatric Institute

If recent headlines about athletes dying by suicide have made you wonder whether progress in brain research can help shed light on the potential role in these suicides of head hits in sport, then you are right—and not just in the case of the athletes. Research on suicide across its spectrum has told us enough about the brain to greatly help in considering whether and how head trauma may have set the stage when an individual dies by suicide.

Most suicides, over 90 percent, occur in the context of a psychiatric illness that, in about four out of five cases, is untreated. In the United States, major depression is the psychiatric illness that accounts for about 60 percent of suicides. The highly publicized suicides in former professional football players illustrate the potential causal contribution of acquired brain disease due to the cumulative effects of repeated head hits damaging the parts of the brain that contribute to the risk for depression and suicide.

In May, 2012, The Washington Post reported: "**Junior Seau**, a linebacker who played in the NFL for 20 seasons and was among the most widely respected players of his generation, was found dead in his California home Wednesday... with a gunshot wound to the chest. There was no suicide note (and) police officials said a gun was found near Seau and his death appeared to be a suicide." The paper also reported that "he had survived a 100-foot fall down a cliff in his car in October 2010, ... and police said it was believed he fell asleep at the wheel." Police seem to have reached this conclusion based on Mr. Seau stating he had fallen asleep at the wheel, but another potential explanation is that this had been a suicide attempt that he was fortunate to survive. The importance of this question is that a nonfatal suicide attempt is associated with a 20- to 50-fold greater risk for suicide compared with the general population.

Two other former NFL players also died by suicide recently. In April, 2012 former Atlanta Falcons safety **Ray Easterling's** death at age 62 was ruled a suicide. And in 2011, former Chicago Bears safety **Dave Duerson** committed suicide. Easterling is reported to have suffered from depression and insomnia, and then dementia that progressively worsened. He and Duerson each died by a self-inflicted gunshot wound. Tellingly, Duerson shot himself in the chest and in his suicide note made it clear that he did so to preserve his brain so that it could be studied by researchers investigating brain damage in NFL players. Like Easterling, Duerson described a progressive deterioration in his memory and difficulty stringing words together. More than 1,500 former players are now suing the league, claiming that, for years, it ignored evidence that repeated blows to the head trigger chronic traumatic encephalopathy, or CTE, a progressive neurodegenerative disease caused by repetitive trauma to the brain which has been linked to dementia and depression.

As of Jan 2009, the Center for the Study of Traumatic Encephalopathy at Boston University School of Medicine had reported six former NFL players with CTE and even a case in an 18 yr. old high school footballer. CTE is characterized by a very high level of a protein called tau that aggregates into neurofibrillary tangles and is found in the brains of individuals engaged in contact sports that have died from other causes such as suicide. It is hypothesized that this abnormal protein, which preferentially accumulates in outer layers of the brain, impairs and eventually kills brain cells. Early on, **CTE causes emotional instability, poor concentration, word-finding difficulties, depression, suicidal thoughts and problems with impulse control.** However, CTE also involves **memory problems** that eventually **progress to dementia.** A key feature is that the illness continues to progress for years after the trauma and concussions. Football players are not alone: sports like ice hockey, soccer and boxing are thought to increase the risk for CTE and soldiers exposed to bomb blasts have developed CTE. All of the first six NFL former players who were found to have CTE by the Boston group had died by age 50 and three were suicides.

Although it seems that dementia and suicide in football players brought this disease to public notice, the pathology is the same as that seen years earlier in boxers, called dementia pugilistica and a variant that causes Parkinson's disease. **Muhummad Ali** is the most famous example of this illness. Although the severity of the brain pathology in boxers is correlated with the number of rounds boxed over a lifetime, no such relationship has been identified with the number of concussive episodes in sport, likely because records of such episodes are highly inaccurate.

We do not understand the reason for the difference in brain pathology seen between acute severe trauma and repeated milder trauma, but the difference implies a different pathogenesis and potential different treatment. Unlike a single severe head injury, since CTE is the result of repeated milder head trauma or hits, it can be prevented by the very simple measure of discontinuing the activity that results in the **repeated head hits** before the illness acquires a momentum that leads it to become progressive in the absence of ongoing trauma to the head. The medical research challenge is to quantify the number and severity of head hits, or their effect on the brain, so as to determine the point in time at which this intervention becomes essential to prevent disease progression.

How big a problem is this?

We are not sure. About 1.5 million Americans suffer minor head injuries annually without loss of consciousness and no need for hospitalization. **Apparently it is the repetitive nature of such injuries, perhaps with yet to be identified vulnerabilities, that cause some individuals to develop CTE.** We do not know the lower limit of severity of head hits that should be counted. A group of Dutch professional soccer players was found to have cognitive deficits in memory and planning in comparison with elite athletes from other sports, and the magnitude of the deficits was in proportion to the frequency of "heading the ball".

Why are suicides and depression so common in the early phase of CTE?

We are not certain but many of these sports involve blows to the front of the head and that part of the brain includes areas such as the prefrontal cortex and anterior cingulate that are required for mood regulation and impulse control. Injuries or strokes in those brain regions can affect mood and impulsiveness. Abnormal input of the neurotransmitter serotonin to those parts of the brain is observed in suicides and in major depressive disorder. Therefore acquired damage to the same brain regions may favor the development of depression and increase the likelihood of acting on depressed and suicidal thoughts and attempting suicide. The same brain regions are also involved in regulating angry feelings and the probability of aggressive acts. **A history of mild head injury resulting in loss of consciousness for a short period is associated with more aggressive behavior following the injury and a greater risk of suicidal behavior.** The increase in aggressive behaviors is greater in those who were more aggressive prior to the injury. Therefore, pre-existing predisposition to aggression and perhaps depression and suicidal behavior, moderates the impact of head injury on future mental health.

What needs to be done next?

We need better methods of measuring the effect on future health of **contact sports and in the military of soldier exposure to the percussion injury of road-side bombs.** Two main approaches involve measuring the number and severity of head hits by helmet monitors and by cognitive tests. Future tests measuring the accumulation of tau protein in the brain may add precision to the determination of the effect on the brain and in particular the cumulative effect. One way to quantify or track the progressive effect of repeated head hits over time is to image the quantity of tau protein just as we can image the amount of amyloid protein that accumulates excessively in Alzheimer's disease and after severe acute head injury. As treatments are developed for CTE we can then use such methods to track the effectiveness of the treatments in lowering levels of tau in the brain.

List of NFL players with chronic traumatic encephalopathy

Jovan Belcher, Forrest Blue, Lew Carpenter, Lou Creekmur, Shane Dronett, Dave Duerson, Ray Easterling, Frank Gifford, Cookie Gilchrist, John Grimsley, Chris Henry, Terry Long, John Mackey, Ollie Matson, Tom McHale, Adrian Robinson, Junior Seau, Justin Strzelczyk, Andre Waters, Mike Webster

Deceased players suspected of having suffered from CTE

Included in the list are players diagnosed with amyotrophic lateral sclerosis (ALS) who were never tested post-mortem for CTE but whose history appears consistent with CTE. A typical diagnosis of ALS has primarily been based on the symptoms and signs the physician observes in the patient and a series of tests to rule out other diseases and therefore, prior to the discovery of CTE as a phenomenon in ex-American football players, many CTE cases were diagnosed as ALS. The testing of CTE in deceased ex-NFL players began only after the disease was first diagnosed, in 2002, in the brain tissue of **Mike Webster**. After then, testing became common practice only gradually. A cohort mortality study run by the National Institute for Occupational Safety and Health (NIOSH) examined 3,349 NFL players who played at least five full seasons from 1959 to 1988. Findings showed that while NFL players lived longer than the average American male, the risk of death associated with neurodegenerative disorders was about three times higher among the NFL cohort. The risk for death from Alzheimer's disease and ALS were about four times higher among the NFL cohort.

Concussions and Chronic Traumatic Encephalopathy

By Conrad Theodore Seitz, 2015-12-27

There is nothing new about the observation that people who have **repeated concussions eventually develop brain damage, altered personalities, mood changes, and mental deterioration.** This is encapsulated in the word "punch-drunk." What is new is that the National Football League (NFL) has seen its financial viability threatened by the repeated **diagnoses of chronic traumatic encephalopathy in some of its most colorful and high-salaried players.**

The NFL's response to this potential threat has been inconsistent, beginning with denial and attempts to marginalize the first pathologist who published these diagnoses: **Dr. Bennet Omalu.**

The diagnostic process and the league's reaction has been dramatized in a movie, Concussion, with Will Smith in the lead role. Mr. Smith is well-practiced in this role, having done a realistic and appealing portrayal of a fictional doctor who diagnoses and treats a fictional epidemic of vampirism in New York City. That movie was a remake of the Charlton Heston classic, The Omega Man, and was titled after the original book: I am Legend. The Charlton Heston movie was actually the second adaptation of the book written by Richard Matheson, the first being The Last Man on Earth, with Vincent Price in the title role.

This post is not about Concussion, which I haven't seen yet. It is about chronic (post)traumatic encephalopathy (CTE) and football. By the time Junior Seau killed himself with a shot to the chest, the problem was well known to football players, and Junior himself thought that he might have it. He didn't specifically request that his brain be studied, but considering the method he used to kill himself, it is likely that he did want that to be done.

ESPN published an article about the struggle over Junior Seau's brain in 2013, entitled *Mind Control*. By the time of Junior's death on May 2, 2012, the NFL had designated Boston University (BU) as the site for CTE research that it would support. However, several researchers and medical examiners were involved in the work, and an unseemly competition developed between the separate researchers over possession and control of the brain tissue. Junior's family members were approached more than once by different people requesting permission to take Junior's brain tissue for study.

The National Institutes of Health was designated as the recipient organization. The NFL had a large part in that final decision, having disbanded its original concussion committee and forming a new committee. The NFL's original stance has been radically changed, an improvement over a policy that the ESPN article described in this way:

The players charge that the league's original concussion committee, which was disbanded in 2009, conducted fraudulent research to hide the connection between football and brain damage. That 15 years of research has been largely discarded, even by the league.

Dr. Rich Ellenbogen is the new committee's co-chairman. The ESPN article states that although the NFL had designated BU as its "brain bank" there were complaints that BU had refused to share its tissue samples with other researchers. Because of these complaints, Ellenbogen and the committee had already tried to steer tissue from the brain of former Chicago Bears safety Dave Duerson to the NIH (unsuccessfully.) In the Seau case, the article describes Ellenbogen's reasoning:

Asked in an interview why they suggested the NIH, Ellenbogen said, "We had been talking about it for a while. My point, for a long time I've been saying… if you've got a problem you want to solve, do you put one university on it or have multiple studies done? **The federal government is very good, in some ways, really good about doing this. They don't have an agenda.**"

When they received Junior Seau's brain, the NIH decided to direct samples to five different research institutions, including BU. This approach ensured immediate replication of the findings by independent groups, none of whom knew at the time the source or name of the deceased. The final diagnosis was no surprise given Junior's symptoms, but it gave vastly more weight to the finding of CTE to have several independent groups all come to the same conclusion. By contrast, a single diagnosis from BU would have been "just one more brain" since they had already made so many diagnoses in former football players.

Four months after **Junior Seau's** autopsy, the NFL donated $30 million to the NIH, an "unrestricted" grant that was the largest it had ever given at that time.

Tyler Seau, Junior's son, got no "closure" from the diagnosis of CTE. In some ways, it made him feel even worse. He had been stressed beyond his limit by his father's erratic behavior; he was then contacted at a particularly sensitive time after his father's death for the necessary procedure of obtaining the family's consent for examination of his brain; and now, with the diagnosis, he realized that, if he had known before his father's death what was happening to him, he could at least have had an understanding of what was going on, even if the condition was untreatable.

The NFL attempted to direct Junior Seau's brain away from researchers who had previously made CTE diagnoses and threatened its livelihood: first, away from Dr. Omalu (by having Dr. Chao, Junior's team physician, bad-mouth Omalu to Tyler Seau), and second, away from BU, which had made so many CTE diagnoses. The end result was the best from a scientific point of view, although **to the NFL, it was no help and may have been even worse because it was independently confirmed by disinterested parties.**

The NFL settled the player's lawsuit in April 2015, offering a projected $1 billion in compensation for head injuries after it agreed to remove the $765 million cap in August 2014. Some parties immediately filed an appeal of the settlement. Others have opted out of the settlement process in advance. Arguments about the fairness or unfairness of the settlement continue, and it won't be finalized until at least early 2016.

New data from PBS' Frontline and BU were released in September, showing that **of 91 former football players who donated their brains for study after death, 87 had signs of CTE.** This is not a random sample, as it is likely that players who suspected they had CTE would donate their brains for study. Nonetheless, it is disturbing to see that so many had the condition, because it suggests that many, or possibly even most, football players have a least some degree of CTE. No further enhancement is likely to occur until a method for diagnosing CTE prior to death is developed. See this International Business Times article for more about the Frontline study.

Junior Seau's symptoms were the most important problem, and this problem should be emphasized to all; a definite diagnosis is not necessary to be on one's guard.

First, he lost what control he had had over his anger and violent tendencies.

Second, he became erratic and prone to mood swings from depression to elation and irritability.

Third, he became inattentive to details that he had formerly taken care to arrange to his satisfaction.

Fourth, frequent was his uncontrolled gambling and sexual behavior. He also was involved in a car crash in 2010 that some believe was a suicide attempt.

The development of these symptoms, particularly personality changes, is a sign of early CTE. People who have symptoms like these should be examined and considered for the diagnosis. Once CTE is suspected, it is possible to control the damage to a person's life and the lives of his family by placing him under observation and using legal means to prevent him from spending all his money or signing contracts that are damaging to him. His driver's license can be taken away; while this does not prevent him from driving, it may reduce the possibility of car crashes.

Some of the behavioral symptoms of CTE may be controlled through the sparing use of what are called "neuroleptic" drugs. This is a controversial practice; the use of drugs to keep patients docile in the nursing home has been shown to reduce their life expectancy, and it is unlikely that the drugs relieve any of the symptoms internally. They only prevent a patient from thinking and planning complex, dangerous behaviors, in my opinion. They likely do not make the patient feel any better.

Thus, the diagnosis of CTE is somewhat like the diagnosis of Alzheimer's disease. There is no cure, not even any partially effective treatment. There are only custodial measures to limit the damaging effects of the patient's behavior. Despite this, the advantages of identifying patients who have CTE are significant: the family can know what to expect and be alert to prevent some of the traumatic behaviors.

There was a curious case that occurred a year ago that has some bearing on the age of development of symptoms of CTE. A 22 year old football player and wrestler with a history of unreported concussions killed himself just before Christmas of 2014. An autopsy showed that he "did not have CTE" but evidence of prior concussions was found. The young man texted his mother just before he died: "I am sorry if I am an embarrassment but these concussions have my head all fucked up," the text said. It is possible that "chronic traumatic encephalopathy" as a tissue diagnosis takes a lot longer to develop than the symptoms of post-concussive encephalopathy.

Further research may identify treatment, but in the meantime, prevention is the only effective approach. This is where the NFL comes in. We can understand their complaint that no-one knows what the incidence of CTE is, that is, how frequently it occurs in people exposed to concussions. This does not excuse the organization from trying to reduce concussions and reduce the forces to which the brain is subjected during the game of football.

At the same time, the way football is played and who plays it have to be changed. Small children to college players should not be subjected to full-contact head-butting without making it clear to the parents and the players that there is a significant risk. **Football is not alone in facing this problem.** Soccer is also the scene of serious head injuries and less obvious concussions. There is little reason for having soccer players wear helmets, but precautions such as increasing time off after a concussion are warranted. There are other sports where the development of CTE is obvious and expected including Boxing, BMX Biking, NASCAR, etc.

BOSTON UNIVERSITY ALZHEIMER'S DISEASE CENTER

The Boston University Alzheimer's Disease Center (BU ADC) was established in 1996 as one of 29 centers in the US funded by the National Institutes of Health to advance research on Alzheimer's disease and related conditions. The BU ADC, through its CTE Center, also fosters and supports high-impact, innovative research on Chronic Traumatic Encephalopathy and other long-term consequences of repetitive brain trauma in athletes and military personnel, including studies funded by the National Institutes of Health, the Department of Veterans Affairs, the Concussion Legacy Foundation formerly known as the Sports Legacy Institute, and the Department of Defense.

CTE Center

The CTE Center is part of the Boston University Alzheimer's Disease Center (BU ADC), established in 1996 as one of 29 centers in the US funded by the National Institutes of Health to advance research on Alzheimer's disease and related conditions. In collaboration with other NIH-funded ADC's and the non-profit , Concussion Legacy Foundation and CTE Center conducts high-impact, innovative research on Chronic Traumatic Encephalopathy and other long-term consequences of repetitive brain trauma in athletes and military personnel. The mission of the CTE Center is to conduct state-of-the-art research on CTE, including its neuropathology and pathogenesis, clinical presentation, genetics and other risk factors, biomarkers, methods of detection during life, and methods of prevention and treatment.

Many organizations, including the NFL and the NFLPA, have voiced support for CTE Center research and encourage athletes to participate when possible. Recently, when asked if league officials' thinking has evolved, NFL spokesman Brian McCarthy said the league has "embraced research, embraced technology when it comes to the safety of our players. We always believe in getting better. We're encouraging players to work with Dr. Cantu and all of the folks at Boston University."

Clinical and pathological research is expensive and requires significant financial support. The CTE Center has made groundbreaking discoveries from relatively little initial funding, so early supporters of the CTE Center research can be sure their financial support will make a big impact.

Donate online by visiting: Support BU CTE Center

Donate to our Clinical Research in Neurodegenerative Disease Research by visiting: Clinical Research in Neurodegenerative Disease Research

Donate to the VA-BU-SLI Brain Bank and Dr. McKee's work directly at Support the Brain Bank

Write a check to the "Trustees of Boston University" with "BU CTE Center" in the memo line and mail it to:

Boston University School of Medicine
Office of Development
72 East Concord Street, L-219
Boston, MA 02118

> "So many of us are better at inflicting pain than we are at feeling it. We push it onto others rather than turning toward it and feeling our way through the darkness. It requires tremendous courage to get curious about our hurt and lean into it, but I believe in our collective ability to do it. In addition to praying and taking action for the folks... this is my commitment today."
>
> Brene Brown

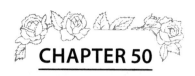

CHAPTER 50

The End of This Book

As of this writing, Barb and I are still moving forward in our recovery. We are gaining strength both physically and spiritually. It was not for me to judge why we survived when others did not.

All I knew was that it was (finally) time for me to get busy doing what God wanted — writing this book! I had to endure the pain, in order to reach out to others, who may have anesthetized their suffering, and help them to find their way,

This book is not a good thing — this book is "a God-thing."

Even Jesus Christ, under the weight of The Cross, fell on the road to his crucifixion. A man along the route was called to help pick up His cross. He helped Jesus with His burden when he was so overwhelmed he could no longer carry it alone.

Sometimes we all need help when we are so overwhelmed we fall and can't go on. There are people in this world who are takers and people who are givers. Sometimes we have to do both. At some point, our spirits need to be replenished as well.

God made it clear to me that my business on this earth was unfinished, and I needed to "love on them some more." I needed to embrace my instincts and teach others how to do this as well.

Nothing happens randomly.

Reach out to your friends
and the people in your life.
Forgive.
If you do not, forgive,
It will destroy you.

Just remember:
To forgive means <u>something has to die</u>.

When all we have in a word from God,
then a word from God is all we need.

Yankee 794 Trauma

Don't give up. This journey is not about the end. It is about the process. It is not about taking shortcuts. Shortcuts don't work in God's World. Just hang on for the ride of your life! Don't despise the process — wait for the full maturity.

You will not have supernatural happen in your life until you walk by Faith. In hard times, it's Faith that will bring the truth of what God wants for you in full measure.

It was the next step in my ultimate recovery, back to an entirely independent life — and to writing this book God kept me alive to write. Hopefully this book will be an inspiration and motivation to others who, up to now, I have yet to meet.

Someday perhaps some will say to me,

"I read your book.
It was like a candle burning in a universe of darkness."

ঽ

When I stand before God at the end of my life,
I would hope that I would not have
a single bit of talent left and could say
"I used everything you gave me."

Erma Bombeck (1927-1996)

ঽ

The purpose of human experience is
to wake up who we really are
and manifest love."

Dr. Maya Angelou

Chapter 50

THIS LETTER IS FROM:
MICHAEL FLUKER, EXECUTIVE DIRECTOR —
Suncoast Center for Independent Living (SCIL)

Barbara (Barb) Scott is a fighter and an inspiration to us all. After her life changing accident, Barb never gave up on living despite the major injuries that she suffered. Re-learning to walk, talk and swallow in adulthood is no small task. Yet, Barb refused to give up on independence without a fight. Her quest to continue making progress eventually led her to Suncoast Center for Independent Living, Inc., (SCIL) where she found additional support from fellow consumers (persons with disabilities) and our staff to aid her on the journey to independence.

SCIL is a non-residential, non-profit 501 (c) (3) federally designated Center for Independent Living (CIL). Centers for Independent Living are cross-disability organizations providing services to people with disabilities so they may lead self-directed lives and fully participate as equal members of society. In addition, SCIL provides a forum where persons with disabilities can develop skills that empower them to independence.

From day one, Barb has consistently attended SCIL classes and support group activities which have provided a social outlet and opportunity to improve her fine motor skills. Although the original intent for attending SCIL was to aid in improving physically, an unforeseen benefit has been the growth in her confidence to advocate for herself and others. Her commitment to advocacy motivated her to volunteer to serve on the SCIL Consumer Advocacy Council where she serves faithfully as Board Secretary. The Consumer Advisory Council (CAC) assists the Suncoast Center for Independent living identify consumer needs for programs, issues of advocacy that require action, and plays an active role in efforts to support the independent living philosophy and uphold the rights of persons with disabilities

Each time she enters SCIL, Barb remains a testimony and inspiration to our consumers that living with a disability is possible and striving for independence is a worthy goal, one worth fighting for.

Michael Fluker
Executive Director
3281 17th Street, Sarasota, FL 34235
Tel: 941-351-9545 ext. 103
Fax: 941-316-9320
A 501 (c) (3) Non-profit

ᘐ

TO MY READERS:

I would love the opportunity and privilege to meet or hear from each of you.

You may wish to send me a personal note and questions:
elizascott6314@gmail com

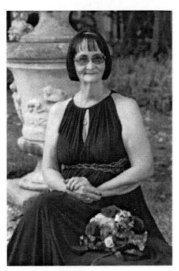

Elizabeth A. Scott
Portrait by Joni Dusek

"If you must look back,
do so forgivingly.
If you must look forward,
do so prayerfully.
However, the wisest thing you
can do is to be present in the
present..........gratefully."

Maya Angelou

"Be the rainbow in
someone else's cloud."

Maya Angelou

"I live a creative life, and you
can't be creative without being
vulnerable. I believe that Creativity
and Fear are basically conjoined
twins; and cannot be separated, one
from the other, without killing them
both. And you don't want to murder
Creativity just to destroy Fear! You
must accept that Creativity cannot
walk ever one step forward except
by marching side-by-side with its
attached sibling of Fear."

Elizabeth Gilbert

Declared Blessing

The Lord bless you and keep you.
The Lord make His face to shine on you.
The Lord turn His face to you
and give you peace.
Numbers 6: 24-26 (NIV)

A blessing is not a blessing until it is declared!

So today,
declare a blessing
over yourself and others.
Speak that blessing in the name of Jesus!

Declare *you are blessed*
with God's supernatural wisdom
and receive clear direction for your life.

Declare today that
you are blessed
with creativity, courage, talent and abundance.

You are blessed
with a strong will,
self-control, and self-dicipline.

You are blessed
with a great family, good friends,
good health, faith, favor and fulfillment.

You are blessed
with success, supernatural strength,
promotion and divine protection.

You are blessed
with a compassionate heart
and a positive outlook on life.

Declare that any curse or negative word
that's ever been spoken over you
is broken right now in the name of Jesus.

Declare that everything
you put your hands to is going to prosper and succeed!
Declare it today and every day.

Deuteronomy 28: 1-14

When I Say I'm A Christian

By Carol Wimmer

When I say, "I am a Christian"
I'm not shouting, "I've been saved!"
I'm whispering, "I get lost!
That's why I chose this way!"

When I say, "I'm a Christian"
I don't speak with human pride
I'm confessing that I stumble –
Needing God to be my guide.

When I say, "I am a Christian"
I'm not bragging of success
I'm admitting that I've failed
And cannot ever pay the debt.

When I say, "I am a Christian"
I don't think I know it all
I submit humbly to my confusion
Asking humbly to be taught.

When I say "I am a Christian
I'm not claiming to be perfect
My flaws are all too visible
But God believes I'm worth it.

When I say, "I am a Christian"
I still feel the sting of pain
I have my share of heartaches
Which is why I seek God's name.

When I say, "I am a Christian"
I do not wish to judge
I have no authority…
I only know I'm loved.

MANIFESTO of the BRAVE and BROKENHEARTED

There is no greater threat
to the critics and cynics and fearmongers
Than those of us who are willing to fall
because we have learned how to rise.

With skinned knees and bruised hearts:
We choose owning our stories of struggle,
Over hiding, over hustling, over pretending.

We will not be characters in our own stories
Not villains, not victims, not ever heroes.
We are the authors of our lives,
We write our own daring endings.
We craft love from heartbreak.
Compassion from shame.
Grace from disappointments.
Courage from failure.
Showing up is our power.
Story is our way home. Truth is our song.
We are the brave and brokenhearted
We are rising strong.

By Brene Brown #RISING STRONG

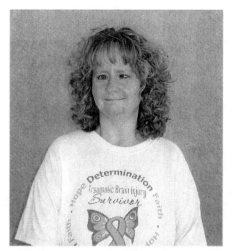

Taken January 4, 2016 – five years
after her accident.

"We delight in the beauty of the butterfly but rarely admit the changes it had gone through to achieve that beauty."

Maya Angelou

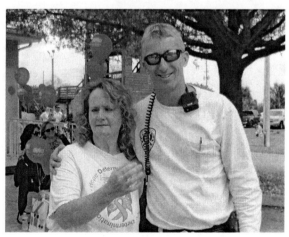

Taken March 2016
Ryan French, one of Barb's 9-1-1 First responders.

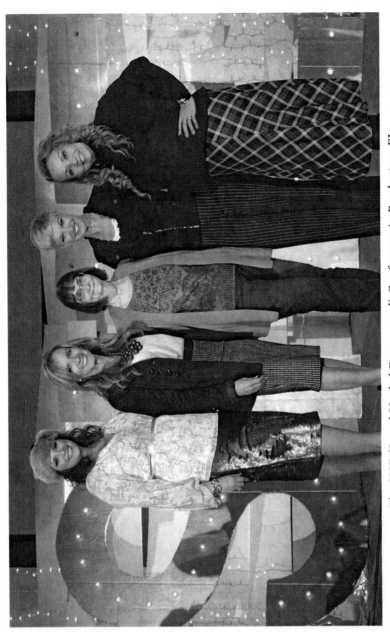

The SHE (Saved Healed Empowered) Conference in Bradenton, FL.
January 22, 2016
(Left to Right) Jeni Cook-Stavale, Joanne Bradford Hoehne,
Elizabeth A. Scott, Tracy Strawberry, Dr. Samantha Phillips

Endorsements

Elizabeth Scott describes in vivid detail the aftermath of her daughter Barbara's tragic accident on December 29, 2010. Her work is both an education and experience in hope and fortitude. It is not often first responders are searched out to thank for their efforts. I am personally and professionally honored the Scott family included Cedar Hammock Fire Rescue, Manatee County EMS, and the crew of Bayflite in their story.

There is no doubt our lives on Earth are short even in times of hardship. Elizabeth provides a chance for the readers to reflect on the delicateness of life as well as the often unknown inner strength we have inside each of us.

Thanks Elizabeth and Barbara for sharing your story...
–Alexander D. Lobeto
Division Chief/Administration, Cedar Hammock Fire Rescue
Alobeto@chfr.org, 941-727-2071 private, 941-737-4057 cell

I proudly endorse Betty (Elizabeth) Scott for the magnificent job in reliving the ordeal her and her wonderful daughter, Barbara endured for these past many years. From the very moment of Barb's horrible accident, Betty (Elizabeth) was by her side doing whatever it took to make sure Barb received the finest attention to help her to her recovery. I am Betty's friend and watched her caring for her daughter. A mothers love for her child was never more apparent than what she went through. Then Betty was struck with cancer and had to battle that malady. I firmly believe that because of her belief in the Lord, her trust and faith was the key for their present health.

Take care my wonderful friend and truly, God Bless you and Barb.
–Ray Driscoll

As a nurse and traumatic brain injury survivor, this is one of the most amazing and critical books of its time. It is a stand-alone, all-encompassing book like no other on each and every subject portrayed. I have read and fully endorse this book, and here is why.

I simply could not put this book down! As the page plot twisted and turned, I was thoroughly riveted by all five senses. You get a book filled with heart, inspiration, recognition of the human spirit, awareness, education, and simply down to earth truth, told in never before mentioned ways.

Each topic, every person, is brought into full bloom by a very talented and creative author, biographer, and autobiographer, with stellar artistic composition. This beautiful story unfolds to include much new understanding and awareness, as well as a full array of many people's lives touched, and melded all into one grand masterpiece.

Elizabeth Scott, author, mother and advocate extraordinaire, brings to us, an interwoven story whose two main characters are nurses, Mother, and daughter, as well as caregivers and survivors. Both, faced with stories within stories of trauma, tragedy, hope, love, faith, miracles, and survival.

Barbara Scott, the daughter, imparts much of herself and her beautiful character here as well. Her severe injury and her miraculous recovery process (which continues to this day and beyond) to a new fabulous version of herself, along with her radiant, if not spunky spirit.

Throughout the pages, healthcare providers are an integral and highly respected part of the story in its whole. Without them, the outcomes would simply never be the possible. As if that is not enough, add to it a brand new awareness of the complexities of multiple kinds of brain injuries, as well as other conditions of life;

Elizabeth's own harrowing journey with death and life... including but not limited to loving, hurting, comforting, sorrow and loss, to healing and faith giving life.

–Stephanie Haggart, RN

About the Author

Elizabeth A. Scott spent her adult life working with a passion for nursing in Missouri (where she was born and raised) and Florida (moving in 1988). It has always been second-nature for her to take on leadership roles when she saw the need and finds a purpose in helping her fellow humans.

After she was widowed at age 30 in 1978, she raised her three children, Andrea, Barbara and Mark, and applied an interest in genetics living on a farm and raising rabbits, cavies, goats and sheep as a hobby and in exhibition.

In the 1980's she was centrally and acutely involved in The American Adoption Congress as a regional director. She published a national newsletter on adoption reform, and held a number of leadership roles.

For 6 years she ran a parrot rescue. She has also volunteered in many forms including homeless shelter and resources, and currently with her church.

She is now an author, speaker and continues to champion work to further education about Traumatic Brain Injury (including CTE and Domestic Violence) as well as encouraging inspiration and hope, and providing resources. She currently lives in Ellenton, Florida, with her husband, and has 5 grandchildren and 3 great-grandchildren.

The Road Not Taken
By Robert Frost (1874–1963)

Two roads diverged in a yellow wood,
And sorry I could not travel both
And be one traveler, long I stood
And looked down one as far as I could
To where it bent in the undergrowth;

Then took the other, as just as fair,
And having perhaps the better claim,
Because it was grassy and wanted wear;
Though as for that the passing there
Had worn them really about the same,

And both that morning equally lay
In leaves no step had trodden black.
Oh, I kept the first for another day!
Yet knowing how way leads on to way,
I doubted if I should ever come back.

I shall be telling this with a sigh
Somewhere ages and ages hence:
Two roads diverged in a wood, and I—
I took the one less traveled by,
And that has made all the difference.

"Tetelestai"

Resources

Brain Injury National Resources
http://www.braininjuryresources.org/

National Resourcs Center for Traumatic Brain Injury
http://www.tbinrc.com/

BRAINLINE.ORG has many resources for people with TBI and their families and caregivers. It is highly recommended. They have listed a state-by-state directory of resources that you can access.

TheSocietyforCognitiveRehabilitation.org is a valuable resource with many resources for TBI survivors and families/caregivers.

CNS — Centre for Neuro Skills
http://www.neuroskills.com/family/family-resources.php
There is an extensive listing of resources for family/caregivers.

AbleData
Phone: 800-227-0216
AbleData provides objective information on assistive technology and rehabilitation equipment available from domestic and international sources to consumers, organizations, professionals, and caregivers within the United States.

America's Heroes at Work
Phone: 1-866-4-USA-DOL (1-866-487-2365)
America's Heroes at Work is a U.S. Department of Labor (DOL) project that addresses the employment challenges of returning service members living with Traumatic Brain Injury (TBI) and/or Post-Traumatic Stress Disorder (PTSD).

American Veterans with Brain Injuries
American Veterans with Brain Injuries (AVBI) is an online resource for American veterans who have suffered a brain injury and their families.

Blinded Veterans Association
Phone: 202-371-8880
The Blinded Veterans Association (BVA) was established specifically to help veterans and their families meet and overcome the challenges of blindness. All legally blinded veterans are eligible for BVA's assistance whether they become blind during or after active duty military service.

Brain Injury Association of America
Phone: 703-761-0750
The Brain Injury Association of America (BIAA) was founded by individuals who wanted to improve the quality of life for patients who had sustained brain injuries and their family members. This organization serves and represents individuals, families and professionals who are touched by a life-altering, often devastating, traumatic brain injury (TBI).

Resources

Brain Injury Network
Phone: 707-544-4323
Founded in 1998, the Brain Injury Network is a non-profit advocacy organization operated for and by survivors of acquired brain injury (ABI).

Brain Injury Partners
The Brain Injury Partners program was created by a team of researchers, software developers and web designers at the Oregon Center for Applied Science, Inc. (ORCAS), in Eugene, Oregon

Brain Trauma Foundation
Phone: 212-772-0608
The Brain Trauma Foundation was founded to improve the outcome of traumatic brain injury (TBI) patients by developing best practice guidelines, conducting clinical research, and educating medical personnel.

CEMM Traumatic Brain Injury
Phone: 719-333-7565
Traumatic Brain Injury: The Journey Home is a CEMM web resource on Traumatic Brain Injury (TBI), including information for patients, family members, and caregivers.

Center for Neuroscience and Regenerative Medicine
Phone: 855-TBI-CNRM (855-824-2676)
The Center for Neuroscience and Regenerative Medicine (CNRM) was established by Congress to bring together physicians and scientists in the National Capital area to develop new approaches to brain injury diagnosis and recovery. They have over 20 active clinical research studies in brain injury and posttraumatic stress disorder. Most of their research takes place at the National Institutes of Health (NIH) and National Naval Medical Center in Bethesda, MD, and Walter Reed Army Medical Center in Washington, DC.

Center on Brain Injury Research and Training
Phone: 541-346-0593
Established in 1993 at the Teaching Research Institute, a division of Western Oregon University, CBIRT conducts research and training to improve the lives of children and adults with traumatic brain injury (TBI). CBIRT's research focuses on developing interventions to improve outcomes related to education, employability, and quality of life. Our training activities promote the use of best practices among educators and other professionals who serve individuals with TBI.

Centers for Disease Control and Prevention
Phone: 800-232-4636
CDC.gov is the Center for Disease Control's primary online communication channel, providing an online source for credible health information.

Commonwealth Community Trust
Phone: 804-740-6930
Commonwealth Community Trust (CCT) is a non-profit, Virginia-based organization established in 1990 by parents of children with disabilities. The CCT provides a convenient and economical way to have trust funds administered for

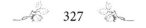

people with disabilities that will supplement the benefits offered by entitlement programs.

**Computer/Electronic Accommodations Program's
Wounded Service Member Initiative
Phone: 703-681-8813**
The Computer/Electronic Accommodations Program (CAP) increases access to information and works to remove barriers to employment opportunities by eliminating the costs of assistive technology and accommodation solutions.

**Defense and Veterans Brain Injury Center National Headquarters
Phone: 1-800-870-9244**
The mission of the Defense and Veterans Brain Injury Center (DVBIC) is to serve active duty military, their beneficiaries, and veterans with traumatic brain injuries (TBIs).

**Defense Centers of Excellence for Psychological Health
and Traumatic Brain Injury Real Warriors Campaign
Phone: 866-966-1020**
The Real Warriors Campaign is an initiative launched by the Defense Centers of Excellence for Psychological Health and Traumatic Brain Injury (DCoE) to promote the processes of building resilience, facilitating recovery and supporting reintegration of returning service members, veterans and their families.

Disability Friendly Colleges
DisabilityFriendlyColleges.com includes interactive charts of more than 75 disability friendly colleges and their services, compiled by the Tiedemann family, who have first-hand experience with the subject.

**Disabled Sports USA
Phone: 301-217-0960**
Disabled Sport USA, a national nonprofit organization, was established in 1967 by disabled Vietnam veterans. DS/USA now offers nationwide sports rehabilitation programs to anyone with a permanent disability.

**Epilepsy Foundation
Phone: 800-332-1000**
The Epilepsy Foundation of America is the national voluntary agency dedicated solely to the welfare of the almost 3 million people with epilepsy in the U.S. and their families.

Directions to Brain Injury Support Group at Bancroft
Affiliated with the Brain Injury Alliance of New Jersey, this support group allows persons with brain injuries and their family members to meet others who are in similar situations, gain valuable emotional support from one another, form friendships, obtain information and resources, and hear speakers discuss a variety of brain-injury topics. The meetings are an opportunity for both persons with brain injuries and their relatives to discuss the difficulties and hardships they face, as well as the accomplishments and joys in their lives.

Resources

Twenty Alliance-affiliated support groups meet in New Jersey, serving 17 counties.
The Alliance monitors the activities of these groups, the qualifications of their leaders, and provides them with information and resources on a regular basis.

Brain Injury Alliance of NJ
The official website of the Brain Injury Alliance of New Jersey, an organization dedicated to bringing "together people with brain injury, their families and friends, and concerned allied health professionals to improve the quality of life people experience after brain injury." The website includes a section on learning about brain injuries as well as programs and services for individuals with brain injuries and their families.

Brain Injury Association of Delaware
The Brain Injury Association of Delaware, affiliated with the Brain Injury Association of America, is a not-for-profit organization whose mission is to create a better future through brain injury prevention, research, education and advocacy.

Brain Injury Association of Pennsylvania
The official website of the Brain Injury Association of Pennsylvania offers information about state programs for brain injured persons, and information on resources, advocacy, research, and prevention.

BrainLine
BrainLine is a national multimedia project offering information and resources about preventing, treating, and living with traumatic brain injuries. BrainLine includes a series of webcasts, an electronic newsletter, and an extensive outreach campaign in partnership with national organizations concerned about traumatic brain injury.

BrainLine Military
This website provides military-specific information and resources on traumatic brain injury to veterans, service members in the Army, Navy, Air Force, Marines, National Guard, Reserve, and their families. Through video, webcasts, articles, personal stories, research briefs, and current news, those whose lives have been affected by TBI can learn more about brain injury symptoms and treatment, rehabilitation, and family issues associated with TBI care and recovery.

Centers for Disease Control & Prevention: Traumatic Brain Injury
CDC's research and programs work to prevent TBI and help people better recognize, respond, and recover if a TBI occurs. Topics in this website include: concussions and mild TBI, serious TBI, concussions in sports, clinical diagnosis and management, statistics, long-term outcomes, causes and risk groups, and prevention.

Defense and Veterans Brain Injury Center
The mission of the Defense and Veterans Brain Injury Center (DVBIC) is to serve active duty military, their beneficiaries, and veterans with traumatic brain injuries (TBIs) through state-of-the-art clinical care, innovative clinical research initiatives and educational programs. DVBIC fulfills this mission through ongoing collaboration with military, VA and civilian health partners, local communities, families and individuals with TBI.

National Institute of Neurological Disorders and Stroke
This website provides detailed information about traumatic brain injuries, including research updates, clinical trial overviews and links to other brain-injury support organizations.

New Jersey Commission on Brain Injury Research
The official website of the New Jersey Commission on Brain Injury Research offers information on Commission's goals and services. The mission of the NJCBIR is "to promote the necessary research that will result in the treatment and cure for traumatic injuries of the brain, thereby giving hope to an ever-increasing number of residents who suffer the debilitating effects of this injury."

Rehabilitation Institute of Chicago
In 2001, the Rehabilitation Institute of Chicago (RIC) set out to build a consumer resource center located on the first floor of its flagship hospital in Chicago, and to provide virtual access to its resource collection through a website. The Center is like a bookstore where all resources are related to persons with disabilities and their families.

Traumatic Brain Injury: The Journey Home
This website provides an informative and sensitive exploration of TBI, including information for patients, family members and caregivers. Topics include types and symptoms of brain injury, TBI treatment and recovery, and helpful insights about the potential long-term effects of brain injury.

U.S. Department of Veterans Affairs
This website offers veterans and service members detailed information about traumatic brain injuries and the rehabilitation process. Topics include the latest news updates and real-life profiles, and videos and documentaries featuring veterans recovering from traumatic brain injuries.

What is TBI
This website is dedicated to providing information and resources to help military personnel who are diagnosed with traumatic brain injuries.

Below are links to searchable directories of organizations, associations, and government agencies.

You can use these directories to find a variety of services and service providers near you.

American Academy of Child & Adolescent Psychiatry
The American Academy of Child and Adolescent Psychiatry (AACAP) is a national professional medical association dedicated to treating and improving the quality of life for children, adolescents, and families affected by mental, behavioral, or developmental disorders. The AACAP's web site has a research tool called the "Child and Adolescent Psychiatrist Finder," which is designed to help parents (and other adults seeking psychiatric care for their children) to locate psychiatrists who specifically provide care for children and adolescents. Any psychiatrist that appears

in the finder has previously reported to AACAP that he/she is a provider of such services.

American Academy of Clinical Neuropsychology
The American Academy of Clinical Neuropsychology (AACN) is an organization for psychologists who have achieved board certification in the specialty of Clinical Neuropsychology, under the auspices of the American Board of Clinical Neuropsychology (ABCN). The AACN's web site provides a directory that lists all current academy members. The directory is searchable by last name, state, country, or languages spoken.

American Academy of Neurology
The American Academy of Neurology (AAN)'s Patients and Caregivers site provides information on neurologic disorders and treatments. The site combines information from such sources as the American Academy of Neurology and the National Institute of Neurological Disorders and Stroke websites into one centralized resource center for patients and their families/caregivers. Among its services is the Find a Neurologist directory, which allows users to locate an AAN member neurologist by city, state/province, and/or country.

American Academy of Physical Medicine and Rehabilitation
The American Academy of Physical Medicine and Rehabilitation (AAPM&R) is the only organization that exclusively serves the needs of practicing Physical Medicine and Rehabilitation (PM&R) physicians. AAPM&R offers Find a PM&R Physician, a searchable database that allows users to locate a PM&R physician in their local area. The database is searchable by last name, state or province, zip/postal code, or telephone area code (US only). Users can also search by country to locate physicians outside the United States. With more than 7,500 members, the Academy represents more than 87 percent of US physiatrists and international colleagues from 37 countries.

American Medical Association
The American Medical Association's (AMA) mission is to unite physicians nationwide to collaborate on the most important professional and public health issues in the United States. The AMA provides DoctorFinder, an online physician locator that provides users with basic professional information on nearly all licensed physicians in the United States. DoctorFinder includes more than 814,000 doctors.

American Occupational Therapy Association
Established in 1917, The American Occupational Therapy Association (AOTA) represents the interests and concerns of occupational therapy practitioners and students of occupational therapy, and improves the quality of occupational therapy services. Current AOTA membership is approximately 39,000, including occupational therapists, occupational therapy assistants, and occupational therapy students. Members reside in all 50 states, the District of Columbia, Puerto Rico, and internationally. AOTA provides a State Associations search tool so that users can find an AOTA affiliated service provider in his/her local area.

American Physical Therapy Association
The American Physical Therapy Association (APTA) is a national professional organization that represents more than 74,000 members. Its goal is to enable

advancements in physical therapy practice, research, and education. APTA's "Find a PT" allows users search a national database of physical therapist members of APTA. Find a PT must be used for the purpose of seeking physical therapy care.

American Psychiatric Association
The American Psychiatric Association (APA) is a medical specialty society with more than 38,000 U.S. and international member physicians. APA's members work together to provide humane care and effective treatment for all persons with mental disorder, including mental retardation and substance-related disorders. APA Members are primarily medical specialists who are psychiatrists or in the process of becoming psychiatrists. The APA provides a District Branches & State Associations directory on its web site.

American Psychological Association
Based in Washington, DC, the American Psychological Association (APA) is a scientific and professional organization that represents psychology in the United States. With 150,000 members, APA is the largest association of psychologists worldwide. The APA provides a search tool, Psychologist Locator, that allows users to find practicing psychologists in their local area.

American Speech-Language-Hearing Association
The American Speech-Language-Hearing Association (ASHA) is the professional, scientific, and credentialing association for 140,000 members and affiliates who are speech-language pathologists, audiologists, and speech, language, and hearing scientists in the United States and internationally. ASHA offers ProSearch, a directory that helps users locate certified audiologist and speech-language pathologists in their local area.

Brain Injury Association of America
Founded in 1980, the Brain Injury Association of America (BIAA) is a national organization serving and representing individuals, families and professionals who are touched by a life-altering, often devastating, traumatic brain injury (TBI). BIAA provides a State Resources Search tool, which includes a range of state agencies that offer information and services to persons with brain injury and their families.

Commission on Accreditation of Rehabilitation Facilities
The Commission on Accreditation of Rehabilitation Facilities (CARF) International family of organizations, including CARF Canada, CARF, and CARF-CCAC, is an independent, nonprofit accreditor of health and human services. CARF International provides an Accredited Provider Search tool so that users can locate a provider in their local area.

Defense and Veterans Brain Injury Center
The mission of the Defense and Veterans Brain Injury Center (DVBIC) is to serve active duty military, their beneficiaries, and veterans with traumatic brain injuries (TBIs) through state-of-the-art clinical care, innovative clinical research initiatives and educational programs. DVBIC provides an Interactive Map that allows users to search for military medical centers, VA hospitals, and other services/partners in their local area.

Resources

Healthfinder.gov
Healthfinder.gov has resources on a wide range of health topics selected from over 1,600 government and non-profit organizations. Healthfinder.gov is coordinated by the Office of Disease Prevention and Health Promotion (ODPHP) and its health information referral service, the National Health Information Center. Healthfinder. gov is supported solely by U.S. government funds. Heathfinder's Services & Information directory helps users find doctors, health centers, and organizations that offer services and support.

Independent Living Research Utilization
Independent Living Research Utilization (ILRU), founded in 1975, provides research, education, and consultation in the areas of independent living, the Americans with Disabilities Act, home and community based services. ILRU also assists people with disabilities and health issues. ILRU provides a Directory of Independent Living Centers & Related Organizations, searchable by state.

National Academy of Neuropsychology
The mission of the National Academy of Neuropsychology (NAN) is to advance neuropsychology as a science and health profession, to promote human welfare, and to generate and disseminate knowledge of brain-behavior relationships. NAN provides a searchable Membership Directory on its web site.

National Board for Certified Counselors
The National Board for Certified Counselors, Inc. and Affiliates (NBCC), an independent not-for-profit credentialing body for counselors, was incorporated in 1982 to establish and monitor a national certification system. NBCC identifies those counselors who have voluntarily sought and obtained certification, and to maintains a register of those counselors. NBCC provides CounselorFind, a voluntary directory that helps individuals, organizations, employers, and the public find a counselor by name, location and/or area of practice.

National Center for Crisis Management
The National Register of Health Service Providers in Psychology, established in 1974, is a national nonprofit organization that is committed to advancing psychology as a profession and improving the delivery of high quality health services to the public. The organization disseminates industry information and news, and supplies self-help resources and a free, unrestricted referral database to consumers. Users can search the Psychologist Directory by city, state, or zip code.

National Dissemination Center for Children with Disabilities
National Dissemination Center for Children with Disabilities (NICHCY) provides information and resources on disabilities in infants, toddlers, children, and youth, as well as public policy related to these issues, including the No Child Left Behind Act. NICHCY provides state specific directory of organizations and agencies that address disability-related issues. The offices listed within this directory are primarily state-level.

National Register of Health Service Providers in Psychology
The National Register of Health Service Providers in Psychology, established in 1974, is a national nonprofit organization that is committed to advancing psychology as a profession and improving the delivery of high quality health services to the public.

The organization disseminates industry information and news, and supplies self-help resources and a free, unrestricted referral database to consumers. Users can search the Psychologist Directory by city, state, or zip code.

Rehabilitation Research Center for Traumatic Brain Injury and Spinal Cord Injury
For the past quarter century Santa Clara Valley Medical Center has been actively involved in the "Model Systems" projects sponsored by the National Institute on Disability and Rehabilitation Research. These projects allowed centers of excellence to expand in the areas of clinical improvement, outcome research, and community programs. The Center's Research Rehabilitation Center provides the Traumatic Brain Injury Resource Directory (TBIRD), which provides information on the range of TBI services in the Santa Clara Valley area (and beyond). This resource is intended for the use of anyone with a TBI, their family and friends, or anyone who works with people with TBI.

Substance Abuse & Mental Health Services Administration: Mental Health
The Substance Abuse and Mental Health Services Administration (SAMHSA)'s mission is to reduce the impact of substance abuse and mental illness on America's communities. SAMHSA's National Mental Health Information Center provides information about mental health via a toll-free telephone number (1-800-789-2647), this web site, and more than 600 publications. The National Mental Health Information Center was developed for users of mental health services and their families, the general public, policy makers, providers, and the media. SAMHSA offers a Mental Health Services Locator, which is searchable by state.

Below are links to international organizations and web resources that offer general information on a range of topics related to traumatic brain injury.

Brain Injury Association of Canada
Phone: 866-977-2492
Founded in 2003, the Brain Injury Association of Canada (BIAC)'s mission is to improve the quality of life for all Canadians affected by acquired brain injury, and promote brain injury prevention. BIAC partners with national, provincial/territorial and regional associations, and other stakeholders, to facilitate post-trauma research, education and advocacy. BIAC is incorporated as a national charitable organization under the Canada Corporations Act and Canada Revenue Agency.

Brain Injury Australia
Phone: +61 2 9808 9390
Founded in 1986, Brain Injury Australia (BIA) represents all Australians with acquired brain injury. BIA represents, through its State and Territory Member Organizations, the needs of people with an acquired brain injury, their families and caregivers. BIA operates at a national level to ensure that all people living with acquired brain injury have access to the supports and resources they need.

Resources

Brain Injury New Zealand
Phone: 09 414 5693
Brain Injury New Zealand (BIANZ) represents the regional Brain Injury Associations around New Zealand. These regional associations provide education, advocacy, support and information to any person with a brain injury and their families and/or caregivers. The national office provides support for the regional associations, national level advocacy, and political review.

European Brain Injury Society
Phone: +32 (0)2 522 20 03
EBIS is a European association that serves traumatic brain injured persons and victims of acquired cerebral lesions: stroke, anoxia, encephalitis, brain tumour. EBIS members have access to a network of brain injury professionals and services. Other benefits include seminars, workshops and advice about relevant activities of the European Union. EBIS has 165 individual and institutional members from all the countries of the European Union, plus Switzerland.

Headway UK
Phone: 0808 800 2244
Headway is a charity set up to give help and support to people affected by brain injury. It does this both locally and nationally. Headway's mission is to promote understanding of all aspects of brain injury and to provide information, support and services to people with a brain injury, their families and carers.

International Brain Injury Association
Phone: 703-960-0027
Founded in 1993, the International Brain Injury Association (IBIA) is dedicated to the development and support of multidisciplinary medical and clinical professionals, advocates, policy makers, consumers and others who work to improve outcomes and opportunities for persons with brain injury.

Shocking Facts About PTSD & TBI

- TBI — 20% of returning Iraq & Afghanistan veterans suffered TBI
- Diagnosed cases of PTSD in veterans have jumped 50%
- More than 200,000 veterans are homeless on any given night.
- 45% of homeless veterans suffer from some mental illness
- Economic impact including medical care, productivity and suicide: $4 to $6 BILLION over two years. These numbers are growing.
- Conservatively 20% of all U.S. combat veterans suffer PTSD
- 20% of the soldiers deployed in the past 10 years have PTSD. (That is well over 300,000 men and women.)
- 17% of combat troops who have been deployed are women.
- 71% of women deployed develop PTSD
- 6 – 11% of returning vets have PTSD (Afghanistan)
- 12 – 20% of returning vets have PTSD (IRAQ)
- 6,912 veterans a year commit suicide (2010)
  22 vets per day commit suicide
  126 vets per week commit suicide
- 55% of women and 38% of men report being victims of sexual harassment (while serving in the military)
- 30% of soldiers develop mental problems within 3-4 months of being home

Dispelling Myths About Posttraumatic Stress Disorder

Combat brings the possibility of losing close friends, bodily harm, exposure to terrifying events, and extended separation from loved ones. As many as 30 percent of service members redeploying from Iraq and Afghanistan can experience stress reactions associated with these situations.[1] Posttraumatic stress disorder (PTSD) may also develop, however, the facts and fiction about PTSD are sometimes hard to tell apart.

While service members may experience stress reactions resulting from a combat deployment, they are not necessarily an indication of PTSD. Common symptoms associated with both combat stress and PTSD, like nightmares, increased anxiety, and reliving the event, could result in a diagnosis of PTSD if there is no noticeable improvement during a short-term period.2 PTSD is a psychiatric condition that requires long-term treatment to deal with symptoms.[2]

Many service members who experience PTSD can benefit from treatment and support, but some fear that they may be considered weak or that peers might lose confidence in their abilities. This is due, in part, to the perception that some service members have about seeking help, as well as the myths surrounding PTSD. Knowing the truth about PTSD can make a real difference in the lives of those who need support. This article debunks some of the common myths about PTSD.

Five Myths and Facts about PTSD

• *Myth: I cannot get or maintain my security clearance if I am diagnosed with PTSD.*

Fact: Getting treatment for PTSD is not necessarily a threat to an individual's security clearance. In fact, mental health counseling can be a positive factor in the clearance process.[3] Army records show that 99.98 percent of cases with psychological concerns obtained/retained their security clearance.[4] Additionally, service members are not required to report some treatments, including those for PTSD, they received due to service in the military when they apply for a security clearance.[5] Factors that could result in clearance refusal include not meeting financial obligations, criminal actions or engaging in activities benefiting a foreign nation.[3]

• *Myth: My military career will end if I am diagnosed with PTSD.*

Fact: Being diagnosed with PTSD in and of itself does not end your military career. There are plenty of examples where service members have sought treatment for various psychological health concerns, including PTSD, and it did not put their careers in jeopardy. In fact, a failure to seek treatment can lead to a more serious psychological condition, and could eventually prevent someone from carrying out some sensitive tasks.[4] Seeking support to address psychological health concerns shows inner strength and is commonly looked on favorably. Check out these video profiles of some service members who have received treatment for psychological health concerns and continue to fulfill their regular duties in uniform, as well as veterans who sought care and continue to serve the military community as civilians.

• *Myth: Service members only experience PTSD symptoms immediately following combat or a traumatic event.*

Fact: Symptoms associated with PTSD usually occur within three months after the traumatic event[6], but symptoms may not appear until six months, or even years later.[7] The types of symptoms can be broken down into four categories: hyperarousal (feeling "keyed up"), avoidance (avoiding reminders of the event), intrusion (reliving the event), and feeling numb or detached.[8] Nightmares, one of the most common symptoms, are experienced by 71–96 percent of those with PTSD.[9] Reaching out for care is an important step since symptoms, such as nightmares, may lessen or disappear and then re-appear later in life. Early intervention can provide the right coping tools to deal with these symptoms, and sometimes even prevent development of chronic PTSD. Visit the National Center for PTSD to learn more about the types of symptoms associated with PTSD.

• *Myth: Service members can never fully recover from PTSD.*

Fact: Successful treatment and positive outcome are greatly enhanced by early intervention. With therapy, and in some cases medication, the symptoms of PTSD can be greatly reduced, even eliminated.[6] Treatment can help you feel more in control and teach effective coping mechanisms to deal with stressful situations when they arise. There are many types of treatment; your medical provider can help you determine which one is best. You can also contact the DCoE Outreach Center 24/7 at 866-966-1020 where highly trained professionals can answer questions and connect you with local resources for support.

Resources

• *Myth: PTSD is a sign of weakness in character.*

Fact: PTSD is a common human reaction to very traumatic situations. PTSD seems to be due to complex chemical changes in the brain when an individual witnesses or experiences a traumatic event. The symptoms of PTSD appear to be frequently experienced in situations where someone perceives they have been exposed to a life-threatening event, although symptoms and reactions vary from person to person.[10] As a service member dealing with PTSD symptoms, seeking help demonstrates strength and will provide benefits to yourself, your family, your unit, and your service. Do not hesitate to seek care – PTSD is treatable and reaching out early often leads to the best outcomes.[7]

Many service members have sought help and continue serving in the military, as shown in these videos. Knowing the facts about PTSD can help you overcome concerns you may have. Visit the following web sites to get additional information and resources on PTSD:

- Defense Center of Excellence for Psychological Health and Traumatic Brain Injury: PTSD Treatment Options
- Center for the Study of Traumatic Stress (CSTS): PTSD
- National Center for PTSD: How Common is PTSD?
- Deployment Health Clinical Center: Mental Health

Sources

[1]Carden, Michael J., Sgt. 1st Class. "Army Works to Expand Combat Stress Detection," American Forces Press Service. Published July 22, 2010.

[2]Combat Stress for Medical Providers [PDF 2.3 MB], Deployment Health Clinical Center, Department of Defense. Published August 2006.

[3]Implementation of Adjudicative Guidelines for Determining Eligibility for Access to Classified Information [PDF 1.1 MB], Department of Defense. Published August 30, 2006.

[4]Haire, Tamara. "Financial Problems or PTSD Need Not Affect Security Clearance," Army News Service. Published July 8, 2009.

[5]Miles, Donna. "Gates Works to Reduce Mental Health Stigma," American Forces Press Service. Published May 1, 2008.

[6]"TBI and PTSD Quick Facts [PDF 28.7 KB]," Deployment Health Clinical Center, Department of Defense. Last accessed June 19, 2014.

[7]Pueschel, Matt. "Combat Exposure Raises PTSD, Smoking, Alcohol Abuse Risks," Force Health Protection & Readiness, Department of Defense. Published May 22, 2009.

[8]"What is PTSD?," National Center for PTSD, Department of Veterans Affairs. Last accessed June 19, 2014.

[9]"Nightmares & PTSD," National Center for PTSD, Department of Veterans Affairs. Last accessed June 19, 2014.

[10]Stress & Trauma, Fact Sheets: A Normal Reaction to an Abnormal Situation, Deployment Health Clinical Center, Department of Defense. Last accessed June 19, 2014.

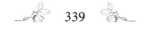

Neuroscience & Neurology

How Does Post-Traumatic Stress Disorder Change the Brain?

by Viatcheslav Wlassoff, PhD | January 24, 2015

Child abuse. Rape. Sexual assault. Brutal physical attack. Being in a war and witnessing violence, bloodshed, and death from close quarters. Near death experiences. These are extremely traumatic events, and some victims bear the scars for life.

The physical scars heal, but some emotional wounds stop the lives of these people dead in their tracks. They are afraid to get close to people or form new relationships. Change terrifies them, and they remain forever hesitant to express their needs or give vent to their creative potential. It may not be always apparent, but post-traumatic stress disorder (PTSD) stifles the life force out of its victims. It is no use telling them to "get over" it because PTSD fundamentally changes the brain's structure and alters its functionalities.

What goes on inside the brains of people with PTSD?

PTSD is painful and frightening. The memories of the event linger and victims often have vivid flashbacks. Frightened and traumatized, they are almost always on edge and the slightest of cues sends them hurtling back inside their protective shells. Usually victims try to avoid people, objects, and situations that remind them of their hurtful experiences; this behavior is debilitating and prevents them from living their lives meaningfully.

Many victims forget the details of the incident, obviously in an attempt to lessen the blow. But this coping mechanism has negative repercussions as well. Without accepting and reconciling with "reality," they turn into fragmented souls.

Extensive neuroimaging studies on the brains of PTSD patients show that several regions differ structurally and functionally from those of healthy individuals. The amygdala, the hippocampus, and the ventromedial prefrontal cortex play a role in triggering the typical symptoms of PTSD. These regions collectively impact the stress response mechanism in humans, so the PTSD victim, even long after his experiences, continues to perceive and respond to stress differently than someone who is not suffering the aftermaths of trauma.

Effect of trauma on the hippocampus

The most significant neurological impact of trauma is seen in the hippocampus. PTSD patients show a considerable reduction in the volume of the hippocampus. This region of the brain is responsible for memory functions. It helps an individual to record new memories and retrieve them later in response to specific and relevant environmental stimuli. The hippocampus also helps us distinguish between past and present memories.

PTSD patients with reduced hippocampal volumes lose the ability to discriminate between past and present experiences or interpret environmental contexts correctly. Their particular neural mechanisms trigger extreme stress responses when confronted with environmental situations that only remotely resemble something from their traumatic past. This is why a sexual assault victim is terrified of parking lots because she was once raped in a similar place. A war veteran still cannot watch violent movies because they remind him of his trench days; his hippocampus cannot minimize the interference of past memories.

Effect of trauma on the ventromedial prefrontal cortex

Severe emotional trauma causes lasting changes in the ventromedial prefrontal cortex region of the brain that is responsible for regulating emotional responses triggered by the amygdala. Specifically, this region regulates negative emotions like fear that occur when confronted with specific stimuli. PTSD patients show a marked decrease in the volume of ventromedial prefrontal cortex and the functional ability of this region. This explains why people suffering from PTSD tend to exhibit fear, anxiety, and extreme stress responses even when faced with stimuli not connected – or only remotely connected – to their experiences from the past.

Effect of trauma on the amygdala

Trauma appears to increase activity in the amygdala. This region of the brain helps us process emotions and is also linked to fear responses. PTSD patients exhibit hyperactivity in the amygdala in response to stimuli that are somehow connected to their traumatic experiences. They exhibit anxiety, panic, and extreme stress when they are shown photographs or presented with narratives of trauma victims whose experiences match theirs; or made to listen to sounds or words related to their traumatic encounters.

What is interesting is that the amygdala in PTSD patients may be so hyperactive that these people exhibit fear and stress responses even when they are confronted with stimuli not associated with their trauma, such as when they are simply shown photographs of people exhibiting fear.

The hippocampus, the ventromedial prefrontal cortex, and the amygdala complete the neural circuitry of stress. The hippocampus facilitates appropriate responses to environmental stimuli, so the amygdala does not go into stress mode. The ventromedial prefrontal cortex regulates emotional responses by controlling the functions of the amygdala. It is thus not surprising that when the hypoactive hippocampus and the functionally-challenged ventromedial prefrontal cortex stop pulling the chains, the amygdala gets into a tizzy.

Hyperactivity of the amygdala is positively related to the severity of PTSD symptoms. The aforementioned developments explain the tell-tale signs of PTSD—startle responses to the most harmless of stimuli and frequent flashbacks or intrusive recollections.

Researchers believe that the brain changes caused by PTSD increase the likelihood of a person developing other psychotic and mood disorders. Understanding how PTSD alters brain chemistry is critical to empathize with the condition of the victims and devise treatment methods that will enable them to live fully and fulfill their true potential.

But in the midst of such grim findings, scientists also sound a note of hope for PTSD patients and their loved ones. According to them, by delving into the pathophysiology of PTSD, they have also realized that the disorder is reversible. The human brain can be re-wired. In fact, drugs and behavioral therapies have been shown to increase the volume of the hippocampus in PTSD patients. The brain is a finely-tuned instrument. It is fragile, but it is heartening to know that the brain also has an amazing capacity to regenerate.

References

Bremner JD (2006). Traumatic stress: effects on the brain. Dialogues in clinical neuroscience, 8 (4), 445-61 PMID: 17290802

Bremner JD, Elzinga B, Schmahl C, & Vermetten E (2008). Structural and functional plasticity of the human brain in posttraumatic stress disorder. Progress in brain research, 167, 171-86 PMID: 18037014

Hull AM (2002). Neuroimaging findings in post-traumatic stress disorder. Systematic review. The British journal of psychiatry : the journal of mental science, 181, 102-10 PMID: 12151279

Koenigs, M., & Grafman, J. (2009). Posttraumatic Stress Disorder: The Role of Medial Prefrontal Cortex and Amygdala The Neuroscientist, 15 (5), 540-548 DOI: 10.1177/1073858409333072

Resources

Nutt DJ, & Malizia AL (2004). Structural and functional brain changes in posttraumatic stress disorder. The Journal of clinical psychiatry, 65 Suppl 1, 11-7 PMID: 14728092

Rocha-Rego, V., Pereira, M., Oliveira, L., Mendlowicz, M., Fiszman, A., Marques-Portella, C., Berger, W., Chu, C., Joffily, M., Moll, J., Mari, J., Figueira, I., & Volchan, E. (2012). Decreased Premotor Cortex Volume in Victims of Urban Violence with Posttraumatic Stress Disorder PLoS ONE, 7 (8) DOI: 10.1371/journal.pone.0042560

Shin LM, Rauch SL, & Pitman RK (2006). Amygdala, medial prefrontal cortex, and hippocampal function in PTSD. Annals of the New York Academy of Sciences, 1071, 67-79 PMID: 16891563

CPSIA information can be obtained at www.ICGtesting.com
Printed in the USA
LVOW11s1056140516

487906LV00004B/5/P